# Early Identification of Children at Risk

## AN INTERNATIONAL PERSPECTIVE

**TOPICS IN DEVELOPMENTAL PSYCHOBIOLOGY**

**Series Editor:** Robert N. Emde
*University of Colorado School of Medicine*
*Denver, Colorado*

---

The Development of Attachment and Affiliative Systems
Edited by Robert N. Emde and Robert J. Harmon

Continuities and Discontinuities in Development
Edited by Robert N. Emde and Robert J. Harmon

Early Identification of Children at Risk: An International Perspective
Edited by William K. Frankenburg, Robert N. Emde, and Joseph W. Sullivan

# Early Identification of Children at Risk

## AN INTERNATIONAL PERSPECTIVE

Edited by
William K. Frankenburg
Robert N. Emde
and
Joseph W. Sullivan
*University of Colorado School of Medicine*
*Denver, Colorado*

Springer Science+Business Media, LLC

Library of Congress Cataloging in Publication Data

Main entry under title:

Early identification of children at risk.

(Topics in developmental psychobiology)
Based on the Fourth International Conference on Children At Risk, held in 1984 at Snowmass, Colo.
Includes bibliographies and index.
1. Developmental disabilities—Diagnosis—Congresses. 2. Developmental disabilities—Prevention—Congresses. 3. Medical screening—Congresses. 4. Child health services—Congresses. 5. Developmental disabilities—Cross cultural studies—Congresses. I. Frankenburg, William K., 1930- . II. Emde, Robert N. III. Sullivan, Joseph W. IV. International Conference on Children At Risk. (4th: 1984: Snowmass, Colo.) V. Series. [DNLM: 1. Child Development Disorders—diagnosis—congresses. 2. Cross-Cultural Comparison—congresses. 3. Mass Screening—congresses. 4. Primary Prevention—congresses. WS 350.6 E123 1984]
RJ135.E26 1985 618.92′0075 85-12340
**ISBN 978-1-4899-0538-3**

**ISBN 978-1-4899-0538-3** **ISBN 978-1-4899-0536-9 (eBook)**
**DOI 10.1007/978-1-4899-0536-9**


**Originally published by Plenum Press, New York in 1985**
**Softcover reprint of the hardcover 1st edition 1985**

# Contributors

**Babiker Badri, Ph.D.** • Department of Psychology and Special Education, Ahfad University College for Women, Omdurman, Sudan

**Kathryn E. Barnard, R.N., Ph.D.** • School of Nursing and Child Development and Mental Retardation Center, University of Washington, Seattle, Washington

**Keith E. Barnes, Ph.D.** • Kelowna Mental Health Centre, Kelowna, British Columbia, Canada

**Helen L. Bee, Ph.D.** • School of Nursing and Child Development and Mental Retardation Center, University of Washington, Seattle, Washington

**Antonio Berdasco, M.D.** • Instituto de Desarrollo de la Salud, Havana, Cuba

**Helga Binder, M.D.** • Department of Physical Medicine, Children's Hospital National Medical Center, Washington, D.C.

**Jeanne Brooks-Gunn, Ph.D.** • Institute for the Study of Exceptional Children, Educational Testing Service, Princeton, New Jersey

**Robert H. Bradley, Ph.D.** • Center for Child Development and Education, University of Arkansas at Little Rock, Little Rock, Arkansas

**David Cadman, M.D.** • Departments of Pediatrics and Clinical Epidemiology and Biostatistics, McMaster University, Hamilton, Ontario, Canada

**Bernard Cats, M.D.** • Department of Neonatology, University of Utrecht, Utrecht, Netherlands

**Larry Chambers, Ph.D.** • Departments of Pediatrics and Clinical Epidemiology and Biostatistics, McMaster University, Hamilton Ontario, Canada

**Wei-ying Chen** • The International Peace Maternity and Child Health Hospital of the China Welfare Institute, Shanghai, People's Republic of China

**Sung Chieh, M.D.** • Section on Intelligence Tests, Research Laboratory of Medical Genetics, Shanghai No. 6 People's Hospital, Shanghai, People's Republic of China

**Yueh-mei Chu, R.N.** • Section on Intelligence Tests, Research Laboratory of Medical Genetics, Shanghai No. 6 People's Hospital, Shanghai, People's Republic of China

**David H. Cooper** • Department of Special Education, University of Maryland, College Park, Maryland

**Margaret Cox, M.D.** • Newfoundland and Labrador Provincial Perinatal Program, The Dr. Charles A. Janeway Child Health Centre, St. John's, Newfoundland, Canada

**M. Ann Easterbrooks, Ph.D.** • Department of Psychiatry, University of Colorado Health Sciences Center, Denver, Colorado

**Robert N. Emde, M.D.** • Department of Psychiatry, University of Colorado Health Sciences Center, Denver, Colorado

**Dale C. Farran** • Center for the Development of Early Education, Kamehameha Schools/Bishop Estate, Honolulu, Hawaii

**Joseph F. Fagan III, Ph.D.** • Department of Psychology, Case Western Reserve University, Cleveland, Ohio

**William Feldman, M.D.** • Children's Hospital of Eastern Ontario, Ottawa, Ontario, Canada

**Ling-ying Feng, M.S.** • Children's Hospital of Shanghai, First Medical College, Shanghai, People's Republic of China

**Sandra G. Funk, Ph.D.** • Department of Pediatrics, Duke University Medical Center, Durham, North Carolina

**William K. Frankenburg, M.D.** • Rocky Mountain Child Development Center, University of Colorado School of Medicine, Denver, Colorado

**Juarlyn L. Gaiter, Ph.D.** • Pediatric Psychology Research Laboratory, Department of Neonatology, Children's Hospital National Medical Center, Washington, D.C.

**Norman Garmezy, Ph.D.** • Department of Psychology, University of Minnesota, Minneapolis, Minnesota

**Amy Goldfarb, M.S.** • Yale University, New Haven, Connecticut

**James A. Green, Ph.D.** • Department of Pediatrics, Duke University Medical Center, Durham, North Carolina

**Edith H. Grotberg, Ph.D.** • Department of Psychology and Special Education, Ahfad University for Women, Omdurman, Sudan

**Julian S. Haber, M.D.** • Miller Speech and Hearing Clinic, Texas Christian University, Fort Worth, Texas

**Mary A. Hammond, Ph.D.** • School of Nursing and Child Development and Mental Retardation Center, University of Washington, Seattle, Washington

**Jo Hermanns, Ph.D.** • Department of Developmental Psychology, University of Utrecht, Utrecht, Netherlands

**Elizabeth Hrncir, Ph.D.** • Child Development Project, Hamilton, Bermuda

**Harry Ireton, Ph.D.** • Department of Family Practice and Community Health, University of Minnesota, Minneapolis, Minnesota

**Ann Johnson, M.D.** • Newfoundland and Labrador Provincial Perinatal Program, St. John's, Newfoundland, Canada

**Deming Jones Leonard** • Center for Marital and Family Studies, University of Denver, Denver, Colorado

**José R. Jordan, D.Sc.** • Instituto de Desarrollo de la Salud, Havana, Cuba

**Zhi-ping Kuo, M.S.** • Children's Hospital of Shanghai, First Medical College, Shanghai, People's Republic of China

**Xiang-yun Liu, M.D.** • Children's Hospital of Shanghai, First Medical College, Shanghai, People's Republic of China

**Philip F. LoPiccolo, M.D., Col. Mc.** • Uniformed Services University of Health Sciences, Bethesda, Maryland; Seventh Medical Command, Heidelberg, West Germany

**Shih-ying Lu, M.D.** • Section on Intelligence Tests, Research Laboratory of Medical Genetics, Shanghai No. 6 People's Hospital, Shanghai, People's Republic of China

**Corazon V. Madrazo, R.N.** • Philippine Nurses' Association, Malate, Manila, Philippines

**Amad Hassan Mahdi, M.D.** • Department of Pediatrics, King Saud University, Riyadh, Saudi Arabia

**Howard J. Markman, Ph.D.** • Center for Marital and Family Studies, University of Denver, Denver, Colorado

**Kathleen McCartney** • Harvard University, Cambridge, Massachusetts

**Edna McKim, R.N., B.N.** • Newfoundland and Labrador Provincial Perinatal Program, St. John's, Newfoundland, Canada

**Tore Mellbin, M.D.** • School Health Service, Uppsala, Sweden

**Sandra K. Mitchell, Ph.D.** • School of Nursing, and Child Development and Mental Retardation Center, University of Washington, Seattle, Washington

**Jeanne E. Montie, R.N., M.A.** • Department of Psychology, Case Western Reserve University, Cleveland, Ohio

**Sharon Murray, Ph.D.** • Department of Hearing and Speech, Children's Hospital National Medical Center, Washington, D.C.

**Cheryl Naulty, M.D.** • Newborn Follow-Up Clinic, Department of Neonatology, Children's Hospital National Medical Center, Washington, D.C.

**Marylee Norris** • Miller Speech and Hearing Clinic, Division of Communication Pathology, Texas Christian University, Fort Worth, Texas

**Lya den Ouden** • Department of Neonatology, University of Utrecht, Utrecht, Netherlands

**Gourdas Pal, M.D.** • Children's Rehabilitation Centre, St. John's, Newfoundland, Canada

**J. Helen Parkyn, B.N., M.P.H.** • South Central Health Unit, Kamloops, British Columbia, Canada

**Stephen L. Rock, M.S.** • Center for Child Development and Education, University of Arkansas at Little Rock, Little Rock, Arkansas

**David Sackett** • Departments of Pediatrics and Clinical Epidemiology and Biostatistics, McMaster University, Hamilton, Ontario, Canada

**Arnold J. Sameroff, Ph.D.** • Institute for the Study of Developmental Disabilities, University of Illinois at Chicago, Chicago, Illinois

**Sandra Scarr** • University of Virginia, Charlottesville, Virginia

**Ying-ying Shih** • The International Peace Maternity and Child Health Hospital of the China Welfare Institute, Shanghai, People's Republic of China

**Linda S. Siegel, Ph.D.** • Department of Special Education, Ontario Institute for Studies in Education, Toronto, Ontario, Canada

**Lynn T. Singer, Ph.D.** • Department of Psychology, Case Western Reserve University, Cleveland, Ohio

**Raymond A. Sturner, M.D.** • Department of Pediatrics, Duke University Medical Center, Durham, North Carolina

**Joseph W. Sullivan, Ph.D.** • Rocky Mountain Child Development Center, Department of Psychology, University of Colorado School of Medicine, Denver, Colorado

**Claes Sundelin, M.D.** • Department of Pediatrics, University Hospital, Uppsala, Sweden

**Salah Ali Taha, M.D.** • Department of Pediatrics, King Saud University, Riyadh, Saudi Arabia

**Tsui-hung Tang** • Section on Intelligence Tests, Research Laboratory of Medical Genetics, Shanghai No. 6 People's Hospital, Shanghai, People's Republic of China

**Reiko Ueda, D.M.S., M.Litt** • Department of Maternal and Child Health, School of Health Sciences, University of Tokyo, Tokyo, Japan

**Jean-Claude Vuille, M.D.** • School Health Service, Bern, Switzerland

**Steven Walter, Ph.D.** • Departments of Pediatrics and Clinical Epidemiology and Biostatistics, McMaster University, Hamilton, Ontario, Canada

**Tze-tsai Wang, M.D.** • Section on Intelligence Tests, Research Laboratory of Medical Genetics, Shanghai No. 6 People's Hospital, Shanghai, People's Republic of China

**Victor Weidtman, M.D.** • Institute for Medical Documentation and Statistics, University of Cologne, Cologne, Federal Republic of Germany

**Phoebe Duaz Williams, R.N., Ph.D.** • The J. Hillis Miller Health Center, University of Florida, College of Nursing, Gainesville, Florida

**Mu-shi Zheng, M.D.** • Children's Hospital of Shanghai, First Medical College, Shanghai, People's Republic of China

**Xi-ying Zhu, R.N.** • Children's Hospital of Shanghai, First Medical College, Shanghai, People's Republic of China

# Preface[1]

This volume contains contributions that are interdisciplinary and international. The editors believe this is an especially timely and promising enterprise, for both sources of diversity are needed for improving our abilities to identify the young child at risk and to prevent disability.

In terms of disciplines, the volume brings together papers by health care providers (such as pediatricians and public health nurses) as well as educators and psychologists. Each of these groups works in dissimilar settings and faces dissimilar problems: Health care providers seek simple identification procedures for use in busy primary care settings; psychologists emphasize well-constructed research designs; and educators reflect the need for early identification and education. Each of these specialist groups has something to offer the other, but too often each tends to limit its publications and readings to its own discipline, thus failing to capitalize on a wider scope of knowledge and practice. We hope that this selection of papers will allow all readers addressing the early identification of children at risk to generate a more integrated interdisciplinary perspective.

We also hope this volume reflects the sense of excitement that we feel from a sharing of international perspectives. There is no single approach to the early identification of children at risk that is universally applicable to all countries. In addition, approaches within each country vary because of availability of financial and human resources and differing expectations of local communities. The readers of this volume will therefore have an opportunity to find reports relevant to their own specific settings and problems.

It is generally agreed that factors determining a given child's development are the result of a series of complex interactions between a child's biological makeup (such as genetic characteristics), biological traits (such as hearing and motor status), and the environment. The environ-

[1]Partial funding for this work was provided by the William T. Grant Foundation of New York.

ment, as perceived by Urie Bronfenbrenner (see his book *Ecology of Human Development: Experiments by Nature and Design*. Cambridge, MA: Harvard University Press, 1979), is analogous to a set of Russian dolls, with one doll (or aspect of the environment) nested inside the other. Contributors to the current volume discuss risk in terms of different aspects of environment–child interaction.

For instance,there is the caregiver–child relationship (as discussed by Emde and Easterbrooks and by Brooks-Gunn in this volume) and there is the nuclear family and interrelationship of parents, as discussed by Markman and Jones Leonard. The degree to which the home environment fosters cognitive development is presented by Bradley and Rock. Still, the family's ability to meet the child's needs is affected by a larger environment; thus, cultural and economic factors are alluded to in chapters by Madrazo and Williams, by Liu and associates, and by Berdasco and Jordan. A comparison of the development of children in different cultures makes it possible to generate and test hypotheses regarding the impact of various environmental factors on child development.

Another reason for focusing on the international aspects of research is the international recognition of the importance of early identification and habilitation of handicapped children. More and more countries recognize that such early habilitation is a preventive approach that seeks to promote the development of all children to their maximum potential. Whereas in the past developing countries have been concerned primarily with keeping children alive through better health care and nutrition, there is increasing recognition that it is in each country's interest to do everything possible to promote the development of its children. These children, after all, will be the country's leaders in later years.

The editors of this book also recognize that the world's population is changing. The degree of mobility of the population and data collection systems vary from one country to the next. Thus, in some countries it is far easier to carry out longitudinal studies than in others. Furthermore, we recognize that the populations of the developing countries far outnumber the populations of the developed countries. Already we have seen that the developing countries are asserting greater control of their own destinies with lesser control by the developed countries. It is our view that this trend will not only continue but will occur at an accelerating pace.

A final reason for the international focus of this volume is that the approaches taken in developing countries, as illustrated in the chapter by Badri and Grotberg regarding the Sudan (a country with a low average per capita income and with a dirth of professional manpower), can suggest approaches that might be adapted to less priviledged sectors of developed countries.

The volume itself results from the Fourth International Conference on Children At Risk, which was held in the fall of 1984. The first such conference, which was held 10 years earlier, concentrated on research covering one of the first developmental screening tests in international use—the Denver Development Screening Test. The following years saw a proliferation of developmental screening activities with the Second International Conference (in 1977) considering a variety of screening tests and the Third International Conference (1981) addressing both screening and diagnostic efforts within at-risk populations. The Fourth International Conference not only updated screening approaches but also examined physical, emotional, and socioeconomic factors that interact to put particular children at risk for later delays, disabilities, and school failure.

## Uniform Terms

One of the difficulties in editing a book of studies designed and implemented throughout the world is that similar terminology and evaluation procedures are not always used. This makes it difficult for the reader to compare studies. Therefore, to assist the reader, the editors have altered papers where necessary to reflect the following terms:

***Screening.*** The application of quick and relatively simple procedures to a relatively asymptomatic population in order to identify persons who have a high likelihood of harboring the problem in question.

***Diagnostic Evaluation.*** The administration of norm-referenced tests and other more lengthy procedures as applied by professionally trained personnel to make a categorical diagnosis.

***Assessment.*** The administration of evaluations to determine current levels of functioning in order to plan the habilitation and/or educational program for the client.

***Screening Test Accuracy: Sensitivity and Specificity.*** Although there are various ways of determining the accuracy of a screening test, we have, whenever possible, used the terms "sensitivity" and "specificity." These terms describe accuracy in identifying all of the diseased or handicapped persons among those screened. *Sensitivity* is the percentage of diseased who are correctly identified as "suspect" on screening. *Specificity* is the percentage of nondiseased correctly identified as "nonsuspect" on screening. The terms "correlation" and "percentage of agreement" do not describe accuracy in identifying all of the diseased or handicapped persons among those screened, and thus are not utilized in this volume except in chapters describing pilot studies.

William K. Frankenburg
Robert N. Emde
Joseph W. Sullivan

# Contents

## *PART IV Regional and National Programs of Early Identification*

PART I

# Early Identification of Children at Risk

## A HISTORICAL PERSPECTIVE

*CHAPTER 1*

# The Concept of Screening Revisited

*William K. Frankenburg*

---

Screening for health problems and handicapping conditions has been recommended as a preventive measure for more than 40 years. Initially, it began in developing countries to identify individuals who constituted a health hazard to others in the community, such as those harboring an infectious disease that, if not isolated or controlled, might spread. An example is the screening for carriers of malaria. This use of screening spread to the United States and other developed countries, which screened for persons harboring tuberculosis and other infectious diseases, such as syphilis. A more recent example of screening to protect the general public is the screening of individuals who may be airplane hijackers and therefore present a threat to other passengers.

## THE SHIFT TO SCREENING TO PREVENT SECONDARY PROBLEMS

Following the Second World War, the emphasis of screening programs shifted from preventing community illnesses (primary prevention) to promoting the health and welfare of the individual. The aim of such screening programs was to move up the time of diagnosis to an earlier stage of the disease process when treatment would be more efficacious. This secondary form of prevention did not attempt the total prevention of a disease, but rather sought to reverse or ameliorate the usual outcome through earlier treatment.

Perhaps the best example of this type of screening was the screening for phenylketonuria (PKU). Prior to legislation mandating that all

---

*William K. Frankenburg* • Rocky Mountain Child Development Center, University of Colorado School of Medicine, Denver, Colorado 80262.

newborns be screened for this condition, the average time of diagnosis of PKU in Colorado was 4 years of age. Since the onset of universal PKU screening in Colorado, the age of diagnosis and treatment has been advanced to less than 4 weeks. Because the critical time to treat this condition is by about 4 weeks of age, the most common result of this condition—mental retardation—has been averted through early treatment (Holtzman, Morales, Cunningham, & Wells, 1975).

Screening that has secondary prevention as its aim is still common, as exemplified by screening for vision and hearing defects, mental retardation, cerebral palsy, and so on. As the world has almost universally embraced such screening, a common misconception has developed; namely, "the earlier the better." Although this situation holds true for many conditions, it is not true for all. For example, there is no benefit from early treatment for color blindness or flat feet, for which screening is commonly conducted. However, although some genetic conditions such as sickle cell disease are generally not considered to benefit from earlier treatment, screening for these conditions is conducted anyway to potentially prevent the occurrence of other affected members through genetic counseling.

Another form of screening that became common in the 1950s was multiphasic screening. This type of screening also embodied the concept of improvement in the welfare of the individual through earlier diagnosis. Pathologists who popularized multiphasic screening typically supervised hospital laboratories and demonstrated that it was more economical to administer several tests at once rather than to perform the tests individually (Holtzman *et al.*, 1975). The result was the proliferation of easily automated screening tests. This approach, which was relatively short-lived, had several basic flaws:

1. Conditions selected for screening were determined by laboratory pathologists on the basis of which tests could be automated rather than on the basis of which conditions would be averted through earlier diagnosis and treatment; and
2. Cutoff points separating nonsuspect cases from suspect cases were selected statistically (i.e., 2 or 3 standard deviations from the mean) regardless of the prevalence of the disease.

The result was that for diseases affecting 30% of the population, cases would be missed; conversely, for relatively rare conditions like PKU (which has a prevalence of 1:15,000) or congenital hearing loss (with a prevalence of 1:1,000 to 1:2,000), there was vast overselection. Under this statistical approach to delineating suspects, Best and colleagues (Best, Mason, Barron, & Shepherd, 1969) have demonstrated that if a healthy individual had 12 independent tests, the likelihood that all tests would fall into the normal range is markedly decreased. Not only did such an application of tests and cutoff points result in excessive anxiety, but it was also expensive, for the individual who was suspect was required to undergo additional, often unnecessary, examinations to rule out disease.

## Problems with Screening Programs for Children

As screening programs involving children have been mandated, a variety of problems have become apparent. The following constitutes but a brief list of such problems:

1. Failure to define in measurable terms what the screening effort is attempting to identify
2. Screening for conditions that will not benefit from early diagnosis and treatment
3. Screening for conditions for which diagnostic and treatment services are not available
4. Failure to obtain informed consent and to ensure complete confidentiality
5. Failure to confine screening to tests having a high degree of validity or accuracy
6. Failure to assure that the screening procedures used will be considered appropriate by those who will provide the diagnosis and treatment
7. Administration of screening tests by poorly trained personnel
8. Administration of screening tests by the same persons who provide diagnosis and treatment
9. Failure to differentiate between a positive screen and a positive diagnosis
10. Failure to monitor screening programs
11. Failure to consider the cost of the entire program and the benefits that will accrue to the population as a whole

A critical aspect of screening programs has been the establishment of a cutoff point on a screening scale that differentiates suspect from nonsuspect individuals. The most widespread approach used to evaluate the accuracy or validity of screening tests is to compare the positives (or suspects) and negatives (or nonsuspects) with the actual presence or absence of the disease in question. This approach is termed *percentage of agreement*. The problem encountered with the percentage of agreement approach is that it is highly related to the prevalence of the problem in the population, and does not specify the accuracy of the screening test in identifying all of the problem cases (Frankenburg, 1975).

For instance, if one were to screen 30,000 children for PKU, which has a prevalence of 1 in 15,000, and if every child were designated by the screening as negative or nonsuspect, the results could be depicted by an agreement of 99.99%. Although this percentage appears to be extremely high, the screening procedure would have failed to identify the two cases of PKU; therefore, the test would have had a 100% error rate in identifying the two children diagnosed as having PKU.

The awareness of the shortcoming of the percentage of agreement approach led to the evaluation of screening tests in terms of sensitivity and specificity. *Sensitivity* is a test's accuracy in identifying all of the diseased individuals (or the percentage of diseased individuals correctly identified). This is calculated as $A/(A + C) \times 100$ in Figure 1.

Because one could achieve 100% accuracy in identifying all of the diseased individuals by designating all screening results as either positive or suspect, use of sensitivity requires that one also determine test accuracy in correctly identifying all of the nondiseased subjects—which is termed *specificity*. In Figure 1, specificity is calculated as follows: $D/(B + D) \times 100$.

For most diseases, there is an overlap between diseased and nondiseased values. For instance, Figure 2 illustrates (in a hypothetical case)

| | | Diagnostic Findings | | |
|---|---|---|---|---|
| | | + | - | |
| Screening Test Findings | + | A<br>Agreement | B<br>Overreferral | A + B |
| | - | C<br>Underreferral | D<br>Agreement | C + D |
| | | A + C | B + D | |

$$\text{Agreement} = \frac{A + D}{A + B + C + D} \times 100$$

$$\text{Sensitivity} = \frac{A}{A + C} \times 100 \qquad \text{Overreferral rate} = \frac{B}{A + B} \times 100$$

$$\text{Specificity} = \frac{D}{B + D} \times 100 \qquad \text{Underreferral rate} = \frac{C}{C + D} \times 100$$

$$\text{Predictive validity of a positive test} = \frac{A}{A + B} \times 100$$

$$\text{Predictive validity of a negative test} = \frac{D}{C + D} \times 100$$

**Figure 1.** Validation of screening tests and calculation of sensitivity and specificity. *Note.* From "Criteria in screening test selection" (p. 30) by W. K. Frankenburg, 1978. In W. K. Frankenburg & B. W. Camp (Eds.), *Pediatric screening tests* (pp. 23–42), Springfield, IL: Charles C Thomas. Copyright 1975 by Charles C Thomas. Reprinted by permission.

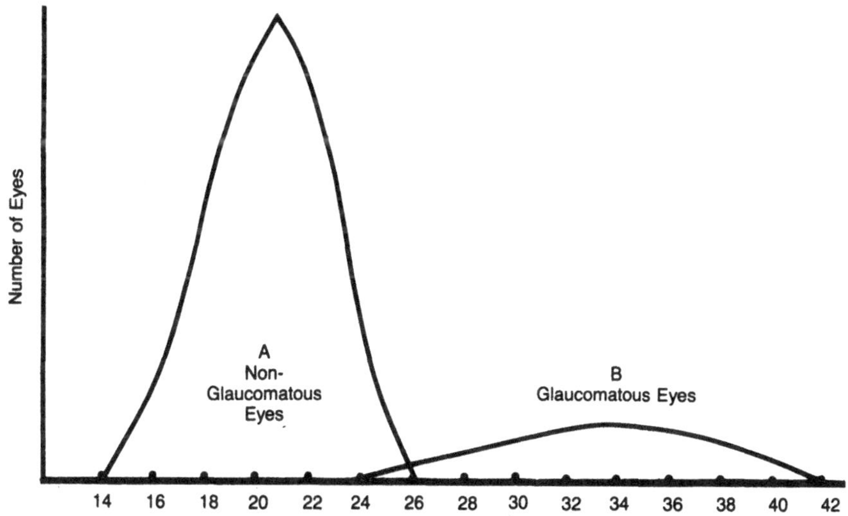


**Figure 2.** Distribution of intraocular pressure: A hypothetical example. *Note.* From "Principles and procedures in the evaluation of screening disease" by R. M. Thorner and Q. R. Remein, *Public Health Monograph No. 67* (PHS Publication No. 846). Adapted by permission.

the overlap between diseased and nondiseased individuals. Figure 3 depicts the interrelationship between sensitivity, specificity, and over- and underreferrals. In a condition where there is an overlap between diseased and nondiseased individuals, any cutoff point will generate errors of over- and underreferrals. For example, selection of a cutoff point at Point A will yield 100% sensitivity, 30% specificity, many overreferrals, and no underreferrals. In contrast, selection of a cutoff point at Point B on the screening scale will yield 18% sensitivity, 100% specificity, many underreferrals, and no overreferrals. Selection of a cutoff point between A and B will be a compromise between the two extremes.

In some cases, screening tests are validated against a criterion test that also may be in error. Buck and Gart (1966) suggested denoting agreement with criterion-referenced tests, which are calculated similar to sensitivity and specificity. A potential problem with this approach is that the screening and criterion tests may evaluate different functions; for instance, the Denver Developmental Screening Test (DDST) may be abnormal for a nonambulatory child, but the criterion measure of the Stanford-Binet, an IQ test, may be normal for that same child. Thus, although there is not agreement between the tests, each test may still be accurate or valid.

A unitary figure—a Youden Index (Youden, 1950)—has been proposed to facilitate validity comparisons of different screening tests.

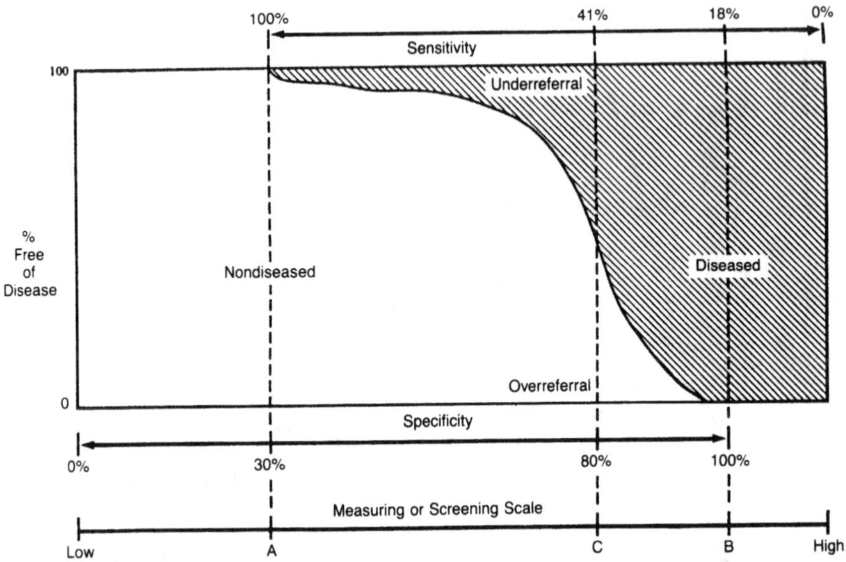


**Figure 3.** Relationship between sensitivity and specificity. *Note.* From "Criteria in screening test selection" (p. 31) by W. K. Frankenburg, 1978. In W. K. Frankenburg & B. W. Camp (Eds.), *Pediatric screening tests* (pp. 23–42), Springfield, IL: Charles C Thomas. Copyright 1975 by Charles C Thomas. Reprinted by permission.

Using this approach, one adds sensitivity and specificity and subtracts 100. The problem with this approach is that it gives an equal weight to sensitivity and specificity. A modification of this approach is to separately weigh sensitivity and specificity depending on the test author's attachment of importance to each.

## Application of Decision Analysis to Cutoff Points

The application of decision analysis (Coons, Gay, & Frankenburg, 1978) to the selection of screening cutoff points is recommended, for it permits selection of cutoff points that maximize benefits while minimizing costs. This approach contrasts the Youden approach, which assumes that errors of over- and underreferral are of equal concern. The method employed in applying decision analysis to screening is to derive a cost and benefit for each of the four cells, A, B, C, and D (as depicted in Table 2 in Frankenburg's "The Denver Approach," Chapter 8). For instance, in the case of cell A, the costs of screening, diagnosis, and treatment would be weighed against the benefits of an increase in lifetime earnings and the decrease in human suffering. After determining a relative value for each of the four quadrants, one moves the cutoff point on the screening test in both directions. As the cutoff point is moved, the number of subjects falling into each of the four cells will vary. For each potential cutoff point, one sums the products (the number of subjects in each cell times its relative value) and thereby derives a total value for each potential cutting point. The optimum cutting point is the one that yields the greatest overall benefit. Sullivan has suggested modification of the decision analysis approach through use of signal detection analysis. This approach would employ both sensitivity/specificity with probabilities (Sullivan, personal communication, May 1984).

### Use of Screening in Locales with Limited Diagnostic Resources

A recent trend utilized where diagnostic services are limited is to apply screening tests to an asymptomatic population and, without providing diagnostic services, to intervene with all children who are suspect on screening. This approach has been implemented independently in Jamaica (Thorburn, 1981) and the Sudan (see Badri and Grotberg, Chapter 24). In both of these developing countries, there are insufficient trained personnel to provide diagnostic services. Instead, all children who are suspect on screening are provided with a "stimulation" program, since it is reasoned that the stimulation will not be harmful, and in the majority of cases where it is applied will be of benefit. Although the reasoning behind this approach may appear to be sound, it would also appear reasonable to monitor the progress of individual children to identify those who may have etiologies for their slowness that require a different type of treatment. An example is the child manifesting a delay in language development who is treated with a language stimulation program. If that child's language delay is due to a hearing loss, language stimulation will not help the child. This approach of treating the most likely cause without further diagnostic investigation can be defended for economic reasons if the majority of children involved suffer from a problem that requires harmless treatment.

Another example of the use of screening procedures as diagnostic procedures has been commonly employed in the People's Republic of China (see Sung, Chu, Lu, Tan, & Wang, Chapter 26). There, children are screened with the Chinese standardized version of the DDST. In that country, such diagnostic tests as the Stanford-Binet and the Bayley Scales of Infant Development have not been restandardized. In addition, there is a lack of clinical psychologists trained in the diagnostic evaluation of infants and preschool-aged children. These realities have prompted Chinese professionals to use the Chinese DDST as an outcome measure when comparing infants of differing risk groups (such as the preterm, eclamptic, and preeclamptic child) (see Chu, Tang, Lu, Chen, & Shih, Chapter 28).

## THE SIMILARITIES OF THE RISK CONCEPT AND SCREENING

The concept of risk, as envisaged by its early proponents, was that it was a type of screening. Similarities were the application of quick and simple procedures to "an asymptomatic population to select out those individuals who were at risk of harboring the problem in question" (Commission on Chronic Illness, 1957, p. 45). Oppé (1967) and Richards and Roberts (1967) have pointed out the major shortcomings of the risk approach in case finding. Whereas it was originally postulated that 20% of the population would harbor 70% of the problems, in reality very few of the population harbored the problems (Richards & Roberts, 1967).

If one seeks reasons for the reversal of the hypothesis through the application of screening criteria, the reasons become obvious:

1. There was use of unreliable (inconsistent) criteria. Hypoxia is one example; what one person interpreted as hypoxia might not be interpreted by another as hypoxia.
2. There was use of unvalidated criteria. Health professionals tended to make up criteria that often lacked a high degree of predictive validity.
3. There was failure to define outcomes in diagnostically measurable terms. Richards and Roberts (1967) called attention to the fact that risk criteria were validated with screening tests and procedures that also generated errors.
4. The work of Drillien (1961) on cerebral palsy and of Lillienfeld and Pasamanick (1955) on mental retardation have demonstrated that many children suffering from these disorders have no history of being at risk of becoming handicapped and therefore would not have been identified with the risk approach.
5. Risk lists or criteria were expanded to the point that the probability of even a healthy individual being designated "at risk" approached 70% (Oppé, 1967). This situation is analogous to the multiphasic laboratory screening in the 1950s.

An additional problem, and one not unrelated to screening, is that previous efforts have concentrated on including an ever larger group of persons in the risk category; efforts at ridding persons of the "risk" title have been largely neglected. It therefore is of little wonder that with increasing age, more and more people are "at risk," even though most turn out not to harbor the problems in question.

## THE POTENTIAL MERGER OF THE RISK CONCEPT AND SCREENING

A relatively new approach to screening has been proposed by public health officials concerned about the allocation of human and financial resources. Their risk strategy is

> to give special attention to those in greatest need within a framework of improved health care for all. Individuals and groups with increased expectation of complications or disease are defined as being "at risk" and the aim of the health services should be to identify them as early as possible and to intervene to reduce the risk. (World Health Organization, 1978)

This approach is a community or population approach, and is therefore less concerned about the individual subject. In this orientation (as opposed to screening), it matters less whether the individual develops the problem in question as long as the *majority* of individuals in the risk group develop the problem.

A potential approach to resolving some of the risk concept problems cited previously is to combine the risk and screening concepts for relatively circumscribed problems that may arise at any time in the life of the child and that benefit from treatment instituted prior to the usual time. This approach would therefore utilize "status" risk factors selected on the basis of validity as being precursors of certain diagnosable diseases or handicaps. Such factors would be either historical (i.e., family history of hearing loss) or biological (the child born with Down's syndrome).

One might disagree with the term *status* for the foregoing risk factors, as these are mediated by changing factors over time. The reason for using the term *status* is that the birth weight, family history, and so on, are fairly constant and therefore are only measured at one point in time. Beginning about 1 year of age, dynamic or changing risk factors might begin to be employed. The term *dynamic* is used to suggest changes over time as noted in growth, development, sensory capacities, and prevalence of illness and accidents. As the name implies, these dynamic risk factors are reevaluated at periodic intervals to determine which child is at risk and which is not. It is suggested that at about 3 years of age, the dynamic risk factors (as opposed to the status factors) will be the main determinants of whether a child is at risk. In this scheme, a child who initially may have been designated at risk due to a low birth weight would no longer be considered at risk at 3 years if growing and developing normally and not suspect on the other dynamic risk factors. Similarily, a child who may not have been initially considered at risk through the use of the status factors may later not develop or grow well due to neglect, and thereby becomes designated

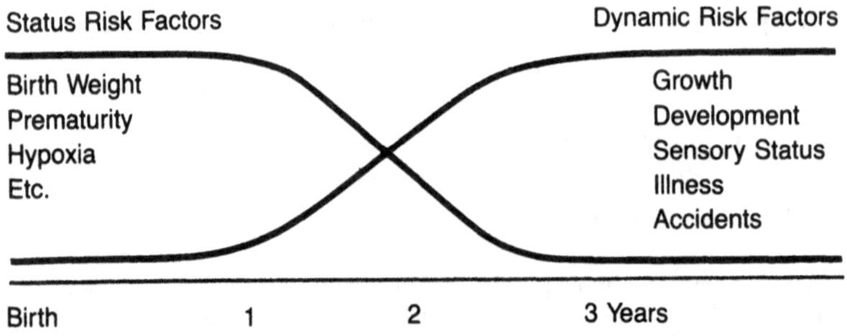


**Figure 4.** Relationship between status and dynamic risk factors.

as at risk. Figure 4 illustrates graphically how the status risk factors merge into the dynamic risk factors. It is important that dynamic risk factors be selected with care so as to limit the number of factors and to avoid having an excessive number of individuals designated at risk (Best *et al.*, 1969).

Criteria for selecting dynamic risk factors may require that the factors be independent of each other, that they be reliable, and that they also have predictive validity. The selection of conditions that would benefit from this approach would have the following characteristics. They would benefit from earlier-than-usual onset of treatment; be relatively prevalent; constitute problems of economic impact; not be predictable on the basis of a single screening procedure or test; be diagnosable with certainty; and have identifiable, valid status and dynamic risk factors.

## CURRENT PROBLEMS WITH SCREENING

Aside from specific problems with current screening programs, a broader problem affecting most screening programs is the current lack of understanding about the pathogenesis of disease.

### Disease Pathogenesis

Without an understanding of the pathogenesis of disease, it is almost impossible to predict with a very high degree of accuracy which individuals will develop the disease in question. This circumstance is particularily true when attempting to predict which of the borderline individuals are destined to become symptomatic. For instance, only 1 out of 100 individuals infected with the tubercle bacillus develops symptomatic pulmonary tuberculosis, yet 100 individuals are treated to prevent the 1 case from becoming symptomatic (Edwards, 1975). In the case of PKU, which has been extensively studied, it is widely recognized that at least 1 out of 100 individuals who appear to have the full disease never become symptomatic (Holtzman *et al.*, 1975). When the criteria for diagnosing the disease are not commonly agreed on, the result is that some borderline individuals (a percentage of whom are probably not destined to become symptomatic) will be treated. When those individuals do not become symptomatic, the results are ascribed to effective screening and treatment, when actually some of the results might have occurred despite treatment. This is the current situation in PKU screening, where different criteria are used in Europe and the United States to decide who will be treated. Thus, part of the problem rests in diagnosing who has the disease in question.

Another problem (related to the first) is identifying and separating those individuals who have a nonprogressive form of the disease, and who therefore do not require treatment, from those who have a rapidly progressing disease and will become symptomatic. An example is differentiating carcinoma *in situ* from the progressive forms of the disease. Other examples are differentiating those cases of bacteriuria that progress to pyelonephritis from those that do not, and differentiating acute hearing losses that are self-limiting from the chronic losses that impair auditory reception and language development. The same holds true in differentiating early developmental problems that are temporary from those that are chronic and therefore have long-term deleterious consequences. As more is learned about disease processes, it may be that Sameroff's transactional model (Sameroff, 1975) will prove most accurate of all developmental models; this would impose limits on the ability to predict disease or handicapping outcomes.

With few exceptions, most diseases are diagnosed with certainty on the basis of the presence of multiple signs and/or symptoms. Frequently each of the signs and symptoms have different times of onset in the disease process (Frankenburg, 1975). This situation is illustrated in Figure 5. As can be seen from this illustration, the more signs and symptoms present, the more certain the professional can be of the diagnosis. The problem arising in screening is that most screens for a disease or handicap measure only one of the multiple signs and symptoms of the disease. For instance, the diagnosis of PKU is based on a minimum of three parameters: an elevated serum phenylalanine level, a normal serum tyrosine level, and the presence of phenylpyryvic acid in the urine. Internationally, screening for PKU is designed to detect only elevated serum phenylalanine levels, which in turn yield 95% false positives (Holtzman *et al.*, 1975). Adding in other screens, such as a serum tyrosine, would increase the cost and generate additional referrals.

A further problem is that each sign or symptom of disease for which

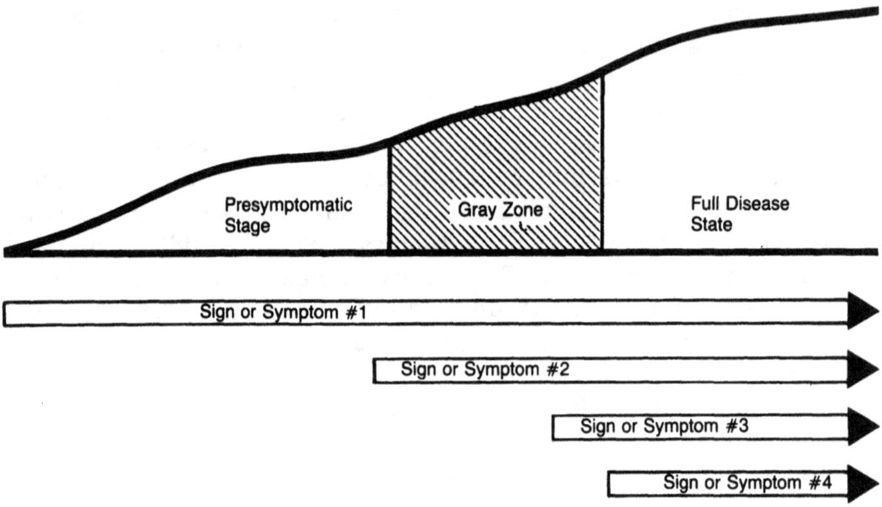


**Figure 5.** The disease process.

one may screen carries a different weight in the diagnosis. In addition, the more aberrant the screening finding, the more likely it is that the diseased or handicapped individual is being identified.

A final problem encountered touches on all of these points. Without a full knowledge of the pathogenesis of diseases and handicapping conditions, professionals may be screening for the wrong condition. For instance, instead of screening for bacteriuria or hearing loss, both of which are mostly transient, screening might be best conducted for the precursors of pyelonephritis and chronic ear infections. To screen for such conditions will require a prior knowledge of the pathogenesis of disease, and may eventually require the application of two or more simultaneous screens in parallel, with only those individuals who are suspect on both the screens being designated as suspect.

### Selection of Cutoff Points

Up to now the major validation criteria in screening test selection has been a dichotomous approach in which everything on one side of the cutoff point is considered to be equally positive and everything on the other side of the cutoff point is considered to be equally negative. Experience in the follow-up of screening results, whether they be for identifying hearing loss, vision defects, developmental status, or infectious diseases like bacteriuria and tuberculosis, demonstrates that this is not appropriate. Instead, the more aberrant the screening finding, the greater the probability the person has the disease in question.

It would therefore be helpful if individuals constructing and validating screening tests developed probability tables to denote the relationships between referral levels and the probability of harboring the problem in question. Because such probabilities (like the predictive value of a positive) are strongly influenced by prevalence rates, tables for two or more prevalence rates might ideally be presented. Local screening program architects, depending on the prevalence of various types of diseases or problems in their community and on the basis of tables like those previously described, could then decide which entities to screen for, which screening test to employ, and which cutoff point might be most appropriate for their community's available resources and priorities.

To overcome some of the foregoing problems, the Denver group has attempted to develop increasingly accurate methods of screening for school problems, such as the use of a combined developmental/environmental screen. The problems encountered include the lack of highly valid concurrent measures. For instance, the predictive accuracy of the criterion-referenced Stanford-Binet has been found to be no better in predicting school problems than the DDST (Camp, van Doorninck, Frankenburg, & Lampe, 1977). Thus, emphasis shifted from concurrent to predictive validity. Attempts to develop even more valid screening procedures lead to the procedures becoming more time-consuming and complex, thereby approximating diagnostic procedures. It therefore appears that it might be useful to operationally define acceptable criteria or limits of criteria for screening and diagnostic tests. This is important, for if screening tests become too complex, they will no longer be quick and simple procedures that can be applied to large masses of the population. Thus, combining developmental screening with the risk approach (as illustrated in Figure 4) warrants further investigation to determine its utility. Although this discussion has been exemplified with developmental screening, the same principles apply to other screening processes as well.

## Advanced Definition of the Disease

Another major problem encountered in many screening programs has been the failure to operationally define, in advance, the disease or problem in question. For instance, a number of countries have restandardized the DDST for use in their own countries; however, they have employed the Denver scoring criteria without first determining which scoring criteria most accurately predicts who will have the problem under their own developmental norms. This is a serious error, because it is more important to have valid scoring criteria than to have local norms.

Local norms designate local tendencies; they differentiate what is common and what is uncommon, but they do not define who needs treatment. It is conceivable that countries having differing prevalences of mental retardation may reach differing decisions as to who should have the highest priority for treatment. Setting treatment priorities is essential in cases where resources are limited.

## RECOMMENDATIONS

Several recommendations regarding screening can be made at this time.

1. The first recommendation is not to mandate more screening programs. To date, a number of screening programs have been mandated that have been difficult to defend. One example is New York State's mandate that all children be screened for adenosine deaminase deficiency. The mandate ignores the fact that the condition is extremely rare (less than a dozen cases have been reported in all the world literature) and efficacious preventative treatment has yet to be demonstrated.

2. The second recommendation is that more large-scale studies be undertaken to identify factors playing relevant roles in the pathogenesis of diseases and handicapping conditions. Once such a better understanding has been obtained, it should be possible to develop better validation criteria that are very much needed for a variety of problems, such as school failure. Then, studies should be undertaken to develop valid and highly accurate screening tests.

3. The third recommendation is to obtain prevalence data for various diseases and handicapping conditions. Such data will make it possible to undertake selective screening for conditions in segments of the population that are known to have a higher-than-usual prevalence rate.

4. The fourth recommendation is that communities establish local oversight committees that would be made up of professionals and lay persons. Such oversight committees would have the responsibility to review the available literature regarding the pros and cons of screening for specific diseases, the selection of tests, and the periodicity of screening. The approval of this committee would be required before any local screening program utilizing public funds would be approved.

## CONCLUSION

Although there is a common assumption that the earlier health problems and handicapping conditions are remediated the better the results, this point of view has not been verified for a variety of health problems and handicapping conditions. A series of longitudinal studies are needed to further clarify the pathogenesis of diseases and handicapping conditions. Particular opportunities for such studies exist in countries such as Cuba and the People's Republic of China, where the population is less mobile than in the United States. Such studies in turn would make it possible for public health planners to conduct screening programs that are both effective and economical, and to allocate a community's resources where they will do the most good.

## REFERENCES

Best, W., Mason, C., Barron, S., & Shepherd, H. (1969). Automated 12-channel serum screening. What is normal? *Pediatric Clinics of North America, 53,* 175.

Buck, A. A., & Gart, J. J. (1966). Comparison of a screening test and a reference test in epidemiological studies. *American Journal of Epidemiology, 83,* 586.

Camp, B. W., van Doorninck, W. J., Frankenburg, W. K., & Lampe, J. M. (1977). Preschool developmental testing in prediction of school problems. *Clinical Pediatrics, 16*(3), 257–263.

Commission on Chronic Illness. (1957). *Chronic illness in the United States: Vol. 1. Prevention of chronic illness.* Cambridge: Harvard University Press.

Coons, C. E., Gay, E. C., & Frankenburg, W. K. (1978, May). *A decision analysis model for choosing optimum test cut-off scores.* Paper presented at the American Association on Mental Deficiency meeting, Denver, CO.

Drillien, C. M. (1961). A longitudinal study of the growth and development of prematurely and maturely born children. *Archives of Diseases in Children, 36,* 233.

Edwards, P. (1975). Tuberculosis. In W. K. Frankenburg & B. W. Camp (Eds.), *Pediatric screening tests* (pp. 147–173). Springfield, IL: Charles C Thomas.

Frankenburg, W. K. (1975). Criteria in screening test selection. In W. K. Frankenburg & B. W. Camp (Eds.), *Pediatric screening tests* (pp. 23–37). Springfield, IL: Charles C Thomas.

Holtzman, N. A., Morales, D. R., Cunningham, G., & Wells, D. G. T. (1975). Phenylketonuria. In W. K. Frankenburg & B. W. Camp (Eds.), *Pediatric screening tests* (pp. 92–118). Springfield, IL: Charles C Thomas.

Lillienfeld, A. M., & Pasamanick, B. (1955). *American Journal of Obstetrics and Gynecology, 70,* 93.

Oppé, T. E. Risk register for babies. (1967). *Developmental Medicine and Child Neurology, 9,* 13.

Richards, I. D. G., & Roberts, C. J. (1967). Search for "suspect" infants. *Lancet, 2,* 711–713.

Sameroff, A. J. (1975). Early influences on development: Fact or fancy? *Merrill-Palmer Quarterly, 21*(4), 267–294.

Thorburn, M. J. (1981). *In Jamaica, community aides for disabled children: Assignment children.* Geneva: United Nation's Children's Fund.

Thorner, R. M., & Remein, Q. R. Principles and procedures in the evaluation of screening for disease. *Public Health Monograph No. 67,* PHS Publication No. 846.

World Health Organization. (1978). *Report of the task force on risk approach* (Publication No. 39). Geneva: World Health Organization.

Youden, W. J. (1950). Index for rating diagnostic tests. *Cancer, 3,* 32.

PART II

# New Perspectives

## THE AT-RISK CHILD IN THE SOCIAL ENVIRONMENT

CHAPTER 2

# Environmental Factors in the Early Screening of Children at Risk

*Arnold J. Sameroff*

The task of developmental screening has been to seek measures that will identify children who are at a high risk for having later problems. Traditional screening measures have focused on child behavior, the rationale being that the best way to predict how children will perform in the future is to examine how they perform in the present. The past and the present may well be the best predictors of the future for individuals with demonstrated stable continuities in behavior. However, when young children are the target, such stabilities are difficult to find (Seifer & Sameroff, 1984), for infancy is a period of transitions. Within the first 3 years of life, the child is transformed from a being who is completely dependent on the caregiving environment to one who has mobility, language, and a sense of self and others.

A first method of predicting later mobility, language, cognition, and social understanding would be to assess early forms of these behaviors. Muscles are necessary for mobility, so early assessments should be directed at the condition of the muscles. Auditory functioning and articulation are necessary for language, so early assessment should be directed at the ability to hear and to make sounds. The ability to think is necessary to understand self and others, so assessments should be directed at early examples of thought.

Although this continuous view of developmental functioning makes intuitive sense, it has not been borne out by empirical investigations. The data of development, especially early development, can be summed up with two principles: divergent development and convergent devel-

*Arnold J. Sameroff* • Institute for the Study of Developmental Disabilities, University of Illinois at Chicago, Chicago, Illinois 60637.

opment. The principle of *divergent development* is that from the same beginnings a multitude of final forms is possible. The principle of *convergent development* is that the same outcome can rise from a multitude of starting points. Infants with the same normal scores on developmental assessments can end up as Nobel prize winners, but also as derelicts. However, infants born very early and with very low birth weights can end up with severe mental retardation, but also with no later deficits.

This chapter attempts to explore the sources of variability in outcome. This exploration moves from assessments of the child to assessments of the child's experience. The case is made that all development follows a similar biological model. In this biological model, outcomes are never a function of the individual or the experiential context taken alone. Instead, outcomes are a product of the combination of an individual and his or her experience. This model presupposes that a singular focus on the characteristics of the individual (in this case the infant) to predict outcome will frequently be misleading. What needs to be added is an analysis and assessment of the experiences available to the child.

## A BIOLOGICAL MODEL FOR BEHAVIORAL DEVELOPMENT

The traditional medical model for understanding the origins of illness has been synonymous with a disease model, in which singular causes are thought to produce singular effects. In this model, prediction of illness is a simple matter of determining whether or not the cause is present. New approaches to biological and behavioral disorders have evolved that base causal analyses on a probablistic interaction of multiple factors. These recent approaches have been required to explain paradoxes that occurred when linear causes failed to explain a variety of disorders. Some cases involve illnesses that were thought for relatively long periods of medical history to have clear presumptive causes, such as turberculosis and phenylketonuria (PKU).

Tuberculosis was initially diagnosed as an environmental disorder. It was thought to be caused by conditions that accompanied poverty (e.g., poor nutrition, poor air, and poor health). To prevent tuberculosis, physicians told the patient to avoid such conditions of poverty and dwell in circumstances of good air, good nutrition, and a life devoid of stress. There were clear data to support the connection between the degree of disorder and the degree of poverty in the population. This analysis, however, was proven to be an artifact when the tubercle bacillus was discovered. A causal mechanism was found whereby the disorder could clearly be attributed to the action of a specific entity. A cure would result from elimination of the entity, a triumph of the disease model of illness.

However, this disease model, although effective in curing some diseases, has not been equally effective in predicting these diseases. Tuberculosis is not caused by the tubercle bacillus. For example, many individuals may carry the bacillus but not have any symptoms of the disorder (Edwards, 1975). The bacillus is a necessary condition for this disorder but not a sufficient condition; something else is also necessary. The additional factor is lowered resistance to disease resulting from poor nutrition, poor health, or poor air, all correlates of poverty. The germ alone cannot cause the disorder; and poor resistance alone cannot cause the disorder; but a combination of the two can. Thus, the disease entity must be viewed in context. If the context were different, the outcome would be different. Prevention of turberculosis can be accomplished with no attention to the specific germ associated with the illness; it can be achieved by eliminating the necessary context for the bacillus (i.e., the factors that lower resistance).

PKU is a disorder closer to this publication's area of concern, developmental disabilities. The discovery of PKU has been seen as a major achievement in the prediction of mental retardation by identifying a singular genetic cause.

In PKU, a gene is missing that affects the rate of conversion from phenylalanine into tyrosine, the next step in a metabolic sequence. The excess of phenylanine negatively affects brain development, so that untreated infants with this disorder become severely mentally retarded. Once a diagnosis is made, treatment is not directed at changing the affected child's genes, but at reducing the level of phenylalanine (Holtzman, Morales, Cunningham, & Wells, 1975). A dietary intervention that reduces the intake of phenylalanine prevents mental retardation. Here, again, a singular causal model is transformed into an interactional one. PKU causes mental retardation only in combination with a diet high in phenylalanine. If either factor were missing, there would be no disability. The anomalous gene alone cannot cause retardation.

Using the presence of PKU to predict mental retardation has additional complications. Adults have been found with the genetic disorder who did not have a dietary intervention, but who show no signs of mental retardation. Conversely, some infants who have had the intervention still became retarded. Other, as yet unidentified, factors besides the level of phenylalanine may be involved.

For both tuberculosis- and PKU-related mental retardation, at least two factors (and probably more) are involved in producing the disorder. Because the combination of these factors varies in each individual, the probability that a disorder will result varies. What appear to be two disorders with clear causes under closer scrutiny can be seen as the result of probabilistic interactions of multiple factors (Gollin, 1981). When applied to the understanding of developmental disabilities, and especially their prediction, what needs to be identified are the multiple factors and the associated probabilities of their interactions.

## REPRODUCTIVE AND CARETAKING CASUALTIES

Early screening is an attempt to identify factors that place a child at risk for developmental disabilities. Initially, the source of that risk was sought exclusively in the medical condition of the newborn infant (Lilienfeld & Parkhurst, 1951). The continuum of reproductive casualty (Pasamanick & Knobloch, 1961) was hypothesized to be a range of conditions that arose from the birth process, that were intrinsic to the child, and that were directly correlated with later outcomes. A major insult was thought to produce a major defect, such as cerebral palsy, whereas a minor insult was hypothesized to produce a minor defect, such as a learning disability. The central theme of this initial view of risk was that the deviation was a characteristic of the child, independent of context.

The reproductive risk concept arose in a medical framework where a disease model was thought to underlie all disorders. According to Engel (1977), the current dominant model of behavioral disorder is still biomedical, leaving little room for social and psychological concepts of illness. The biomedical model is reductionist in that all behavioral aberrations are explained on the basis of disordered somatic structure and function.

The contribution of the concept of reproductive casualty was to focus attention on the birth process as a source of development disabilities. However, the unexpected consequence of this attention was that major revisions were found to be necessary in the underlying biomedical model. Sameroff and Chandler (1975) attempted to find the etiological links hypothesized between reproductive factors and later psychological symptoms. In an extensive review of longitudinal studies of the consequences of birth complications, they were unable to discover deviant developmental consequences that could be linearly related to biological risk factors:

> Retrospective studies often gave the impression of having established clear relationships between pregnancy and delivery complications and later deviance. Prospective studies of the same variables have, however, not succeeded in demonstrating the predictive efficiency of these supposed risk factors. Most infants who suffer perinatal problems have proven to have normal developmental outcomes.
>
> The large role given to socioeconomic and familial factors in producing

> emotional difficulties and intellectual retardation (in children) tends to overshadow the effects of early perinatal difficulties. The environment appears to have the potential of minimizing or maximizing such early developmental difficulties. High socioeconomic status dissipates the effects of such perinatal complications as anoxia or low birth weight. Poor social environmental conditions tend to amplify the effects of such early complications. Since the caretaking environment plays such a major role in determining developmental outcomes, a "continuum of caretaking casualty" [is] hypothesized to describe the range of deviant outcomes which would be attributed to poor parenting. (p. 236)

The implications for models of developmental risk were that the characteristics of the child, especially the biomedical characteristics, could not be given sole status as causative factors in deviancy. The focus on "caretaking casualty" was the result of an emphasis on deviant outcomes for children. However, for the vast majority of children who suffer reproductive problems, behavioral outcomes are normal. To understand this discontinuity between biological and behavioral functioning, one must study the compensating aspects of the caretaking system, the environmental characteristics that move children from abnormal biological states to normal behavioral ones.

Sameroff and Chandler suggested that the self-righting tendencies that operated biologically in the embryological system to produce a physically normal infant (Waddington, 1966) might operate postnatally through social systems to produce a psychologically normal child. The biological self-righting tendencies are coded in a genetic system that monitors biochemically the status of the developing embryo and introduces regulatory processes to maintain a normative condition. Sameroff (1982) suggested that similar self-righting tendencies are located in the caregiving environment organized around behavioral norms and coded into social institutions and cultural heritages. In any society that endures over several generations, there must be a codified system of childbearing and socialization into appropriate roles to assure the continuity of that society.

In defining the developmental risk associated with any specific child, one must relate the characteristics of the child to the ability of the environment to regulate the development of that child toward social norms. In extreme cases of massive biological abnormality, such regulations may ineffectual. At the other extreme, disordered social environments might convert biologically normal infants into caretaking casualties.

The Kauai study of Werner and her colleagues (Werner, Bierman, & French, 1971; Werner & Smith, 1977; Werner & Smith, 1982) provides a good description of the interplay among risk factors in the child and those in the environment. A sample of children were followed from birth through adolescence. Assessments were made of the birth condition of the children and their developmental progress at 2, 10, and 18 years of age. From the predominantly lower socioeconomic (SES) sample, more than half had learning or emotional problems by 18 years of age. The first two books reporting this study (Werner et al., 1971; Werner & Smith, 1977) helped to dispel the notion that birth complications had a determining effect on behavioral outcomes. Children with severe early trauma frequently showed no later deficits unless the problems were combined with persistently poor environmental circumstances, such as chronic poverty, family instability, or maternal mental health problems.

In the third report of the Kauai study, Werner and Smith (1982) divided all the children who had been at a high clinical risk at 2 years of age into three groups: those who developed problems by 10 years of age, those who did not develop problems until 18 years of age, and those who did not develop problems at all. This latter "resilient" group was the target of analyses to determine what factors in development protected them from disorders. Most of the protective factors that were identified were not surprising: good temperament, favorable parental attitudes, low levels of family conflict, counseling and remedial assistance, small family size, and a smaller load of stressful life experiences. What was surprising was the variety of interactions among the factors and the degree of complexity of analysis needed to match the complexity of variables that affected the course of a child's development. For example, Werner and Smith attempted to separate those factors that led to healthier outcomes both in the presence or absence of risk conditions from those factors that only had an interactional effect (i.e., a positive impact in the presence of risk factors but no impact when risk factors were absent). These latter protective factors were not found to discriminate between positive and negative outcomes for middle-class children whose lives were relatively free of stress, but they were very important in the lives of children who were growing up in poverty and subject to a large number of negative life events.

The Kauai study is in tune with many others (Sameroff & Chandler, 1975) in targeting SES and family mental health as important moderators of child development. Both mental health and social status are summary variables that incorporate a wide range of factors that may interfere with optimal child rearing. The child could be passively affected through a withdrawn parent who is unavailable for the affective exchanges necessary for healthy emotional development, or through an impoverished environment where a limited range of stimulating experiences inhibits intellectual growth. On the other hand, the child could be actively affected through disorganizing experiences with abusive and intrusive parents, or through trauma and the increased number of stressful life events associated with lower SES existence.

The next section of this chapter explores the various factors that play a role in shaping the experience of the child. To the extent that experience is a necessary ingredient in the developmental equation, an assessment that can screen the experience of a child for risk factors would be an important additional tool for the clinician.

## ENVIRONMENTAL RISK ASSESSMENT

Since 1970, my colleagues and I have been conducting a longitudinal study that investigates the role of parental mental illness, social status, and other family cognitive and social variables that might be risk factors in the early development of children from birth through 4 years of age. The Rochester Longitudinal Study (RLS) was explicitly concerned with the impact of parental factors on the development of children. Recently, we reported findings from this longitudinal study through $2\frac{1}{2}$ years of age (Sameroff, Seifer, & Zax, 1982). This report also will include analyses of factors contributing to child outcomes at age 4 (Sameroff & Seifer, 1983). Of specific relevance are analyses of the relative impact of a variety of risk factors, especially the parental perspectives we believe mediate much of early child development.

In previous analyses comparing children from various groups of mothers, we demonstrated that both parental mental illness and social status factors were directly related to child performance (Sameroff *et al.*, 1982). Although these results are meaningful, they do not fully address the issue of what psychological mechanisms are responsible for the individual and group variation observed in the children's development. As the next step in addressing the complex interactions of risk factors, we examined additional groups of measures that might explain broader social status and mental illness factors (Sameroff & Seifer, 1983). These included the cognitive capacities, attitudes, beliefs, and values of the mother, as well as the stresses that have impact on the family. The measures used in these multivariate analyses and the characteristics of the RLS sample are summarized below.

### Rochester Longitudinal Study

When the children of the RLS were 4 years of age, 215 families were participating in the study. These families were heterogeneous on many dimensions. In fact, all five of Hollingshead's (1957) SES levels were represented. There were white, black, and Puerto Rican families with 1 to 10 children. Most of the women were married when their child was born, but 37 were single (i.e., had never married), and 17 were separated or divorced. The mothers' ages ranged from 15 to 40, and their educational attainment varied from completion of the third grade to advanced degrees.

The two outcome-criterion measures of child performance used were the Wechsler Primary and Preschool Scales of Intelligence (Wechsler, 1967) and Verbal IQ (WPPSI-VIQ), and the Rochester Adaptive Behavior Inventory (RABI), a measure of social-emotional competence (Seifer, Sameroff, & Jones, 1981). The RABI was developed during the course of the RLS and consisted of a 90-minute interview of the mother by a trained interviewer about the adaptive behavior of her child. A global rating was used, which is a summary score given by the interviewer on a 5-point scale where 1 point indicates superior adjustment and 5 points indicates clinical disturbance.

### *Risk Variables*

From the set of variables assessed during the RLS, 11 variables hypothesized to be related to either cognitive or social-emotional competence were selected (Sameroff & Seifer, 1983). These variables were

1. severity of maternal mental illness,
2. chronicity of maternal mental illness,
3. maternal anxiety,
4. parental perspectives,
5. maternal interactive behaviors,
6. maternal education,
7. occupation of head of household,
8. minority group social status,
9. family social support,
10. stressful life events, and
11. family size.

Each of these variables was used to form a low-risk group and a high-risk group as described below and in Table 1.

***Severity of Maternal Mental Illness.*** The categories of maternal mental illness in the RLS were determined from two psychiatric interviews (one when the mother was pregnant and one when the child was 30 months of age), and information obtained from a local psychiatric registry.

***Chronicity of Maternal Mental Illness.*** The chronicity of mothers' mental illness was derived from the same sources as the severity measure.

***Maternal Anxiety.*** The severity and chronicity of mental illness scores described above were most sensitive to variation in the clinical range of mental functioning. In contrast, the anxiety measures de-

**Table 1.** Summary of Risk Variables

| Risk variable | Low risk | High risk |
|---|---|---|
| Severity of illness | No mental illness | Some mental illness |
| Chronicity of illness | 0-1 psychiatric contacts | 2 or more psychiatric contacts |
| Anxiety | Low 75% | High 25% |
| Parental perspectives | High 75% | Low 25% |
| Interaction | High 75% | Low 25% |
| Education | High school | No high school |
| Occupational level | Skilled labor or higher | Semi-skilled or unskilled labor |
| Minority status | White | Non-white |
| Family support | Father present | Father absent |
| Life events | Low 75% | High 25% |
| Family size | 1–3 | 4 or more |

scribed here were more sensitive to variation in the subclinical range. Three measures of maternal anxiety were used: the total score from the Institute for Personality and Ability Testing (IPAT) Anxiety Scale developed by Cattell and Scheier (1963), the Neuroticism scale from the Eysenck and Eysenck (1969) personality inventory, and the Malaise Inventory (Rutter, Tizard, Yule, Graham, & Whitmore, 1976) in the Isle of Wight studies. These three measures were standardized and then averaged using unit weights.

***Parental Perspectives.*** For this dimension we chose measures that reflected rigidity versus flexibility in parental attitudes, beliefs, and values regarding children. The hypothesis was that in situations that called for adaptive behavior on the part of parents (e.g., environmental stress in the form of life changes or family stress in the form of mental illness or a child's handicap), parents with limited flexibility would be unable to buffer the child or be buffered from the child. We thought rigidity would be reflected in a combination of three measures that scored categorical interpretations of child behavior, conforming values to external norms, and an authoritarian orientation to child rearing.

The Concepts of Development Questionnaire (CODQ) (Sameroff & Feil, 1984) evaluates parents' understanding of development on a scale ranging from *categorical* to *perspectivistic*. At the categorical end, child development is seen as a determined expression of single causes like constitution or environment. At the perspectivistic end, child behavior is seen as the outcome of complex, transactional processes. The CODQ will be described more fully in a later section of this chapter.

The Kohn (1969) Parental Values Scale measures the values that parents believe are important for their children. This measure differs from the CODQ in that it taps specific values of parents for their own child. The main factor derived from this scale is a measure of conformity where parents value qualities of obedience, neatness, good manners, and appropriate sex role higher than qualities of responsibility, consideration of others, and curiosity.

The third measure used was the Parental Attitude Research Instrument (PARI) developed by Schaefer and Bell (1958). This measure is more directed at specific parenting styles than either the CODQ or Kohn measures described above. The authoritarian-control scale (Becker & Krug, 1965) accounts for most of the variance in the 115 PARI items. This scale indicates acceptance of parenting styles that emphasize parental control and minimize child-directed behavior. These three scales were standardized and summed using unit weights.

***Mothers' Interactive Behaviors.*** Direct observations of mother-child interactions to measure the way that mothers actually behaved with their children were done in the home when the study children were 4 months of age and again when they were 12 months old. The data at each age were factor analyzed, and in both cases the most compelling variable was found to be the amount of spontaneous behavior exhibited by the mother toward her child. A composite variable was created by standardizing the mothers' spontaneous measure at both ages and summing them with unit weights.

***Maternal Education.*** The level of mothers' education was determined during the prenatal interviews.

***Occupation of Head of Household.*** The occupation(s) of family members was also determined during the prenatal interviews. Although occupational status in itself is not a risk factor, to the extent that it reflects the financial resources of the family it can be interpreted as one. This information was coded in terms of Hollinghead's (1957) index of social position. The father's occupation was used if he was present in the household; otherwise the mother's occupation was used.

***Minority Group Social Status.*** The sample consisted of white, black, and Puerto Rican families. The low-risk group consisted of the white families. The high-risk group was formed from the minority group families since lack of equal opportunity independent of education has been shown to be related to less successful outcomes in these groups (Jencks, 1972).

***Family Social Support.*** Additional variables are necessary to describe specific qualities of any individual family in addition to the more general family demographic characteristics. The amount of family support the mother has in raising her children was considered an important variable. Our low-risk group consisted of those families where the father was present during the entire course of the study, while the high-risk group included families where the father was absent or where the parents separated during the 4 years in question.

***Stressful Life Events.*** During the 4 years of the study, mothers were questioned about events that affected the child and family. A measure of stressful negative life events was developed (Rosenzweig, Seifer, & Sameroff, 1983) that was patterned after the inventories of Holmes and Rahe (1967). Events such as loss of job, death in the family, or physical illness were included in the scale.

***Family Size.*** The final risk variable used was the size of the family. The presence or absence of other children determines the degree to which there is competition for social and physical resources that are at a premium in at-risk famlies.

## Effects of Single Risk Factors

The low-risk and high-risk groups for all 11 risk variables were compared on the two outcome criteria of WPPSI-VIQ and RABI global rating.

All comparisons for the VIQ scores were significantly different, and in all cases the low-risk group had higher scores than the high-risk group. The largest absolute difference was for minority status (about 18 points), but most differences were about 7 to 10 IQ points (about one-half to two-thirds of a standard deviation).

On the RABI global rating, the low-risk group performed significantly better than the high-risk group for all but one of the comparisons. This exception was for mother–child interaction, where no difference was found. The differences between groups on these comparisons were generally about one-half of a standard deviation.

## Effects of Multiple Risk Factors

Although there are many differences on individual risk factors, there are two major shortcomings in such analyses. First, any one particular risk group consists of a relatively large number of individuals, and the discrimination between the two groups is not large enough to accurately predict poor outcome based on risk status alone. Second, it is not clear if the many risk factors are totally overlapping in their effects or if there are additive components when these risk variables are viewed in unison.

A multiple risk score was created to alleviate these shortcomings that consisted of the total number of risk groups of which any individual family was a member. The actual scores ranged from 0 to 9 (out of a possible 11), and the sample was well distributed between scores of 0 and 8. Only 1 family had a multiple risk score of 9, and it was combined in all analyses with families whose score was 8. The largest re-

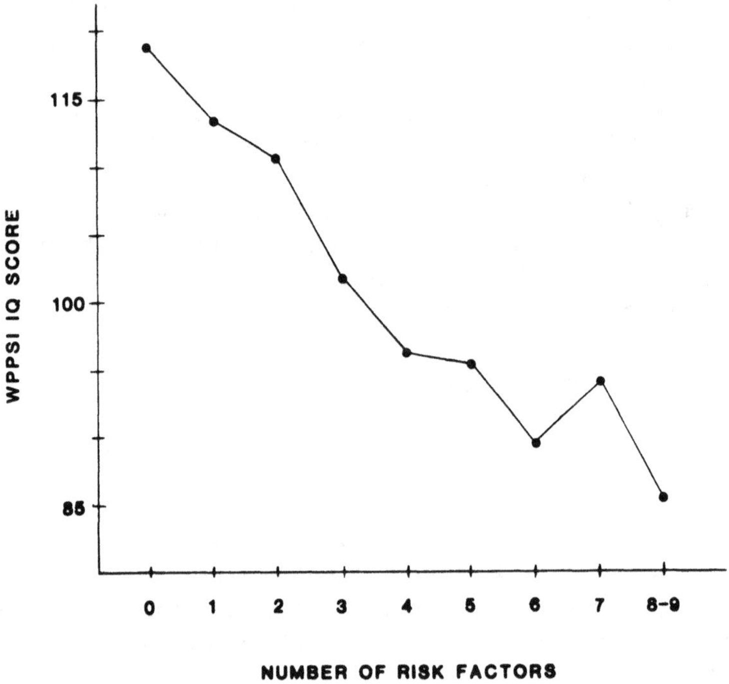


**Figure 1.** Relation between number of multiple risk factors and WPPSI verbal IQ performances at 4 years.

sulting group contained 36 families, and the smallest group had 10 families.

## Multiple Risk Scores and Outcomes

The relation between the multiple risk classification and the 4-year IQ outcome criterion is summarized graphically in Figure 1. It is clear from this figure that the effect of combining the 11 risk variables was to accentuate the differences noted for the individual scores described above. As the number of risk factors increases, performance decreases for children at 4 years of age.

In addition to the clear downward linear trend, the size of the effect for multiple risk factors was much larger than for individual risk factors. For the IQ scores, the difference between the lowest and highest groups was about 2 standard deviations (*SD*s). This compares with a difference of less than 1 *SD* for most of the individual risk factors.

The relation between the total risk scores and the RABI is shown in Figure 2. For the RABI, the difference in the multiple risk analysis was about 1.33 *SD*s compared with the .5 *SD* differences found in the

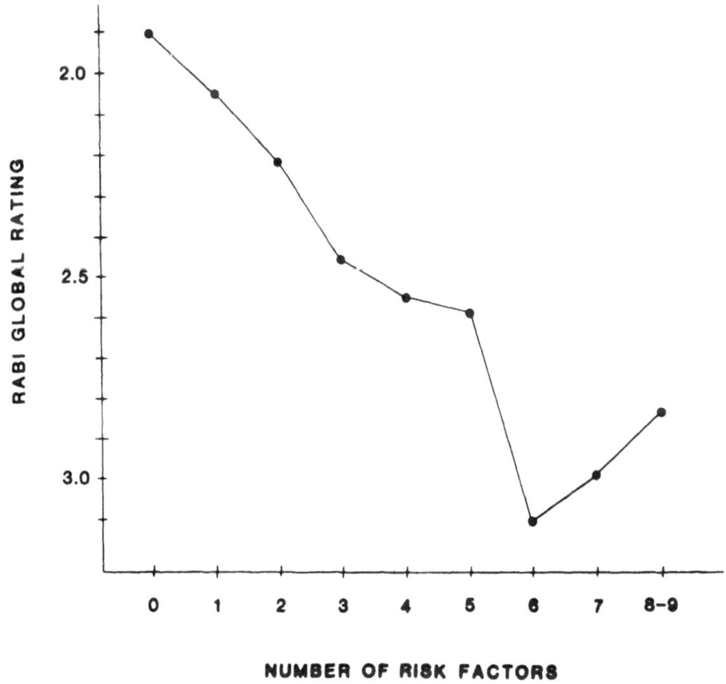


**Figure 2.** Relation between number of multiple risk factors and RABI global rating of social-emotional competence at 4 years.

single risk analyses. Thus, the combination of risk factors results in a nearly three-fold increase in the magnitude of differences found among groups of children.

## Risk and Outcome

Increased levels of risk have a linear effect on child competence. However, presentation of results in this form obscures the impact that multiple risk has on individuals. To clarify such individual effects, the same data are presented in terms of the proportion of good versus poor outcomes for high-risk, moderate-risk, and low-risk groups of children (see Figures 3 and 4).

In the high-risk group (6 to 9 risk factors) only 2% of the children had superior IQ scores of 116 to 150, while 29% had very low scores that ranged from 50 to 84. In contrast, in the low-risk group (0–2 risk factors) only 1% of the children had very low IQs, but 51% had scores in the highest range (see Figure 3). A similar pattern was obvious for social-emotional competence. In the high-risk group, only 2% had superior global ratings while 36% were rated in the poorest category. The situa-

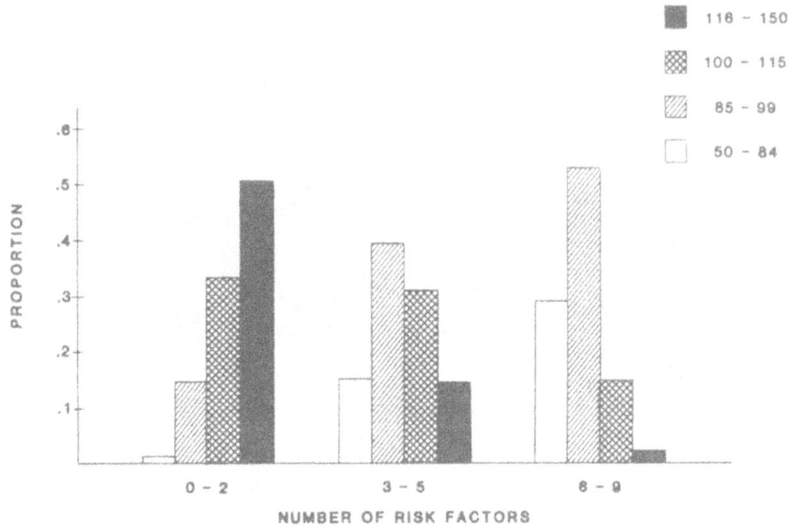


**Figure 3.** Proportion of children in four categories of WPPSI-VIQ performance within three multiple risk groupings at 4 years.

tion was reversed in the low-risk group—26% were rated superior and only 5% were rated poor (see Figure 4). For both the IQ and RABI scores, the moderate-risk group had patterns midway between the high- and low-risk children.

Thus, when these data are viewed from the perspective of individual predictions, the probability of very poor outcome is 30 times greater

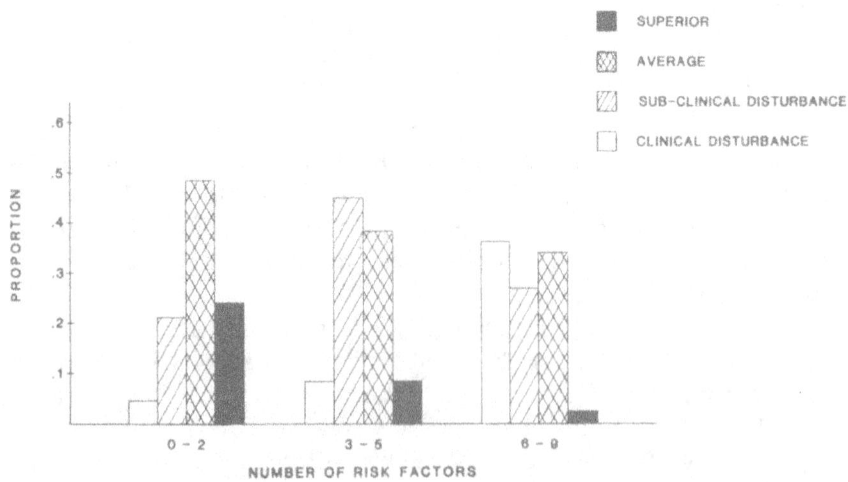


**Figure 4.** Proportion of children in four categories of RABI global rating of social-emotional competence within three multiple risk groupings at 4 years.

for cognitive competence and 7 times greater for social-emotional competence as one moves from low-risk to high-risk status. Conversely, the probability of superior outcomes are 25 times less likely for cognitive competence and 13 times less likely for social-emotional competence in the high-risk group.

The combination of risk factors into a single score has shown the strongest relationship to child intellectual and social-emotional competence. The more risk factors, the heavier the load on the developmental system. By examining a population that is biased toward developmental problems, one can examine a large array of risk factors that would not be evident in a more homogeneous sample. What is clear is that there are many children who are suffering severe deficits in competence. To the extent that any one of the identified risk factors is increased in the general population, increases in the number of children who will suffer the consequences can be expected.

Prediction of developmental outcome has been demonstrated to be a complex enterprise. Because of the dynamics of the developmental system, the effects of single risk factors can be moderated by other positive aspects of the child rearing environment. Where there is economic deprivation, competent, interactive parents can make up for the deficit. Where there is a high level of environmental stress, parental coping skills can reduce the impact on the child; and where there is a low level of stressful events, poor parental coping may be irrelevant. However, where compensating mechanisms are deficient and stress levels are high, problems for the child will be much more likely.

There is little that the clinician can do to alter a family's demographic characteristics or to reduce the number of stressful life events. An area where there is some possibility of change is in the family's ability to cope with stress. An aspect of coping that my colleagues and I have focused on in our research is the ability of parents to understand the development of their child. If a parent is capable of a perspectivistic view of the child, then the parent can also think of alternative ways of dealing with not only the child, but with other life problems as well.

## CONCEPTS OF DEVELOPMENT

Theories of development have been frequently based on what are seen as the determinants of a child's outcome. As with scientists, parents can differ in the importance they give to influences arising from the child's nature (a constitutional approach), to the child's nurturing (an environmental approach), or to some combination of the two (an interactive or transactional approach) (Sameroff & Chandler, 1975). However, the degree to which parents can hold a complex theory of development will depend on the degree to which they can deal with complexity in general. For example, if parents cannot consider two variables in the same context, they will be unable to have an interactional view of development. In short, the limitations in the formal complexity of parental thought will limit the range of contents in their developmental theories.

Models for the organization of thought typically deal with a dimension running from the immediacy of "here and now" experiences to successively removed levels of abstraction. Sameroff (1975) made an initial attempt to formulate steps along this dimension based on a Piagetian view of cognition. The application of a Piagetian analysis to social thought is not a new enterprise and has given rise to the field of social cognition (Chandler, 1977). Kohlberg (1969) was one of the first to elaborate on Piaget's own work in the area of moral reasoning. Selman (1980) expanded this work in the direction of interpersonal understanding, which was then specifically adapted to parents' concepts of children by Newberger (1980).

The stages in the parent's construction of the child were formulated at four levels analogous to Piaget's "sensory-motor," "pre-operational," "concrete operational," and "formal operational" levels. These were the symbiotic, the categorical, the compensating, and the perspectivistic levels.

At the *symbiotic* level, the parent is concerned primarily with the immediate relationship to the child. Parents will respond in a here-and-now fashion to the child's behavior. Their emotional response is directly related to how successful they are at ministering to the child. In a sense they do not see themselves as separate from the child, since they interpret the child's behavior as being directly tied to their own activity. Symbiotic parents are basically atheoretical in their understanding of development. If, for example, breastfeeding feels good for the mother, then it is good for the baby. Lack of differentiation between self and child makes the ability to reflect on the developmental process impossible.

At the *categorical* level, parents are able to see their children and themselves as separate entities such that the children's actions can be viewed as being intrinsic characteristics of the child and not only the result of the parent's activity. A consequence of this objectification of the world is that labels can be applied to these objects. The parent who has had a successful experience with his or her child assigns positive labels (for example, the good child, the pretty child, or the bright child). Once labels are assigned, however, they may become permanent in the parent's mind. Even though infants may outgrow the behavior that caused them to be labeled as difficult in the first place, the perceptions and reactions of the parent restricted to the categorical level will continue to be dominated by the original label. Furthermore, parents at this level tend to see behavior as having single causes, for example, any specific developmental outcome will have had either a constitutional or an environmental determinant.

At the *compensating* level, parents are able to view their child as having an existence not only apart from the parent's activities as at the symbiotic level, but also apart from their labels as at the categorical level. For example, the behavior of a child can now be related to age. Infants cry, toddlers are hyperactive, whereas adolescents sulk. The positive achievement at this higher level is that the behavior of the infant that could have given him or her a life-long label of "difficult" is seen as age-specific. Moreover, the parent sees that the child will probably behave quite differently at later ages. The parent is able to use a much broader context for valuing the child. No single label can typify the entire range of the child's behavior. At the compensating level, the normative behavior at each age is considered a characteristic of human development that finds its source in the child. It takes an advance to the next level for the parent to appreciate the complex relationship between the behavior of the child and the way he or she was reared.

Additional context is provided when the parent can view the child from the *perspectivistic* level. At this level the particular child and the particular caregiving situation can be placed in a hypothetical context of any child in any caregiving situation. The concrete situation at hand is only one of a multitude of possibilities. The parent is able to see the child's behavior as stemming from individual experience with a specific environment. The parent at this level can understand that if the experience had been different, the child's characteristics would be different. Deviancies in the child are now perceived as being deviancies in the relation of a particular child to a particular context, rather than as concrete expressions of the essential nature of the child. Remediation can be proposed by altering the experience of the child through environmental change.

In sum, the way a parent interprets the behavior of his or her child is related to the parent's complexity of developmental thought. From the most simple level of here-and-now interaction with the child, the parent is able to place the elements of the interaction into an increasingly broader context, advancing to being able to separate children from their labels, and eventually to being able to separate children from the particular life circumstances in which they were raised. If these circumstances had been or would become different, children with different behaviors would result.

### Assessing Concepts of Development

Once a sequence of levels of parental thinking had been defined, it was possible to devise screening measures to assess these levels. The first measure was in the form of a questionnaire in which the respondents were asked to rate a series of statements on a 4-point scale from *strongly agree* to *strongly disagree*. Forty-four items were constructed to tap the four levels.

Symbiotic-level items were based on immediate affective reactions to the child. Examples of these items are "A mother is very happy when she can get her baby to smile" or, the opposite, "Mothers feel upset if they can't get their babies to look at them."

Categorical-level items focused on identification of people with their role labels or on single explanations of behavior based on either environment or constitution alone. An example of a constitutional item would be "Premature babies will have a lot of problems later on," and an example of an environmental item would be "Parents have to be strict with their young children or else they'll turn out badly." A role–stereotype item would be "Boy babies are more active than girl babies."

Compensating-level items attempted to tap age–behavior coordinations and an awareness of the interaction of constitution and environment in producing developmental outcomes. Examples of such items include "Children have to be treated differently as they grow older" and "Difficult babies will grow out of it."

Perspectivistic-level items were more difficult to formulate. These items defined any specific developmental outcomes as an instance of a set of possible outcomes, and also described the family as a system of dynamic reciprocal relationships. Examples are "It is generally better for the father and mother to share responsibility in the home for disciplining and taking care of their children" or "Children's problems never have a single cause."

All items were treated as a single scale and a Cronbach's (1950) alpha was calculated as were part–whole correlations for each item. An alpha of .71 was obtained. Items with low part–whole correlations were dropped from the scale. We were disappointed because this procedure eliminated all the symbiotic items. The scale was further reduced until 20 items remained, the 10 categorical and the 10 compensating-perspectivistic items with the greatest part-whole correlations. The alpha for the final 20-item scale was .82. Three scores are produced. These are a categorical score, which is the mean of the 10 categorical items, a perspectivistic score, which is the mean of the 10 compensating and perspectivistic items, and a CODQ total score, which combined the amount of agreement to the compensating-perspectivistic items and the amount of disagreement to the categorical items.

### *Concepts of Development Vignettes*

An issue with which we were concerned was that item construction was based on our interpretation of what parents were thinking about development, rather than on their actual thoughts. In a pilot study, a number of parents were interviewed about their ideas, but it was found difficult to elicit their theories without asking about specific examples. Based on this exploratory work, we wrote a series of Concepts of Development Vignettes (CODVs) about a variety of developmental problems and then asked parents to explain the various developmental outcomes.

In a second pilot study, my collegues and I examined parental responses and found it possible to conduct a formal analysis of the answers along the concepts of development dimension. We hoped that somehow a symbiotic level of responding would emerge to make up for the failure to find this level in our questionnaire results. A scoring manual was written for the analysis of the vignettes and is summarized below.

*Level 1—Nonreflective (Symbiotic).* As with the CODQ, we were unable to get a positive expression of the symbiotic level with the CODV—and for the same reasons. As soon as people are asked a question about their thinking, they must move to a conceptual level that removes them from the here-and-now lack of differentiation we believe characterizes the symbiotic level. However, a complement of the symbiotic view was found in the inability of the parent to produce a reflective answer.

Responses at this level are atheoretical in that influences and outcomes are not differentiated. In other words, development or change is not acknowledged. Developmental influences such as environment or constitution are not mentioned, and individual characteristics, behaviors, or events are not considered to have causal or even temporal antecedents. Discussion is here-and-now oriented (e.g., "They're just listening to their parents fighting. I just don't know why" or "He's just not a contented baby. I don't know why.").

*Level 2—Categorical.* At this level, the parent is able to state a cause or a determinant of developmental outcomes. However, only one influence for a particular situation is considered, or only one developmental course to a particular outcome is described. For example, if parental attention is viewed as the determinant of success in school, then any child with a lot of parental attention should do well in school. Either constitutional or environmental factors (or an aspect of these) can be explained as determining development. Explanations are situation-specific and uncoordinated across different problems. "IQ is inherited" may be stated in one context, and "You need to give children attention so that they can be smart" may be stated in another. Other examples are "She's never had no one to play with so she hasn't learned how to play" or "She couldn't take the pressure from her husband's job."

*Level 3—Compensating.* At this level, two or more influences are discussed and coordinated for single developmental outcomes. These may involve constitutional and environmental influences, two constitutional influences, or two environmental influences. Additionally, if one environmental influence is said to affect two children differently, then the response is scored at this level. An example that has multiple influences and coordinates past and present is "It may be a combination of lack of stimulation and possible poor nutrition to the mother prenatally. She might have a learning disability related to trauma at birth." Also at this level would be an explanation based on birth order, such as "Possibly since she is the second child the parents aren't spending as much time helping her with her homework as they did her brother."

*Level 4—Perspectivistic.* A comprehensive explanation of the developmental process is given. Multiple influences on developmental outcomes are considered and any particular developmental equation is understood within the set of the all-hypothetical examples. Parent–child relations are presented as transactions, with parents affecting the child's behavior and the child affecting parental behavior. The child's development is viewed as taking place within the context of a dynamic system of relationships, and parents may be described as changing as well as their children. Generally these responses lack the static character seen in responses at lower levels. An example follows:

> Probably mounting tension with frustration of the children fighting and everything piling up. Probably just took it out in this form. She probably took it out on Billy because of his past behavior, because he was a demanding child. Probably just assumed that it was his fault. Result of inner turmoil. Maybe hostility due to money problems and maybe she resented him subconsciously. I don't know if it could be a subconscious feeling that it was her husband or something

### *Studies of Developmental Concepts*

In order to test our assessments, we tried to find samples in which there would be a broad range of responses as well as identifiable groups that we could predict would score differently on the measures. A series of studies were performed using various combinations of our measures on samples that varied in social and cultural characteristics. The large differences in child outcomes found between groups differing in social status raised the question of whether parents from these differing social levels differed in their concepts of development. Kohn's (1969) report of the high correlation between conforming values and lower social status stimulated this hypothesis. In addition, we wanted to see if any relationship found between concepts of development and social status was culture specific. To this end, samples from the United States and England, from both higher and lower social status groups (Sameroff & Feil, 1984), were studied.

***English-American Study.*** For a pilot study of the CODQ, a sample of mothers was recruited in England and in the United States. Families were classified into 4 subgroups according to SES. Significant differences were found for both nationality and SES effects; the United States sample scored as more perspectivistic than the English sample, and the high SES mothers scored as more perspectivistic than the low SES mothers. However, when the means in the 4 subgroups were examined, only the United States high SES group was different from the other 3. The high SES English group had the same mean as the 2 low SES groups. Although of higher intelligence, this high SES English group is imbued with a cultural tradition of inherited social position and an accompanying belief that individuals should "stay in their place;" they agreed more with categorical concepts of development than an American high SES group whose cultural heritage is based more on social mobility than stasis.

***Standardization study.*** The data from the English-American study were collected using a pilot form of the CODQ. After this version of the CODQ was refined and the COD vignettes prepared, a study was designed to obtain normative data on the instruments as well as to compare their scores in a local sample. Eighty mothers of preschool children were recruited in such a way that the five Hollingshead (1957) SES groups were represented. In addition, about half the sample had only one child, whereas the rest had larger families.

The SES differences found in the English-American study were replicated in the standardization study. There were strong linear effects on each of the concept of development measures. In addition, the CODQ and CODV scores were strongly intercorrelated (Sameroff & Feil, 1984).

Several conclusions emerge from an examination of data. The first is that the majority of responses were at the compensating level. Most parents have a good basic understanding of development that should permit them to adequately interpret the problems they may have with their children. The second conclusion is that there are strong SES differences. The SES-I gave no categorical or lower responses, while 42% of the SES-V responses fell below the compensating level. The final point is that in a socially stratified sample, such as was used in the standardization study, only 3% of the responses were at the perspectivistic level. These data make it clear that there is a great deal of room for change in the way our society views development.

## Determinants of Concepts of Development

The several studies that have been described have allowed identification of a number of factors that limit levels of understanding. Constraints have been found from life in lower SES environments, from adherence to traditional culture systems, from a life course that makes no demands for perspective-taking, and from an individual's general lower level of cognitive functioning.

In every culture tested, we have found simpler concepts of development in lower SES groups. This SES difference could be attributed exclusively to the lower level of intelligence generally found in such groups; however, Kohn's (1969) work has made a strong case for an explanation based on the constrictions of thought produced by lower SES existence. The need for conformity as an adaptive value for people with fewer choices in life has been well documented in Kohn's analyses of the relationship between low SES and working conditions.

My colleagues and I have hypothesized that the way parents understand development is important because it should influence the way their children are raised and, consequently, how their children will turn out. We have presented some data to support this view, but it must be noted that strong correlations between such variables have not been found in the past and should not be expected in the future. The complexity of parental thought only has meaning when entered into the same equation with the specific contents of that thought and the characteristics of the children being raised (Sameroff & Chandler, 1975; Sameroff & Seifer, 1983). A healthy, happy child can be raised relatively easily by a parent at any level of developmental understanding. The child will make the symbiotic mother feel effective, will get positive labels from the categorical mother, and will fit into the compensating mother's scheme of development. Being perspectivistic allows a parent the widest range of adaptive thought. However, there can also be negative consequences associated with such complex thinking because parents can think about all the things that might go wrong, despite the fact that their child is doing very well at the time.

## CONCLUSIONS

The way parents interpret the behavior of their children is related to the parents' level of understanding development. However, parents' ability to place a child in a developmental context is only one dimension of the complex matrix necessary to chart the child's course through life. Many other dimensions are intertwined and must be understood in their interconnectedness if individual developmental predictions are to be successful. Escalona (1968) noted that although we may be very good at assessing the current behavior of the child, we are very bad at explaining how the child got to be that way or predicting what the child will be like in the future. Child development must be viewed from a systems perspective that integrates many necessary factors (Sameroff,

1982, 1983). Focusing on the characteristics of the child is not predictive unless the characteristics of the caregiving environment are included in the equation. Moreover, we are beginning to realize that the characteristics of the environment must be interpreted in complex terms (Bronfenbrenner, 1979).

The analysis of risk factors within the family and social environment is an example of such an interpretation. Just as children are screened for developmental risk, environments can be screened. Environments with large numbers of risk factors will produce few competent children. High levels of stress and low levels of social support are ingredients in the risk equation, but of equal importance is the ability of parents to understand and cope with developmental problems. The addition of environmental screening measures to developmental screening measures of the child will maximize the probability of correctly identifying those children in need of intervention.

## REFERENCES


Becker, W. C., & Krug, R. S. (1965). The parent attitude research instrument: A research review. *Child Development, 36*, 329–365.

Bronfenbrenner, U. (1979). *The ecology of human development.* Cambridge: Harvard Univ. Press.

Cattell, R. B., & Scheier, I. H. (1963). *Handbook for the IPAT anxiety scale questionnaire* (2nd ed.). Champaign, IL: Institute for Personality and Ability Testing.

Chandler, M. J. (1977). Social cognition: A selective review of current research. In W. F. Overton & J. M. Gallagher (Eds.), *Knowledge and development: Advances in research and theory* (Vol. 1). New York: Plenum Press.

Cronbach, L. J. (1951). Coefficient alpha and the internal structure of tests. *Psychometrika, 16*, 297–334.

Edwards, P. Tuberculosis. (1975). In W. K. Frankenburg & B. W. Camp (Eds.), *Pediatric screening tests.* Springfield, IL: Charles C Thomas.

Engel, G. L. (1977). The need for a new medical model: A challenge for biomedicine. *Science, 196*, 129–136.

Escalona, S. K. (1968). *The roots of individuality.* Chicago: Aldine.

Eysenck, H. J., & Eysenck, S. B. G. (1969). *Personality structure and measurement.* San Diego: Robert R. Knapp.

Gollin, E. S. (1981). Development and plasticity. In E. S. Gollin (Ed.), *Developmental plasticity.* New York: Academic Press.

Hollingshead, A. B. (1957). *Two factor index of social position.* Mimeograph. (Available from Sociology Department, Yale University, New Haven, CT.)

Holmes, T. H., & Rahe, R. H. (1967). The social readjustment rating scale. *Journal of Psychosomatic Research, 11*, 213–218.

Holtzman, N. A., Morales, D. R., Cunningham, G., & Wells, D. G. T. (1975). Phenylketonuria. In W. K. Frankenburg & B. W. Camp (Eds.), *Pediatric screening tests.* Springfield, IL: Charles C Thomas.

Jencks, C. (1972). *Inequality.* New York: Basic Books.

Kohlberg, L. (1969). Stage and sequence: The cognitive developmental approach to socialization. In D. Goslin (Ed.), *Handbook of socialization theory and research.* Chicago: Rand-McNally.

Kohn, M. L. (1969). *Class and conformity: A study in values.* Homewood, IL: The Dorsey Press.

Lilienfeld, A. M., & Parkhurst, E. (1951). A study of the association of factors of pregnancy and parturition with the development of cerebral palsy: A preliminary report. *American Journal of Hygiene, 53,* 262–282.

Newberger, C. M. (1980). The cognitive structure of parenthood: Designing a descriptive measure. In R. R. Yando (Eds.), *New directions for child development: Clinical development research* (Vol. 7). San Francisco: Jossey-Bass.

Pasamanick, B., & Knobloch, H. (1961). Epidemiological studies on the complications of pregnancy and the birth process. In G. Caplan (Ed.), *Prevention of mental disorders in children.* New York: Basic Books.

Rosenzweig, L., Seifer, R., & Sameroff, A. J. (1983). *The impact of stressful life events on high-risk families.* Unpublished manuscript. (Available from authors, Illinois Institute for Developmental Disabilities, 1640 W. Roosevelt Road, Chicago, IL 60608.)

Rutter, M., Tizard, J., Yule, W., Graham, P., & Whitmore, K. (1976). Research report: Isle of Wight studies, 1964–1974. *Psychological Medicine, 6,* 313–332.

Sameroff, A. J. (1975). Transactional models in early social relations. *Human Development, 18,* 65–79.

Sameroff, A. J. (1982). Development and the dialectic: The need for a systems approach. In W. A. Collins (Ed.), *Minnesota symposium on child psychology* (Vol. 15). Hillsdale, NJ: Lawrence Erlbaum.

Sameroff, A. J. (1983). Systems of development: Contexts and evolution. In W. Kessen (Ed.), *History, theories, and methods* (Vol. 1), of P. H. Mussen (Ed.), *Handbook of child psychology* (4 vols.). New York: Wiley.

Sameroff, A. J., & Chandler, M. J. (1975). Reproductive risk and the continuum of caretaking casualty. In F. D. Horowitz, M. Hetherington, S. Scarr-Salapatek, & G. Siegel (Eds.), *Review of child development research* (Vol. 4). Chicago: Univ. of Chicago Press.

Sameroff, A. J., & Feil, L. A. (1984). Parental concepts of development. In I. Sigel (Ed.), *Parental belief systems: The psychological consequences for children.* Hillsdale, NJ: Lawrence Erlbaum.

Sameroff, A. J., & Seifer, R. (1983). Familial risk and child competence. *Child Development, 54,* 1524–1268.

Sameroff, A. J., Seifer, R., & Zax, M. (1982). Early development of children at risk for emotional disorder. *Monographs of the Society for Research in Child Development, 47,* (Serial No. 199).

Schaefer, E. S., & Bell, R. Q. (1958). Development of a parental attitude research instrument. *Child Development, 29,* 339–361.

Seifer, R., & Sameroff, A. J. (1984). Multiple determinants of risk and vulnerability. In E. J. Anthony & B. J. Cohler (Eds.), *The invulnerable child.* New York: Guilford.

Seifer, R., Sameroff, A. J., & Jones, F. H. (1981). Adaptive behavior in young children of emotionally disturbed women. *Journal of Applied Developmental Psychology, 1,* 251–276.

Selman, R. L. (1980). *The growth of interpersonal understanding: Developmental and clinical analyses.* New York: Academic Press.

Waddington, C. H. (1966). *Principles of development and differentiation.* New York: Macmillan.

Wechsler, D. (1967). *Wechsler preschool and primary scale of intelligence manual.* New York: Psychological Corporation.

Werner, E. E., Bierman, J. M., & French, F. E. (1971). *The children of Kauai: A longitudinal study from the prenatal period to age ten.* Honolulu: Univ. of Hawaii Press.

Werner, E. E., & Smith, R. S. (1977). *Kauai's children come of age.* Honolulu: Univ. of Hawaii Press.

Werner, E. E., & Smith, R. S. (1982). *Vulnerable but invincible: A longitudinal study of resilient children and youth.* New York: McGraw Hill.

*CHAPTER 3*

# Broadening Research on Developmental Risk

## IMPLICATIONS FROM STUDIES OF VULNERABLE AND STRESS-RESISTANT CHILDREN

*Norman Garmezy*

Risk research, with its roots in epidemiology, is concerned with the identification of factors that accentuate or inhibit disease and deficiency states, and the processes that underlie them. Risk studies run the gamut from individual case histories to cross-sectional, and short-term and lengthier longitudinal investigations. The studies traverse the entire life span from birth to old age, with foci that include a broad range of risk factors. These include etiological studies emphasizing potential biological and behavioral precursors; personal positive and negative predispositional attributes; genetic and environmental influences on disorder; the actualizing power of stressful experiences; the ameliorating force of identifiable "protective" factors; the study of coping patterns, including their origins, development, and situational contexts; and the evaluation of outcomes ranging from signs of severe biobehavioral and social deficits to patterns of resilience and adaptation amid disadvantage.

The chapters in this volume reflect many of these areas. A large number are focused on the identification and screening of infants and children who are defined by biological, cognitive, or sensory factors as being at risk. In many instances, correlates of such vulnerabilities as pre-

*Norman Garmezy* • Department of Psychology, University of Minnesota, Minneapolis, Minnesota 55455. Preparation of the chapter was facilitated by grants from the William T. Grant Foundation, the National Institute of Mental Health, and a Research Career Award (NIMH-USPHS).

maturity, poor nutritional status, low birth weight, organic brain damage, and physical handicap implicate a variety of psychosocial stressors. These include the disadvantaged socioeconomic status of many at-risk children; they frequently have mothers who are young, unmarried, and poor, or they may come from disorganized urban or rural families. Numerous outcome studies (typically short-term) are also in evidence in the present volume.

From a historical perspective, the emphasis on infants and young children with developmental disabilities reflects a pioneering area of risk studies that clearly has retained its vitality through research on screening and intervention. In recent years new areas have come to be identified with such risk research, broadening the groups of children included in research studies and the types of research conducted with them.

This trend is illustrated by a University of Minnesota risk research program, Project Competence, and its different phases of activity over the past 15 years. Initially the program involved children presumed to be vulnerable to psychopathology on the basis of possible genetic and environmental influences. Included in these studies were children whose at-risk status implicated a variety of disordered psychiatric states, including schizophrenia, depression, antisocial disorder, hyperactivity, and socially isolative behavior (Garmezy & Devine, 1984). A second, more recent direction of the program's research has been the attempted identification of stress-resistant or resilient children, as reflected in signs of continued competence despite the presence of adverse circumstances (Garmezy, Masten, & Tellegen, 1984; Garmezy & Tellegen, 1984).

## CHILDREN VULNERABLE TO PSYCHOPATHOLOGY

Risk studies of children vulnerable to schizophrenia (Watt, Anthony, Wynne, & Rolf, 1984), affective disorders (Beardslee, Bemporad, Keller, & Klerman, 1983; Weissman, 1979), and antisocial disorders (Patterson, 1982; Robins, 1966; West & Farrington, 1973) have tended more toward the inclusion of older children rather than infants and toddlers. There are several reasons for such age selectivity. First, in the search for precursors to later behavioral disorders, the general research set of risk investigators has been to analyze complex behavioral processes (e.g., deficits in attention and information-processing, deviant social-emotional behaviors, poor peer interaction, disturbed parent-child relations, states of psychophysiological arousal, and so on). Such procedures require a level of cooperation that only older children can provide. (An exception to this general statement involves significant longitudinal research programs that take pregnant women with a known history of psychopathology as their starting point and follow the "at risk" offspring from birth onward (e.g., Marcus, Auerbach, Wilkinson, Maeir, Mark, & Peles, 1984; McNeil, Kaij, Malmquist-Larsson, Naslund, Persson-Blennow, McNeil, & Blennow, 1983; Sameroff, Seifer, & Zax, 1982).

## A Multimethod, Multivariate Approach

One example of developmental-clinical research of a high order and the utilization of varied research procedures in the evaluation of risk status in the very young is provided by Sameroff, Seifer, and Zax (1982). They demonstrate the importance of a multimethod, multivariable approach to assessment of child competence and related maternal attributes for investigators concerned with the early course of children with developmental disabilities. Such extensive evaluations are more likely to prove fruitful in understanding the adaptive potential of such children than would be the use of simpler, single-method screening techniques.

The multiple assessment approach utilized by Sameroff *et al.* (1982) reveals a broad-band sophisticated approach to unraveling the identification of potential precursor states. Initially a careful evaluation was made of the psychiatric status of mothers in the study using diagnostic psychiatric interviews; several comparison groups of mothers were formed from these interviews. The groups included mothers diagnosed as having schizophrenia, neurotic depression, personality disorder, and a control group which had no mental illness.

With the birth of the babies, data were collected on the course of labor and delivery, and the status of the newborn. The babies' minor physical anomalies were recorded, heart-rate measures were taken when they were 3 days old, and behavioral assessments were made. To insure reliability of observations, Sameroff *et al.* (1982) required multiple judges trained in scoring observation protocols.

Of particular interest to investigators of early disability are the multiple behavioral measures that Sameroff *et al.* (1982) used to provide cognitive, psychomotor, social, emotional, and psychophysiological assessments of the offspring of the disordered and normal mothers at birth, 4, 12, and 30 months of age. When the infants were 4 months of age, new observations were conducted of mother and baby in both home and laboratory. Psychometric tests of infant development were administered, and mothers provided ratings of their infants' temperament. At 12 months the home observations were repeated, attachment processes were studied, and additional measures of the infants' developmental status were made. At $2\frac{1}{2}$ years, the mothers described and rated their children's adaptive behavior, a social-medical history was obtained, prenatal attitudes toward the child were measured, and developmental assessments were continued (including IQ and social maturity ratings). At this point, a psychiatric interview with the mothers was administered in an effort to note the presence or absence of disorder, and the severity of disturbance (if present).

In this ongoing longitudinal study, evaluations of the subject children have been continued during childhood. Today studies of the members of the risk cohort are being carried forward into the early adolescent years.

## Risk Studies of Schizophrenia

In several ways the task of those who study developmental disabilities is somewhat easier than the research path that must be followed by investigators of children at risk for later psychopathology. Studies of children at risk for schizophrenia illustrate this point. In this disorder, risk status traditionally (if one can use the word for an emergent area of research) has been defined by the criterion of a present or previous diagnosis of disorder in a biological parent. Genetic studies supportive of such a criterion include the following: High concordance rates for schizophrenia have been found in monozygotic as opposed to dizygotic twin pairs; family pedigree studies show a genetic tendency toward the disorder; there are higher incidence rates of schizophrenia for adopted-away offspring of schizophrenic patients when compared with adoptees of parents without a history of mental illness; a heightened incidence of schizophrenia in first- and second-degree relatives of a schizophrenic proband has been found; there is a greater morbidity risk for schizophrenia in children born of a schizophrenic parent relative to offspring of normal parents; and the highest morbidity risk is for children of dual mated schizophrenic parentage.

Because of these genetic studies, risk researchers were moved to select as an at-risk population the biological offspring of adults who had been diagnosed as schizophrenic. They made this selection despite their awareness of a difficult problem: The genetic studies clearly suggested that the future incidence rate for such a cohort would be comparatively small (approximately 10% to 12% of reasonably large samples), and that the onset of disorder would be likely to extend upward into the early 20s and even the mid-40s. The specter of attrition in both the experimental samples and the investigators did not deter the growth of risk studies, but the reality was a discomforting one.

Researchers of developmental disability already evident in infancy face far less strenuous problems in identifying and selecting their samples, whereas maintaining a cohort over time is aided by parental concern over the well-being of the child and the necessity for continued medical surveillance. Such factors support in-depth research studies that extend the development of adequate screening techniques into broadly based, multimethod, and longitudinal investigations of the adaptive qualities of children in various contexts (the home, school, neighborhood, work environment, etc.).

### Competence and Adaptation

If there is a lesson to be learned from those who have studied children vulnerable to psychopathology, it is the importance of developing a broad set of variables that tap various dimensions of competence. Because this construct is central in evaluating developmentally disabled children, it may be of interest to cite the various aspects of competence functioning that researchers on risk for schizophrenia have brought to their investigations. These include neurological assessments; measures of attention, vigilance, and information processing; intellectual and school evaluation; the assessment of children's social behavior; teacher and peer (sociometric) ratings; measures of mother–child play and social interactions; personality measures and family process interaction variables; parental rearing patterns; home observations; and tests of developmental, cognitive, social-emotional, and work skills.

In addition, many early factors that may influence later competence have been assessed in different research programs. These include medical record contents related to prenatal and perinatal complications, pregnancy and birth difficulties, low birth weight status, and the like. Other relevant aspects evaluated in some studies (Watt *et al.*, 1984) include careful evaluations of family social class status, the caretaking effectiveness of mothers who had suffered a recent mental breakdown, the post-partum mental status of mothers during the 6 months following a child's birth, and the foster home experiences of some children. Examples such as these point to the importance of using a broad-gauged set of competence indicators rather than relying on a single assessment instrument.

Within the laboratory, there have been interesting efforts to use complex analytical tools for detecting underlying processes when cognitive deficits are evident. A study by Nuechterlein (1983) is an instructive example drawn from the important area of attentional deficit. He used signal detection theory to contrast the attentional deficits exhibited by children of schizophrenic mothers with those of hyperactive children on the Continuous Performance Test (CPT). Analysis demonstrated that differing processes underlie the attentional deficits in subsets of the two groups of children. The children at risk for schizophrenia revealed a deficit based on their lack of a sensitive-discriminative ability, whereas the comparison group of hyperactive children provided deficits that arose out of their incautious style of responding to the visual stimuli.

Because attentional parameters are so significant in the investigation of developmental defects, researchers in this area may find it valuable to examine exciting advances made in recent years in understanding the basic mechanisms underlying human information processing.

## Multiple Comparison Groups

An additional characteristic of many of the studies of children at risk for schizophrenia and related psychopathologies has been the use of multiple comparison groups. Researchers often take comfort in having available a single normal control group. Often *control* is a misnomer for a comparsion group, as the multiple controls over highly relevant subject and situational variables often cannot be captured by inclusion of a single group matched to the experimental cohort. This is particularly true of risk studies. For example, in evaluating the correlates of developmental disability, one must consider control of numerous factors such as mental age, IQ, socioeconomic status, specificity of handicap, family intactness, minority status, and other potentially influencing factors. The use of multiple subject groups may help to establish the necessary comparisons against which the performance of disabled index children can be evaluated.

An example drawn from the University of Minnesota's research program on stress-resistant children may help to illustrate this problem. O'Dougherty, Wright, Garmezy, Loewenson, and Torres (1983) studied a group of children who in early childhood had survived the life-threatening cyanotic heart defect of transposition of the great arteries (TGA) by successful open heart surgery. Because these children had undergone varying degrees of hypoxia as a result of their congenital defect, O'Doughtery (1981) evaluated the attentional behavior of the children, using the CPT as modified by Nuechterlein (1983) for his signal detection analysis. O'Dougherty quickly became aware that although the CPT had been widely used for clinical neurological assessments of children there existed no systematic normative data available against which to compare assessed performance. (Nuechterlein had derived a limited normative sample by testing classroom controls of his index cases, but O'Dougherty's sample characteristics differed so markedly from Nuechterlein's that new normative data had to be secured.) Therefore, O'Dougherty preceded her experimental investigations with a major normative study of CPT performance by testing representative samples of children of both sexes enrolled in kindergarten through 6th grade

(O'Dougherty, 1981). Only when these data were available was she able to proceed with studies of the TGA children.

One additional observation related to O'Dougherty's study is worthy of mention. Brooks-Gunn (Chapter 6) has suggested that instead of traditional studies of between-group differences ( handicapped vs. nonhandicapped children) use be made of differences within groups of handicapped children on competence measures.

> An even more fine-tuned individual difference approach might involve comparing infants with similar diagnostic classification who differ with respect to some specific competency. For example, cerebral palsied infants with intact informational processing skills and those with delays might be compared. (p. 105)

This suggestion had been incorporated by O'Dougherty *et al.* (1983), who carried the strategy an important step further. Using medical data obtained from hospital records of the TGA neonates, they created a model of multiple risk factors to predict the later adaptation of the children studied. These specific factors included (a) associated heart defects; (b) the need for the Blalock–Hanlon as a further palliative procedure; (c) congestive heart failure in the first month of life; (d) the child's height and weight immediately prior to open heart surgery as an index of duration of hypoxia; (e) seizures during or following open heart surgery; (f) cerebrovascular stroke syndrome; (g) duration of cardiac repair with cardiopulmonary bypass; and ( h) duration of hospitalization following open heart surgery. A cumulative risk index built around these medical variables was combined with family socioeconomic status and the current level of family stress as possible moderator variables with the potential to affect the child's level of current adaptation. Results supported a relationship between variations in levels of cumulative risk and later neurological and psychological outcomes for the children. If similar forms of predictive models of risk in developmental disability could be developed, they too might be used as a framework for testing interrelationships between medical and psychosocial variables with current and future adaptational outcomes.

## STRESS-RESISTANT CHILDREN: RISK AND PROTECTIVE FACTORS

In O'Dougherty's study (1981), the socioeconomic status of the family bore a modest relationship to the later verbal abilities of TGA children deemed to be at risk. Levels of current family stress were also shown to have a significant relationship to psychological outcome. High family stress constituted a risk factor, whereas low family stress had the coloration of a protective factor that tended to moderate potential negative outcomes in the children.

This conception of a protective factor is relatively new in the medical and psychological literature on stress and stress responsivity (Garmezy, in press; Garmezy & Rutter, 1985; Rutter, 1979), but it begins to assume greater prominence in the search for familial and situational attributes that correlate with adaptive patterns in handicapped children.

One can speculate about the nature of some nonmedical factors that may be protective. These may include positive parent and child temperaments that provide a good fit, a benign family environment marked by cohesion, warmth, positive parental values and aspirations, parental reinforcement of the child's self-help activities, external supports to assist a family with a handicapped child, and the presence of supportive teachers, school administrators, and peer group.

A fine line may separate variables initially perceived as protective, but of heightened risk when present in the extreme. For example, Schaffer (1964) described 13 out of 30 families of cerebral palsied children under age 6 which he described as "too cohesive." These families, he believed, directed excessive attention to the handicapped child.

Low socioeconomic status is considered to be a major risk factor, but this view, too, can obscure protective components within a social class. Pavenstedt (1965, 1967) has provided a striking analysis of the child-rearing environments of upper-lower and low-lower class families. She clearly demarcates the protective factors that exist in the former group, and the risk factors that characterize the latter.

In part, the problem lies in the failure to "psychologize" the social class variable. Block (1971) once observed that "indices of socioeconomic status relate in non-chance ways to a great variety of psychological variables" (p. 271), including IQ, character structure, child-rearing practices, etc. But such relationships are often inconsistent and associatively weak. The issue is one of defining the stimulus variables and environmental patternings that exist within different social classes and are, in part, instrumental in the formation of personality structure within class categories. Such knowledge requires greater specificity than does mere categorization, and it is specificity that is demanded when assigning risk or protective status to a given attribute.

### Family Attributes

In a broader sense, risk or protective status may be ascribed to the rearing environments of handicapped children.

As part of our research program with stress-resistant children, Silverstein (1982) studied a cohort comprised of severely handicapped children who were subjected to the stress of being mainstreamed in regular classrooms. Through 6 hours of semi-structured interviewing, she sought to identify family background factors and parental coping strategies that were related to the handicapped child's manifest competence in the mainstreamed classroom. The study provided intensive clinical descriptions of 27 families, their backgrounds, and the methods they used in rearing their handicapped offspring (including their modes of seeking available medical and educational services needed by the children).

On the basis of family ratings by clinical judges, several protective factors were identified in families with high scores on coping and resource scales constructed by Silverstein. These included

1. a stable marriage;
2. well-educated parents;
3. father's interest in the child;
4. membership in a support group related to the child's handicap; and
5. good parental coping as rated on scales of (a) information-seeking to secure educational and medical assistance for their child, and (b) direct actions taken by parents to secure such services.

By contrast, the identifiable risk factors in other families were (a) unmarried parents, (b) mother unmarried at the time of her baby's birth, (c) poorly educated parents, (d) alcohol or substance abuse problem in the family, and (e) inadequate coping by the parent.

### Categorizing Protective Factors

Silverstein's (1982) findings are supported by a recent review (Garmezy, 1985) of other research areas in which protective factors were identified. Three broad classes of variables appear to accompany the maintenance of competence in children exposed to a variety of different stressors. First, there are the personal dispositional attributes of the child, including such positive temperament characteristics (Rutter, 1979) as social responsiveness, active participation, intelligence, a sense of autonomy, health, and positive self-esteem (see Block & Block, 1980; Wallerstein & Kelly, 1980; Werner & Smith, 1982). The second involves patterns evident in those children's families, which are marked by cohesion, warmth, and an absence of discord. The third relates to the availability and utilization of support systems both within the family and external to it (Garmezy, 1985; Garmezy & Rutter, 1985).

At present, the study of protective factors is more a future promise rather than a present achievement. But I venture to predict that the study of the strengths and protective factors in children who are at risk will prove to be a vital research enterprise in the decade ahead. One impetus for further research is the growing awareness that knowledge of individual differences in children who are disadvantaged by biological, cognitive, and social realities is essential to the development of rational prevention efforts. If we are unable to specify risk and protective factors, we can only engage in interventions based largely on those obligations that a decent-minded society owes its citizens. However, greater specificity than this is required for developing rational patterns of prevention. Only systematic programs of research on the normative and nonnormative aspects of biological and psychological development will provide the essential understanding of differential outcomes in children at risk—maladaptation and reduced effectance motivation in some, retained or enhanced competence and successful coping in others.

This general theme urges on all risk researchers a recurrent, systematic examination of the range of adaptations that characterize their cohorts. The essence of risk research requires an investment not solely in those who seem to fit predictions of subsequent vulnerability, but (of equivalent or even greater importance) also in others who show unexpected strengths. Often positive outcomes—so inconsistent with earlier deficit states—can best be evaluated in a child's workplace, the school.

**Studies in the Classroom**

An example of such an effort can be seen in a parallel investigation conducted by Raison (1982) in conjunction with Silverstein's study of the coping patterns of parents of mainstreamed, physically handicapped children. Raison used an ethological observational system (Problem Behavior Analysis) that had been developed by Charlesworth and associates (Charlesworth & Spiker, 1975; Charlesworth, LaFrenier, Nemcek, & Clark, 1980). This technique is designed to provide information about the problem-solving behavior used by children in everyday situations. Specifically, the analysis focuses on the child's reactions following disruptions or blocks to ongoing behavior.

Raison compared the responses made by the handicapped children in both their mainstreamed and special schools. In the former, the behavior of nonhandicapped peers provided the comparison performance. A total of 105.7 hours of observation were made, the majority of these taking place in the mainstreamed school (94.7 hours). Interobserver agreement was satisfactorily achieved and was later checked weekly. Ratings were based on a rotational schema; the target child's behavior was observed for 5 minutes; observation was made, in turn, of a nonhandicapped child of the same sex who has in closest proximity to the index child; then the observer returned to the handicapped child for 5 additional minutes, followed by observation of the next (nearest) comparison child, and so on. The data on each handicapped child were summed and averaged; all comparison children's problem-solving behavior was also averaged. A variety of responses to blocks encountered in the school setting were coded (seeks help, demands, complies, refuses, asks questions, searches, volunteers information, etc.). The prime issue posed by the response was whether it successfully removed or failed to remove the block or obstacle confronted by the child.

In addition to the foregoing, observations were made of other activities of the child in 30-second observation periods (e.g., interacts with peers, plays, talks with teacher, attends, fails to attend, etc.). Academic, behavioral, and social competence measures were also taken for each child based on peer, teacher, and achievement ratings.

Raison found "a surprising lack of group differences" in how the handicapped students responded to problems when compared with the nonhandicapped students:

> They were no more or less compliant, unless directions were given which were quite hard to follow because of their physical limitations. They answered group and individual questions just as accurately as the non-handicapped group. Their needs, cognitive and social, directed to peers or adults were met with the same frequency and they sought help and information in the same proportion as did the non-handicapped group. The only major difference was that their physical needs were met more often. The salience of their handicap and the presence of aides in the room would seem to account for this difference. (Raison, 1982, p. 137)

In sum, the handicapped children, in terms of social needs and physical impositions, were not more needy or dependent as is sometimes supposed, nor did they have difficulty with physical obstacles because of their handicaps. (These findings were not lost on the teachers, who came to view mainstreaming more positively.)

Now being planned is an integration of the Silverstein–Raison studies in an effort to learn whether competence in the classroom is correlated with parental attitudes toward their handicapped child, and with parents' active intervention efforts to secure needed assistance for their child.

## Ongoing Studies

Recent articles (Garmezy, Masten, & Tellegen, 1984; Garmezy & Tellegen, 1984) present an overview of the third and largest cohort studied by the University of Minnesota's Project Competence. The cohort is a community-based group comprising approximately 200 children drawn from two centralized urban school samples, whose parents have contributed information about the children's specific exposure to a heterogeneous sampling of stressful life events. Because the methods used with this large cohort have been described in the citations above, they will not be repeated here. These describe the techniques used to derive composite competence scores for the children, the nature of the interviews conducted both with mothers and children, and the three generic models of stress resistance that will be tested in multivariate regression data analysis.

The three models are these

1. A *compensatory* model in which stress factors and personal attributes are seen as combining additively to predict competence;
2. A *challenge* model in which stress, if not excessive, has the potential of enhancing competence; and
3. An *immunity versus vulnerability* model in which personal attributes modulate the impact of stress, with protective factors providing a possible immunity against stress, whereas more negative factors may add to the vulnerability of persons exposed to a similar stress experience.

The central theme of the Minnesota research program remains the difficult one of searching out the components of stress resistance in children and their families. The effort is an exploratory one that likely will be followed by a new generation of studies in other laboratories. These will be focused on comparisons implicating risk, protective, and competence factors in different cohorts of children ranging from those already disordered, to others who are at risk but are as yet asymptomatic, and to those adaptive children who reveal competencies despite adversity.

Researchers into developmental disability are part of the overall risk research movement in this and other countries. Their work, important in and of itself, has implications that reach far beyond the field of developmental disabilities. Their exchange of findings with scientists in other areas of risk can help to insure progress in identifying the broad bands of outcomes that characterize virtually all children exposed to disadvantaging life circumstances.

## REFERENCES

Beardslee, W. R., Bemporad, J. Keller, M. B., & Klerman, G. L. (1983). Children of parents with major affective disorders: A review. *American Journal of Psychiatry, 140*, 825–832.

Block, J. *Lives through time.* (1971). Berkeley, CA: Bancroft Books.

Block, J. H., & Block, J. (1980). The role of ego-control and ego-resiliency in the organization of behavior. In W. A. Collins (Ed.), *Development of cognition, affect, and social relations: The Minnesota symposium on child psychology* (Vol. 13). Hillsdale, NJ: Lawrence Erlbaum.

Charlesworth, W. R., LaFreniere, P., Nemeck, D., & Clark, P. (1980). *Asking and answering questions: Observations of preschoolers and their teachers in various sized lesson groups.* Unpublished paper. Minneapolis, MN: Institute of Child Development, University of Minnesota.

Charlesworth, W. R., & Spiker, D. (1975). An ethological approach to observation in learning settings. In R. A. Weinberg & F. W. Wood (Eds.), *Observations of pupils and teachers in mainstream and special education: Alternative strategies.* Minneapolis, MN: University of Minnesota.

Garmezy, N. (1985). Stress-resistant children: The search for protective factors. In J. E. Stevenson (Ed.), *Recent research in developmental psychopathology. Journal of Child Psychology and Psychiatry,* Book Supplemental No. 4. Oxford: Pergamon Press.

Garmezy, N., & Devine, V. (1985). Project Competence: The Minnesota studies of children vulnerable to psychopathology. In N. Watt, E. J. Anthony, L. C. Wynne, & J. E. Rolf (Eds.), *Children at risk for schizophrenia.* Cambridge: Cambridge Univ. Press.

Garmezy, N., Masten, A. S., & Tellegen, A. (1984). The study of stress and competence in children: A building block for developmental psychopathology. *Child Development, 55,* 97–111.

Garmezy, N., & Rutter, M. (1985). Acute reactions to stress. In M. Rutter & L. Hersov (Eds.), *Child psychiatry: Modern approaches* (2nd ed.). Oxford: Blackwell Scientific Publications.

Garmezy, N., & Tellegren, A. (1984). Studies of stress-resistant children: Methods, variables, and preliminary findings. In F. Morrison, C. Lord, & D. Keating (Eds.), *Advances in applied developmental psychology* (Vol. 1). New York: Academic Press.

McNeil, T. F., Kaij, L. Malmquist-Larsson, A., Naslund, B., Persson-Blennow, I., McNeil, N., & Blennow, G. (1983). Offspring of women with nonorganic psychoses. *Acta Psychiatrica Scandinavica, 68,* 234–250.

Marcus, J., Auerbach, J., Wilkinson, L., Maeir, S., Mark, A., & Peles, V. (in press). Infants at risk for schizophrenia: The Jerusalem infant development study. In N. F. Watt, E. J. Anthony, L. C. Wynne, & J. Rolf (Eds), *Children at risk for schizophrenia.* Cambridge: Cambridge Univ. Press.

Nuechterlein, K. H. (1983). Signal detection in vigilance tasks and behavioral attributes among offspring and schizophrenic mothers and among hyperactive children. *Journal of Abnormal Psychology, 92,* 4–28.

O'Dougherty, M. M. (1981). *The relationship between early risk status and later competence and adaptation in children who survive severe heart defects.* Unpublished doctoral dissertation. Minneapolis, MN: University of Minnesota.

O'Dougherty, M., Wright, F. S., Garmezy, N., Loewenson, R. B., & Torres, F. (1983). Later competence and adaptation in infants who survive severe heart defects. *Child Development, 54,* 1129–1142.

Patterson, G. R. (1982). *Coercive family process.* Eugene, OR: Castalia.

Pavenstedt, E. (1965). A comparison of the child-rearing environment of upper-lower and very low-lower class families. *American Journal of Orthopsychiatry, 35,* 89–98.

Pavenstedt, E. (1967). *The drifters: Children of disorganized lower-class families.* Boston: Little, Brown & Co.

Raison, S. B. (1982). *Coping behavior of mainstreamed physically handicapped students.* Unpublished doctoral dissertation. Minneapolis, MN: University of Minnesota.

Robins, L. N. (1966). *Deviant children grown up.* Baltimore: Williams & Wilkins.

Rutter, M. (1979). Protective factors in children's responses to stress and disadvantage. In M. W. Kent & J. E. Rolf (Eds.), *Primary prevention of psychopathology* (Vol. 3). Hanover, NH: Univ. Press of New England.

Sameroff, A. J., Seifer, R., & Zax, M. (1982). Early development of children at risk for emotional disorder. *Monographs of the Society for Child Development,* 47(7, Serial No. 199).

Schaffer, H. R. (1964). The too-cohesive family: A form of group pathology. *International Journal of Social Psychiatry, 10,* 266–275.

Silverstein, P. R. (1982). *Coping and adaptation in families of physically handicapped school children.* Unpublished doctoral dissertation. University of Minnesota, Minneapolis, MN.

Wallerstein, J. S., & Kelley, J. B. (1980). *Surviving the breakup.* New York: Basic Books.

Watt, N., Anthony, E. J., Wynne, L. C., & Rolf, J. (Eds.). (1984). *Children at risk for schizophrenia.* Cambridge: Cambridge Univ. Press.

Weissman, M. M. (1979). Depressed parents and their children: Implications for prevention. In J. D. Noshpitz (Ed.), *Basic handbook of child psychiatry* (Vol. 4). New York: Basic Books.

Werner, E. E., & Smith, R. S. (1982). *Vulnerable but invincible: A study of resilient children.* New York: McGraw-Hill.

West, D. J., & Farrington, D. P. (1973). *Who becomes delinquent?* London: Heinemann.

*CHAPTER 4*

# Marital Discord and Children at Risk

## IMPLICATIONS FOR RESEARCH AND PREVENTION

*Howard J. Markman and Deming Jones Leonard*

The reader may initially wonder why a chapter on marriage is included in this book on children at risk. The reason for our focus on marriage stems from research indicating that marital conflict and dissolution pose a serious threat to the cognitive and emotional adjustment of children of these couples. The basic premise of this chapter is that growing up in a dysfunctional family environment is one of the major risk factors for future child psychopathology. The quality of parental relationship may cause, exacerbate, or heal child problems. Thus, the study of why marriages succeed and fail and how to prevent marital discord should be directly relevant to risk researchers.

The goal of this chapter is to consider the implications of recent marital interaction research for the early identification of and intervention in marriages that pose risk for children. Focus on the marital dyad is consistent with a trend by risk researchers toward a "more total ecological assessment of the family" (Anastasiow, 1982, p. xiii).

## OVERVIEW OF RISK ASSESSMENT IN FAMILIES

There are many ways to assess families for risk. The first involves a demographic assessment, including social class, number of members, number of parents, and so on. Because these factors are known to be

***Howard J. Markman and Deming Jones Leonard*** • Center for Marital and Family Studies, University of Denver, Denver, Colorado 80302.

associated with risk for psychopathology, this appears to be the most economical way to assess families for risk. A second approach includes an evaluation of the home environment with an instrument like Caldwell's Home Observation for Measurement of the Environment (HOME) Inventory (Bradely, 1982). The HOME evaluates physical features of the home and quantitative aspects of the mother–child relationship, but qualitative aspects are not assessed. A third approach is to assess the *quality* of the personal relationships among family members. Evidence is converging from diverse sources that the quality of one's personal relationships is an important determinant of mental (and physical) health (Notarius & Pelligrini, 1984). For young children, the family (or family-substitute) is the major source of personal relationships (Furman, 1981).

With these assessment issues in mind, we discuss in this chapter research into family functioning that focuses on the interrelationship between the marital dyad and child behavior problems. First, the implications of the research on the marital dyad and the importance of the understanding and prevention of marital distress to risk research are emphasized. Second, findings from our research at the University of Denver on the prediction of marital distress and our recent attempt to apply the results of this research to understanding how marital problems affect children are summarized. Finally, we review the results of studies investigating the possibility of preventing marital distress, and discuss how efforts to strengthen marriages can have preventative effects on children.

## MARITAL DISCORD AND CHILD BEHAVIOR PROBLEMS

### Rates of Marital Discord: A National Problem

U.S. Government figures indicate that approximately 4 out of 10 first marriages (more than one million per year) end in divorce (National Center for Health Statistics, 1983). Because over 60% of divorces involve couples with one or more children, an estimated one million children per year are directly affected by divorce (Cherlin, 1981; Glick and Norton, 1976). Furthermore, the decision to divorce is often the result of many years of marital distress and conflict. Because the divorce rate represents only a portion of the population of couples who experience marital distress, the incidence of such distress is significantly greater than that of divorce.

The negative impact of marital distress and divorce can only be estimated. There have been two distinct areas of research on the negative effects of marital discord on mental health. One has linked marital disruption to increased risk of psychopathology in the partners (Bloom, Asher, & White, 1978; Stroebe & Stroebe, 1983), and the other has linked it to increased risk of behavioral and emotional problems in children who grow up in these families (Emery, 1982; Hetherington, 1979; Wallerstein & Kelly, 1980). The present chapter focuses on discord in marriage as a potential risk factor for children.

## Research into Marital Discord and Child Problems

The strongest evidence that there is a relationship between marital discord and child behavior problems comes from studies of children of divorce and of conflicted marriages. These studies demonstrate that high levels of marital discord are correlated with high levels of child disturbance (see Emery, 1982, for a review). Because child problems are found in discordant intact marriages (Emery & O'Leary, 1982; Oltmanns, Broderick & O'Leary, 1977; Porter & O'Leary, 1980) as well as divorced samples (e.g., Anthony, 1974; Hetherington, 1979; McDermott, 1968, 1970; Wallerstein & Kelly, 1980; Westman, Cline, Swift, & Kramer, 1976), the correlation cannot be simply explained by parental separation due to divorce. In fact, conflict—not separation—seems to be most closely associated with child behavior problems (Emery, 1982). For example, investigators comparing children from homes broken by divorce as compared to death found more behavior problems in children of divorce (Douglas, Ross, Hammond, & Mulligan, 1966; Gibson, 1969). In addition, children from broken but conflict-free homes have been found to have fewer behavior problems than children from conflictual, unbroken homes (Gibson, 1969; McCord, McCord, & Thurber, 1962; Power, Ash, Schoenberg, & Storey, 1974). Many of the problems in children from broken homes are evident before separation from the parent (Lamberg, Essen, & Head, 1977). Children from high conflict homes who were placed in high conflict foster homes still expressed the behavior problems that were evident at the time of separation. Those children who were placed in conflict-free foster homes demonstrated fewer behavior problems (Rutter, 1980). Thus, conflict appears to be a prime factor related to child behavior problems, whether it occurs within intact or dissolved marriages.

Recent studies have shed light on other, more specific factors that may be involved in marital discord and child disturbances. Several studies have examined the nature of the marital conflict and found that openly hostile conflict (Porter & O'Leary, 1980; Rutter, Yule, Quinton, Rowland, Yule, & Berger, 1975) and continuing conflict (Rutter, 1980) are highly correlated with child behavior problems. When the types of behavior problems most commonly associated with marital discord are examined, problems of undercontrol are more frequently found than problems of overcontrol (Emery & O'Leary, 1982; Oltmanns *et al.*, 1977; Rutter, 1971). Studies examining sex differences have found that boys seem more vulnerable to the negative effects of marital discord than girls (Emery, 1982). This difference is more clearly understood in the light of a recent study indicating that boys and girls are affected differently by parental disagreement over discipline (Block, Block, & Morrison, 1981). Specifically, boys living in families with high levels of parental disagreement tend to have lowered impulse control (i.e., undercontrolled), whereas girls tend to have heightened impulse control (i.e., overcontrolled). Finally, buffering effects have also been found, with a good relationship with at least one parent tending to protect children from the negative effects of marital conflict (Heatherington, Cox, & Cox, 1979; Hess & Camara, 1979).

To summarize, the available data indicate that marital discord poses a threat to the adjustment of children of these marriages, particularly threatening cognitive functioning, physical health, and emotional functioning (Garbarino, 1982). This suggests that having parents in conflict is a major risk factor for children. However, less is known about why this is the case.

### Proposed Mechanisms Relating Marital Discord to Child Problems

Studies in this area have typically relied on correlational designs; therefore, there is uncertainty about causality of the co-occurrence of marital distress and child behavior. Because the families studied were experiencing both marital distress and child behavior problems, the direction and mechanisms of causality are unclear. Nevertheless, several mechanisms have been proposed to explain why marital distress is related to behavior problems in children. Four of these are reviewed. The mechanisms have in common the general assumption that marital discord causes child behavior problems. This assumption is based on the findings that marital influences on child behavior are more pervasive than vice versa (Oltmanns *et al.*, 1977; Rutter, 1980).

One proposed mechanism that has been investigated more than most is that marital discord leads to altered discipline practices by parents, which in turn leads to child behavior problems. This alteration could be inconsistency from each parent, inconsistency between parents, or an alternation of the intensity or frequency of discipline (Becker, Peterson, Luria, Shoemaker, & Hellmer, 1962; McCord, McCord, & Howard, 1961; Patterson, 1977). For example, Heatherington and her associates (Hetherington, 1976; Hetherington *et al.*, 1979) investigated changes in post-divorce discipline by comparing a sample of divorced parents and a sample of parents from intact marriages. The divorced parents were found to make fewer maturity demands, have poorer communication, be less affectionate, and be more inconsistent with their children. In addition, the children from the divorced sample, especially the boys, were less compliant in response to parental commands than were the children from intact marriages. Although this study indicates that discipline differs as a function of marital turmoil, it is unclear when the changes in discipline began (i.e., before or after the divorce) and if the changes in discipline caused the changes in the child's behavior.

Block *et al.* (1981), in a longitudinal study, provide evidence that disagreement over discipline may be causally related to future behavior problems. Using independent ratings of child adjustment and an index of parental disagreement about child rearing obtained from parents of normal preschool children, they found that parental disagreement about child rearing was related to subsequent divorce and to undercontrolled behavior in boys and overcontrolled behavior in girls one year later. Inconsistency in discipline can thus be seen as related to marital turmoil as well as a potential precursor to problems in children.

A second proposed causal mechanism focuses on modeling. Interparental conflict is thought to interfere with normal imitation of the same-sex parent, due to the approach–avoidance situation set up in aligning with one parent (Schwartz, 1979). One possible result of disruption in modeling is the rejection of the same-sex parent as a role model. As a result, alternative and perhaps more deviant models may be sought, or the child's development may be impaired due to the lack of an appropriate model. A second possibility is that hostile, aggressive behaviors of conflict-ridden parents may be imitated. The finding of increased negativity displayed by conflicted parents toward their children (e.g., Johnson & Lobitz, 1974) lends support to this view.

A third proposed mechanism is that children refocus parental conflict by developing behavior problems, and thus "take on the symptom" of the family. Minuchin and others (Minuchin, Rosman, & Baker, 1978), using a family systems approach, have suggested that children serve the function of redirecting parental concerns by developing a problem themselves. Thus, behavior problems are seen as functional adaptation to a distressed family system. Family systems theorists have been among the most prominent in linking marital conflict and child problems. As Framo (1975) succinctly puts it: "Whenever you have a disturbed child, you have a disturbed marriage" (p. 22). Within the family systems perspective, numerous mini-theories have been proposed to explain this outcome. They range from low parental self-esteem (Satir, 1974), to dysfunctional family alliances (Minuchin *et al.*, 1978), to dysfunctional parent–child communication (e.g., double-bind messages, negativity, and unclear communication). However, most early research has focused on the role of dysfunctional family or parent–child interaction rather than directly on the disturbed marriage (Markman & Notarius, in press).

Finally, a fourth mechanism is that parents in conflict have lower levels of emotional availability for their children (see Emde & Easterbrooks, Chapter 5, for discussion of emotional availability).

## The Marital Dyad and Risk Research

These four mechanisms have in common the hypothesis that marital discord has its negative effect on children through dysfunctional family interaction. Unfortunately, few studies have directly assessed marital interaction, parent–child interaction, and child adjustment in the same study. Those that have assessed interaction have come from the developmental literature on normal families (e.g., Belsky, Gilstap, & Rovine, 1984; Golberg & Easterbrooks, 1984) and therefore do not focus on the potential negative effects of disturbed parental interaction on child adjustment. The studies reviewed above have used the construct of marital conflict without directly examining the *process* of this conflict. Instead, marital conflict has commonly been measured by assessing marital satisfaction and/or marital agreement. These are static measures that do not allow tests of the process-oriented theories of how marital discord is related to child adjustment (and to determine how marital adjustment influences child development). Adequate tests require direct examination of marital interaction in a family context. Thus, there is need to directly examine marital interaction in relation to child adjustment. This need is amplified by findings from the marital literature that strongly indicate that dysfunctional marital interaction may be causally related to marital discord and, by implication, to child behavior problems (Markman, 1979, 1981).

This is a particularly exciting time to be involved in risk research, for researchers are just beginning to understand how the marital dyad may influence subsequent emotional problems in childhood. There are several reasons why the marital dyad has begun to gain prominence in this field.

First, there has been increasing attention paid to the importance of longitudinal versus cross-sectional research in understanding the development of child problems and risk conditions. It makes sense from a longitudinal perspective to give attention to the prior condition of the marital relationship as a possible determinant of future child behavior problems.

Second, there has been an increasing focus on the importance of interactional versus static variables. This has led researchers to examine the nature of the marital exchange and how it might influence children.

Finally, there has been a decrease in gaps between traditionally isolated fields of inquiry. For example, developmental psychologists have turned from focusing on just mother–infant interaction to now include the father. Similarly, family interaction researchers have recognized that in spite of their focus on the family, their previous work has either studied parent–child interaction or marital interaction (Markman & Notarious, in press). Attention has thus been recently directed to understanding how these different subcomponents of the family influence each other.

Currently, risk status for families is assigned based on three types of characteristics: (a) demographic indicators associated with psychological disorders (e.g., poverty, quality of family environment); (b) parental characteristics (e.g., schizophrenia, affective disorder); and (c) child characteristics (e.g., prematurity, biological handicap). We propose that marital discord should be an additional indicator when assessing families for risk, and that marital discord adds to the amount of risk presented by the three traditional indicators. An overview of our own research, which has investigated the role of dysfunctional interaction patterns between couples in the development and maintenance of marital conflict, is presented next.

## RESEARCH ON THE MARITAL DYAD: ILLUSTRATIONS FROM THE DENVER LONGITUDINAL STUDY OF FAMILY DEVELOPMENT

Our research and clinical experience has led us to the conclusion that the interaction process between spouses is the most proximal cause of marital distress (Notarious & Pelligrini, 1984). We suggest that the assessment of marital interaction not only will help identify couples who are distressed or at risk for marital distress, but will also identify risk conditions for current or future children of these couples.

Because interaction patterns once formed are generally stable, it is likely that the same characteristics that influence the premarital dyad or couples in the early stages of family development will influence future marital, parent–child, and family interactions. Therefore, we should be able to intervene early in deviant marital interactions to prevent future marital and child problems. Alternatively, intervention can begin at points of family transitions, when couples or families are most receptive to intervention attempts. This strategy is likely to change communication or interaction patterns in a way that will enhance the marital, parent–child, and family relationships.

Although preventative efforts need not wait for a full understanding of how parental interaction and conflict negatively affect children, the more that is known about the mechanisms underlying this covariation, the more effective prevention efforts ought to be. Thus, it is important to devote attention to research on how and why parental conflict influences child development and child adjustment. We have developed a model that attempts to integrate basic research into both treatment and prevention. In the next section, our approach to prevention and a brief overview of our research model are described.

### A Behavioral-Competency Model for Prevention Research

We have developed and implemented a behavioral-competency model of prevention research. The model stresses the importance of basing preventive interventions on theoretical and empirical foundations laid by cross-sectional and longitudinal research (Markman, Floyd, & Dickson-Markman, 1982; Markman, Jamieson, & Floyd, 1983). The first step in a model involves cross-sectional studies assessing the behavior of groups independently identified as either competent or incompetent, in specific transition periods (defined as times of increased stress when one or more family members are called on to discard old roles and assume new ones). These behaviors are then measured during transition periods (before distress develops) and their predictive validity is assessed through longitudinal studies. Comparisons of the predistress behavioral characteristics of population members who go on to develop disordered behaviors with those who do not generate variables that can then be used as behaviors to be modified in preventive intervention programs. Note that the model emphasizes examining how couples and families *behave* (interact) in situations common to the transition periods. Behavioral indexes are used rather than personality or demographic indexes, which are not easily modifiable in interventions.

The theoretical framework guiding our prevention research program is a broadly defined cognitive-behavioral model of marriage. According to cognitive-behavioral theorists, marital distress results from the distressed couple's reliance on negative reinforcement strategies (e.g., coercion) or dysfunctional communication patterns (e.g., cross-complaining) to change each other's behavior, which produces an exchange of unsatisfying outcomes (Jacobson & Weiss, 1978; Lazarus, 1968). Furthermore, the quality and frequency of interaction decline as the exchange of negative outcomes increases. Nondistressed couples, on the other hand, learn to use positive reinforcement strategies to effect change. Hence, they minimize negative interaction cycles and increase the exchange of positive outcomes (Jacobson & Weiss, 1978; Stuart 1969). The cognitive-behavioral model emphasizes the couple's interaction as the key determinant of marital distress. Moreover, the model maintains that distressed couples are deficient in skills needed to resolve marital problems that all couples encounter. Skills have both behavioral and cognitive components and function to help couples and families cope with the stresses of marital and family life (Markman, 1984).

## Cross-Sectional Research on Communication and Marital Discord

One major ongoing aspect of our research has been to investigate the interactional patterns associated with marital distress. The results of these studies have indicated that distressed couples were characterized by more negative interaction (e.g., negative affect, mind reading, cross-complaining) from both couples' own perspectives and the perspective of objective observers. Sequential analyses of marital interactions revealed strong evidence of negative reciprocity in distressed relationships (e.g., wife negative leads to husband negative leads to wife negative and so on) (Gottman, Markman, & Notarius, 1977). Although the interactions of nondistressed couples were characterized to a degree by negative communications (e.g., negative effect, mind reading), wives (not husbands) tended to break the negative cycle. We speculate that wives in distressed relationships have stopped doing this relationship work of de-escalating negative communications (Notarius, Markman, & Gottman, 1983).

In a recent study (Floyd & Markman, 1983), we attempted to combine objective rating and couple self-rating to compare distressed and nondistressed couples. Consistent with previous studies, the results indicated that distressed wives' ratings of their husbands' interactions were significantly more negative than nondistressed wives' ratings. Also, observers rated distressed wives much more negatively than they rated nondistressed wives. The most important finding was that distressed husbands viewed their wives' behaviors significantly more positively than observers, and that distressed wives viewed their husbands' behavior significantly more negatively than observers. These findings were interpreted as preliminary evidence of an observer bias operating in distressed relationships, with the husbands having a positive bias (positive screen) and the wives having a negative bias (negative screen). No such evidence of bias was found in nondistressed couples.

The next section reviews how this observer-bias model can be applied to understand the ways that dysfunctional marital interaction may cause dysfunctional parent–child interactions and subsequent child adjustment problems.

### *Marital Interaction and Child Behavior Problems*

The observer-bias model, when applied to the parent–child relationship, suggests that dysfunctional parent–child interaction could occur through parents' altered perception of child behavior as a result of marital discord. For example, parents with a distressed marital relationship may experience their children's behavior more negatively than would an objective observer.

An alternative explanation would be that parents in a distressed marital relationship may experience their children's behavior more positively than would an objective observer. They may become overly invested in the parent–child relationship to compensate for the lack of rewards in the marital relationship. In this case, the observer bias for the parents would be in the positive direction. Despite this positivity bias, there may still be dysfunctional parent–child interactions if the bias is extreme. Thus, there are two directions in which observer bias may contribute to dysfunctional parent–child interaction and may then lead to child behavior problems. Future research (Jones Leonard, 1984) will test these hypotheses.

## Longitudinal Study of Marital and Family Distress

Research in the marital field traditionally relies on cross-sectional designs that do not allow a test of the etiological importance of negative communication patterns. A plausible alternative hypothesis of the results reviewed above is that the negative communication is an outcome rather than a cause of distressed relationships. Thus, another major component of the research program has been the assessment of the extent to which premarital communication patterns are predictive of future outcomes. A longitudinal study of premarital couples provided evidence that supported the social exchange theory prediction that perceptions of the positivity of communication would be predictive of future relationship satisfaction (Markman, 1979, 1981). The results strongly indicated that the more positively couples rated each other's interactions before marriage, the more satisfied they were $2\frac{1}{2}$ and 5 years later. These findings thus link actual (as opposed to self-reported) communication to future distress and satisfaction. Currently, we are conducting a longitudinal study of family development with larger and more heterogeneous samples.

In addition, we are extending our research aims to examine the

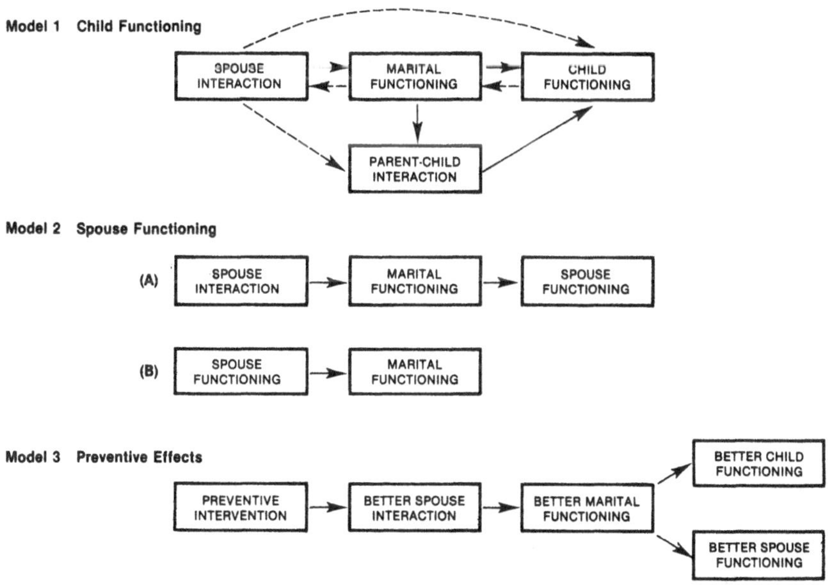


**Figure 1.** General longitudinal models.

negative mental health consequences of marital distress on spouses and children. To date, both lines of research (e.g., spouse psychopathology, child psychopathology) have been based primarily on cross-sectional or retrospective studies, which limit the understanding of etiological relationships. For example, no study to date has adequately tested the hypothesis that disturbed parental communication leads to increased risk of child psychopathology. Thus, appropriate intervention to prevent negative effects has not yet been identified.

The three general models that we will be testing are presented in Figure 1. Model 1 describes the relations between spouse interaction, marital functioning, parent–child functioning and child functioning. On the basis of available cross-sectional research (e.g., Aldous, 1977; Belsky *et al.*, 1984), we predict that the quality of spouse interaction over time is related to marital functioning and parent–child interaction. In turn, marital functioning and parent–child interaction are related to child functioning. It is also possible that the quality of spouse interaction directly affects child adjustment (Heatherington *et al.*, 1979; Minuchin, *et al.*, 1978).

Model 2 describes the relations between spouse interaction, marital functioning, and spouse functioning. On the basis of available cross-sectional research (Bloom *et al.*, 1978; Stroebe & Stroebe, 1983), we predict that the quality of spouse interaction over time is related to marital functioning, and both are related to spouse functioning. Finally, we will test whether our preventive intervention program is related to better couple interaction, which in turn should lead to better marital functioning, parent–child interaction, and child functioning. It is also possible that improved couple interaction and marital functioning should lead to improved spouse functioning (see Model 3).

In addition, our behavioral-competency model of prevention will be applied to the study of transition to parenthood. This should make it possible to identify the behavioral competencies of couples associated with, for example, (a) retention of high degree of marital satisfaction after childbirth, (b) good social and developmental functioning of the child, (c) low levels of anxiety in parents, and (d) increased agreement concerning child rearing, etc.

One specific question that we have already started to investigate is to what extent are levels of spouses' psychological adjustments related to current and future relationship quality? We have found that individual adjustment is positively correlated with both current and future levels of communication positivity and relationship satisfaction (Markman *et al.*, 1982). These relationships are particularly strong for males. The data support previous studies with divorced, separated, and widowed populations that found correlations between individual adjustment and relationship status. The longitudinal stages of the study will enable tests of the competing hypotheses that individual maladjustment causes marital distress or vice versa. The higher correlations for males as compared to females are consistent with data from other studies showing that males' needs may be better met in relationships than females' and that males may suffer more when relationships dissolve or their spouse dies (Stroebe & Stroebe, 1983).

Other questions that will be addressed as the study continues include (a) what is the role of parental conflict in the development of child behavior problems? (b) can a good relationship buffer members from negative psychological and health effects? (c) what are the sources of family stress (e.g., having a handicapped child) and how do families cope with these stresses? and (d) what role do male and female differences in such areas as expectations or intimacy skills have in the development of marital and family problems?

## Prevention of Marital and Family Distress

In light of the severe negative consequences of marital distress and divorce, there is a clear need to prevent problems rather than treat them after they occur (Schofield, 1966). The obvious rationale for such prevention is that early change in a couple's interaction, at a point when their behavior patterns are not well established, may decrease the probability of developing problems later on (Markman *et al.*, 1982). The times in a couple's relationship when they are most amenable to intervention are transition periods (e.g., planning marriage, birth of the first child) (Bloom, 1977; Markman *et al.*, 1982). During such times, the couple encounters new situations and role demands for which they may be unprepared, making them more amenable to interventions that help them cope with these changes. For marital problems, the logical time for intervention is before the couple is married; for child problems, the logical time for intervention is before the child is born.

A review of the prevention literature indicates that interventions are designed without much attention to etiological or conceptual considerations (Heller & Monahan, 1977). Typically, work is begun on a problem without prior research to suggest possible intervention strategies. This is the case for the small literature on prevention programs for couples and families, which is based on common sense and clinical experience rather than empirical data (Markman *et al.*, 1982).

Based on our previous research, a prevention program was developed. The Premarital Relationship Enhancement Program (PREP) is aimed at helping couples increase their competencies for developing a well-functioning, happy marriage (Markman & Floyd, 1980). The components of the program have been designed to counteract known or suspected causes of marital and family distress, and enhance the couples' abilities to develop and maintain intimacy. Implicit in the theory is the idea that couples should learn to be as flexible as possible in responding to the stresses and strains encountered in marital and family interactions.

To adequately evaluate any preventative program, longitudinal studies are necessary. Earlier studies evaluating PREP indicated that couples receiving PREP intervention (as compared to control couples) had declining levels of relationship satisfaction from pre- to post-tests (Markman and Floyd, 1980). However, 1 year later, PREP couples showed significant increases in satisfaction, whereas control couples showed significant declines (Markman *et al.*, 1982). Thus, the intervention may initially "shake things up" in the relationship (e.g., by bringing potential conflict areas to the forefront), but it may be successful in the long run. The data suggest further that the intervention may be preventing declines in satisfaction that typically start in the first year of marriage, and continue thereafter (or at least until the children leave home).

In our current study the results of the PREP evaluation have shown that intervention couples were more satisfied with their relationship and improved their level of communication skills as measured by objective observer's evaluations and when compared to matched controls. Preliminary longitudinal results indicate that these changes are maintained

1 year later. We are also planning to develop and evaluate other short-term intervention programs delivered at other transition periods, as we learn more about how families cope (and do not cope) with these life transitions.

Next, we briefly review two examples of the direction that our future prevention research will follow.

### *Lamaze Childbirth Preparation*

Recent research has documented what first-time parents have long known: Having a first child is an anxiety-producing experience that may have negative effects on the marital relationship (e.g., Cowan & Cowan, 1978). These results suggest that intervention during the "transition to parenthood" stage may prevent the negative effects on couples commonly reported in the literature. Although there are no widely available interventions designed to prepare couples specifically for the transition to parenthood, childbirth preparation classes have become readily available in recent years. Originally these courses were introduced to give women more control during labor and delivery and to reduce fears and pain. Recently more emphasis has been placed on the potential impact this preparation has on the marital relationship (Bean, 1974; Chabbon, 1966; Ewy & Ewy, 1976). Advocates of the Lamaze childbirth preparation claim that by having the husband and wife share in the preparation for and in the process of childbirth, a sense of family can be strongly established and the marital relationship strengthened and enhanced (Tanzer & Block, 1972).

Thus far, we have conducted one preliminary study in this area. We compared couples who were having their first child and who participated in Lamaze childbirth preparation with a group who did not participate in Lamaze (Markman & Kadushin, 1984). The results indicated that 3 months after childbirth the Lamaze group maintained previously high levels of marital satisfaction and low levels of anxiety, whereas the non-Lamaze group demonstrated striking increases in anxiety and decreases in marital satisfaction. Although self-selection into the Lamaze group raises several alternative explanations of the findings (see Markman, & Kadushin, 1984, for a discussion), this study suggests that Lamaze training may be serving as an effective primary preventive intervention for young couples. Longitudinal studies are necessary to assess the potential preventive effects on children.

### *Strengthening Families of Handicapped Children through Parent Communication-Skill Training*

One important application of the PREP program is to strengthen at-risk families by enhancing parental communication. Currently we are focusing attention on one type of at-risk family, those with a handicapped child, in collaboration with the Rocky Mountain Child Development Center and the Colorado Department of Health. The rationale for our project is based on four related research findings:

1. A major determinant of a child's future cognitive, emotional, self-help and social development is the family's ability to meet that child's needs. This is true for children with handicapping conditions as well as for children without special needs (Garbarino, 1982).

2. A major cause of separation and divorce is parental inability to communicate effectively (Markman *et al.*, 1982).

3. When families are stressed, the need for effective communication becomes even more important (Gottman, Notarius, Gonso, & Markman, 1976).

4. The learning of a diagnosis of a child with a handicap is a crisis in a family that produces stress so severe that the handicapped child and siblings may be negatively affected, and the parents may even separate or divorce (e.g., Kazak & Marvin, 1984).

Despite these findings, most developmental evaluation clinics and crippled children's programs have generally failed to address the need for systematically training parents in communication skills. In fact, although a recent issue of the journal *Family Relations* (January, 1984) was devoted to families with handicapped children, not one out of 22 articles dealt with interventions with parents. In fact, only a few articles discussed interventions of any type. This is unfortunate because parental inability to communicate effectively and the dissolution of families can be detrimental to the development of all the children in the family, and can lead to the handicapped child's not reaching his or her fullest potential (Kazak & Marvin, 1984).

The major goal of this project is to apply the PREP program to families serviced by Colorado's diagnostic and evaluation clinics, and to expand the program to meet the unique needs of this population. The results of an informal needs assessment based on the perceptions of the staff of the clinics indicated that the following should be addressed in our intervention:

1. Lack of parental acceptance of the diagnosis (denial)
2. Anger and frustration over the diagnosis
3. Guilt and blaming
4. Inability to understand the problem
5. Lack of follow through of referrals
6. Conflict between parents

The PREP program is relatively short and thus can be used with families in crisis situations. In such situations, crisis intervention theory and research strongly suggest it is best to intervene during the crisis period, not after (Bloom, 1977). Moreover, during periods of crisis families are generally more accessible to outside help.

These two projects illustrate the importance of forging links with community groups to help couples and families pass through predictable and unpredictable crises in their lives. Other community groups that also deserve attention include churches and synagogues, and primary health care givers.

## CONCLUSION

We have argued that marital distress is a significant mental health problem. More specifically, we have reviewed research that suggests that marital conflict has negative effects on children and therefore should be considered a risk factor for children. However, little attention has been given to the marital dyad by risk researchers or early intervention programs (even home-based programs). The marital research literature highlights two directions for future research and intervention. First, it provides a rich source of hypotheses concerning the possible pathways linking marital distress and child problems. Second, it provides suggestions for preventive intervention that focus on the marital dyad.

Our emphasis on the role of marital discord in causing child problems is consistent with the current ideology concerning mental health and mental illness. For instance, Bloom *et al.* (1978) state,

> When the history of Twentieth Century efforts to control mental disorders is written, the great contribution of the last third of the century may well be seen in the movement away from consideration of predisposing factors in mental illness toward the concern with precipitating factors. The growing concern with current reality, with those factors which precipitate significant psychopathology, is an act of great affirmation. It recognizes what John F. Kennedy in early 1963 called the "harsh environmental conditions" which often are associated with mental illness. It legitimizes the search for effective primary preventions. (p. 889)

Applied to our current topic, efforts to strengthen marriages should go a long way toward elimination of children's suffering.

## REFERENCES

Aldous, J. (1977). Family interaction patterns. *Annual Review of Sociology, 3,* 105–135.

Anastasiow, N. (1982). Preface in N. Anastasiow, W. Frankenburg, & A. Fandal (Eds.), *Identifying the Developmentally Delayed Child.* Baltimore: University Park Press.

Anthony, E. J. (1974). Children at risk from divorce: A review. In E. J. Anthony & C. Koupernik (Eds.), *The child in his family III.* New York: Wiley.

Bean, C. A. (1974). *Methods of childbirth.* New York: Doubleday.

Becker, W. C., Peterson, D. R., Luria, Z., Shoemaker, D. J., & Hellmer, L. A. (1962). Relations of factors derived from parent interview rating to behavior problems of five-year-olds. *Child Development, 33,* 509–535.

Belsky, J., Gilstrap, B., & Rovine, M. (1984). Stability and change in mother-infant and father-infant interaction in a family setting: One to three to nine months. *Child Development, 55,* 692–705.

Block, J. H., Block, J., & Morrison, A. (1981). Parental agreement-disagreement on child-rearing orientations and gender-related personality correlates in children. *Child Development, 52,* 695–974.

Bloom, B. (1977). *Community mental health: A general introduction.* Monterey, CA: Brooks-Cole.

Bloom, B., Asher, S., & White, S. (1978). Marital disruption as a stressor: A review and analysis. *Psychological Bulletin, 85,* 867–894.

Bradley, R. (1982). The Home Inventory: A review of the first fifteen years. In N. Anastasiow, W. Frankenburg, & A. Fandel (Eds.), *Identifying the Developmentally Delayed Child.* Baltimore: University Park Press.

Chabbon, I. (1966). *Awake and aware.* New York: Delocorte Press.

Cherlin, A. J. (1981). *Marriage, divorce, remarriage.* Harvard Univ. Press, Cambridge, MA.

Cowan, C., & Cowan, J. (1978). Preparation for parenthood. *Marital and Family Review, 3,* 5.

Douglas, J. W. B., Ross, T. M., Hammond, W. A., & Mulligan, D. G. (1966). Delinquency and social class. *British Journal of Criminology, 6,* 294–302.

Emery, R. (1982). Interparental conflict and the children of discord and divorce. *Psychological Bulletin, 92,* 310–330.

Emery, R. E., & O'Leary, K. D. (1982). Children's perceptions of marital discord and behavior problems of boys and girls. *Journal of Abnormal Child Psychology, 10,* 11–24.

Ewy, D., & Ewy, R. (1976). *A Lamaze guide: Preparation for childbirth.* New York: Signet Books.

Floyd, F., & Markman, H. J. (1983). Observational biases in spouse observation: Toward a cognitive/behavioral model of marriage. *Journal of Consulting and Clinical Psychology, 51,* 450–457.

Framo, J. (1975). Rationale and techniques of intensive family therapy. In I. Boszormenyi-Nagy and J. L. Framo (Eds.), *Intensive Family Therapy.* New York: Hoeber Medical Division.

Furman, W. (1981). Qualitative features of sibling relationships. Unpublished manuscript, University of Denver.

Garbarino, J. (1982). *Children & Families in the Social Environment.* NY: Aldine Press.

Glick, P. C., & Norton, A. J. (1976). Number, timing, and duration of marriages and divorces in the United States: June, 1975. U.S. Bureau of the Census, *Current Population Reports,* Series p. 20:297, U.S. Government Printing Office, Washington, D.C.

Gibson, H. B. (1969). Early delinquency in relation to broken homes. *Journal of Child Psychology and Psychiatry and Allied Disciplines, 10,* 195–204.

Goldberg, W. A., & Easterbrooks, M. A. (1984). The role of marital quality in toddler development. *Developmental Psychology, 20* (3), 504–514.

Gottman, J. G., Markman, H. J., & Notarius, C. I. (1977). The topography of marital conflict: A sequential analysis of verbal and nonverbal behavior. *Journal of Marriage and the Family, 39,* 461–478.

Gottman, J. G., Notarius, C. I., Gonso, J., & Markman, H. J. (1976). *A couple's guide to communication.* Champaign, IL: Research Press.

Heller, K., & Monahan, J. (1977). *Psychology and community change.* Homewood, IL: Dorsey Press.

Hess, R. D., & Camara, K. A. (1979). Post-divorce family relationships as mediating factors in the consequences of divorce for children. *Journal of Social Issues, 35,* 79–96.

Hetherington, E. M. (1979). Divorce: A child's perspective. *American Psychologist, 34,* 851–858.

Hetherington, E. M., Cox, M., & Cox, R. (1976). Family interaction and the social emotional and cognitive development of children following divorce. In V. Vaughn & T. Brazelton (Eds.), *The family: Settling priorities.* New York: Science and Medicine.

Jacobson, N., & Weiss, R. (1978). Behavioral marriage therapy: The contents of Gurman et al. may be hazardous to our health. *Family Process,* 149–164.

Johnson, S. M., & Lobitz, G. K. (1974). The personal and marital adjustment of parents as related to observed child deviance and parenting behaviors. *Journal of Abnormal Child Psychology, 2,* 193–207.

Jones Leonard, D. (1984). *Observer bias as a possible mechanism in the relationships between marital discord and child behavior problems.* Unpublished Masters Proposal, University of Denver, Denver, CO.

Kazak, A., & Marvin, R. (1984). Differences, difficulties and adaptation: Stress & social networks in families with a handicapped child. *Family Relations, 33,* 67–77.

Lambert, L., Essen, J., & Head, J. (1977). Variations in behavior ratings of children who have been in care. *Journal of Child Psychology and Psychiatry and Allied Disciplines, 18,* 335–346.

Lazarus, A. A. (1968). Behavior therapy and marriage counseling. *Journal of the American Society of Psychomatic Dentistry and Medicine, 15,* 49–56.

Markman, H. J. (1979). The application of a behavioral model of marriage in predicting relationship satisfaction of couples planning marriage. *Journal of Consulting and Clinical Psychology, 4,* 743–749.

Markman, H. J. (1981). The prediction of marital distress: A five year follow-up. *Journal of Consulting and Clinical Psychology, 49,* 760–762.

Markman, H. J. (1984). The longitudinal study of couples' interaction: Implications for cognitive/behavioral, social exchange, and social skills models of relationship development. In K. Hahlweg & N. Jacobson (Eds.), *Marital interaction: Analysis and modification.* New York: Guilford Press.

Markman, H. J., & Floyd, F. (1980). Possibilities for the prevention of marital discord: A behavioral perspective. *American Journal of Family Therapy, 8,* 29–48.

Markman, H. J., Floyd, F., & Dickson-Markman, F. (1982). Toward a model for the prediction and prevention of marital and family distress and dissolution. In S. Duck (Ed.), *Personal relationships 4: Dissolving personal relationships.* London: Academic Press.

Markman, H. J., Jamieson, K., & Floyd, F. (1983). The assessment and modification of premarital relationships: Implications for the etiology and prevention of marital distress. In J. Vincent (Ed.), *Advances in family intervention, assessment and theory.* Greenwich, CT: JAI Press.

Markman, H. J., & Kadushin, F. S. (1984). The preventive effects of Lamaze training on first-time parents: A longitudinal study. Under editorial review.

Markman, H., & Notarius, C. (in press). Coding marital and family interaction: Current Status. In T. Jacob (Ed.), *Family interaction and psychopathology: Theories, methods, and findings.* New York: Plenum.

McCord, J., McCord, W., & Thurber, E. (1962). Some effects of paternal absence on male children. *Journal of Abnormal and Social Psychology, 64,* 361–369.

McCord, W., McCord, J., & Howard, A. (1961). Familial correlates of aggression in nondelinquent male children. *Journal of Abnormal and Social Psychology, 62,* 79–83.

McDermott, J. F. (1968). Parental divorce in early childhood. *American Journal of Psychiatry, 124,* 1424–1432.

McDermot, J. F. (1970). Divorce and its psychological sequelae in children. *Archives of General Psychiatry, 23,* 421–427.

Minuchin, S., Rosman, B. L., & Baker, L. (1978). *Psychosomatic families: Anorexia nervosa in context.* Cambridge, MA.: Harvard Univ. Press.

National Center for Health Statistics. (1983). Births, marriages, divorces, and deaths for November, 1982. *Monthly Vital Statistics Report 31, No. 11. DHHS Pub. No. (PHS) 83-1120.* Public Health Service, Hyattsville, MD.

Notarius, C. I., Markman, H. J., & Gottman, J. (1983). The Couples Interaction Scoring System: Clinical issues. In E. Filsinger (Ed.), *Marital measurement sourcebook.* Beverly Hills: Sage.

Notarius, C., & Pelligrini, D. (1984). Marital processes as stressors and stress mediators: Implications for marital repair. In S. Duck (Ed.), *Personal relationships, 5: Repairing personal relationships.* London: Academic Press.

Oltmanns, T. F., Broderick, J. E., & O'Leary, K. D. (1977). Marital adjustment and the efficacy of behavior therapy with children. *Journal of Consulting and Clinical Psychology, 45,* 724–729.

Patterson, G. R. (1977). Accelerating stimuli for two classes of coercive behaviors. *Journal of Abnormal Child Psychology, 80,* 287–295.

Porter, B., & O'Leary, K. D. (1980). Marital discord and childhood behavior problems. *Journal of Abnormal Child Psychology, 80,* 287–295.

Power, M. J., Ash, M., Schoenberg, E., & Storey, E. C. (1974). Delinquency and the family. *British Journal of Social Work, 4,* 17–38.

Rutter, M. (1971). Parent-child separation: Psychological effects on the children. *Journal of Child Psychology and Psychiatry and Allied Disciplines, 12,* 233–260.

Rutter, M. (1980). Protective factors in children's responses to stress and disadvantage. In M. W. Kent & J. E. Rolf (Eds.), *Primary prevention of psychopathology: III.* Hanover, NH: Univ. Press of New England.

Rutter, M., Yule, B., Quinton, D., Rowland, O., Yule, W., & Berger, M. (1975). Attainment and adjustment in two geographic areas: III Some factors accounting for area differences. *British Journal of Psychiatry, 125,* 520–533.

Satir, V. (1974). *Conjoint family therapy.* Palo Alto, CA: Science and Behavior Books.

Schofield, W. (1966). *Psychotherapy: The purchase of friendship.* Englewood Cliffs, NJ: Prentice-Hall.

Schwartz, J. C. (1979). Childhood origins of psychopathology. *American Psychologist, 34,* 879–885.

Stroebe, M. S., & Stroebe, W. (1983). Who suffers more? Sex differences in health risks of the widowed. *Psychological Bulletin, 93,* 279–301.

Stuart, R. B., (1969). Operant-interpersonal treatment for marital discord. *Journal of Consulting and Clinical Psychology, 33,* 675–682.

Tanzer, D., & Block, J. L. (1972). *Why natural childbirth? A psychologists' report on the benefits to mothers, fathers and babies.* New York: Shocken Books.

Wallerstein, J. S., & Kelly, J. B. (1980). *Surviving the breakup.* New York: Basic Books.

Westman, J. D., Cline, D. W., Swift, W. J., & Kramer, D. A. (1976). The role of child psychiatry in divorce. *Archives of General Psychiatry, 23,* 416–420.

CHAPTER 5

# Assessing Emotional Availability in Early Development

*Robert N. Emde and M. Ann Easterbrooks*

---

It is not difficult to designate high-risk groups for infants and young children likely to have emotional and social problems in their development. Such groups can be designated according to (a) handicapping and health factors in the child (e.g., prematurity, major sensory motoric deficits, malformations, disfigurements, and multiple hospitalizations); (b) handicapping and health factors in the parent (e.g., major mental illness, such as severe depression, sociopathy, or schizophrenia); and (c) general social and economic factors (e.g., low socioeconomic status, but also including factors such as infants and young children with teenage parents, single parents, and parents with poor marital adjustment) (see Markman & Jones Leonard, Chapter 4). When one is planning intervention, however, designating high-risk groups is an inefficient way of screening. As Frankenburg points out in this volume, there are too many individuals in high-risk groups who do not require intervention—that is, who are not disordered and who are not in the process of becoming disordered. The problem for screening, therefore, is the early identification of those *individuals* (including those within high-risk groups) who are needing of intervention.

In spite of need, we do not yet have screening devices for early identification of individuals at risk for emotional and social disorders. Still, the field of emotion research is a burgeoning one, and there is a

---

***Robert N. Emde and M. Ann Easterbrooks*** • Department of Psychiatry, University of Colorado Health Sciences Center, Denver, Colorado 80262. Preparation of this paper was facilitated by grants from the National Institute of Mental Health (project grant 22803) and Research Scientist Award MH 36808 to Dr. Emde, and from the John D. and Catherine T. MacArthur Foundation grant to the Network on the Transition from Infancy to Early Childhood.

sense of optimism that accurate screening tools in these disorders may soon emerge. In this chapter, we propose that assessment be guided by a mediating variable we refer to as *emotional availability*. We believe that identifying individual differences in emotional availability holds special promise for screening.

## SOME PRACTICAL CONSIDERATIONS: EMOTIONAL AVAILABILITY AND COMING TO GRIPS WITH THE PAINFULLY OBVIOUS

What is emotional availability? This is a relational concept based on the fact that, in any caring relationship, a certain range of organized emotions is associated with continued involvement, intimacy, and developmental change. Thus, although the clinician can begin to assess emotional availability in the child alone or in the parent alone, emotional availability is most appropriately assessed with the child and parent together. Emotional availability will, therefore, refer to the degree to which each partner expresses emotions and is responsive to the emotions of the other.

Clinical experience demonstrates that emotions are apt to be a sensitive barometer of early developmental functioning in the child–parent system (Emde, Gaensbauer, & Harmon, 1982). If the relationship is going well, there should be some indication of sustained pleasure and mutual interest, as well as a well-modulated range of emotional expressions, both negative and positive. One expects to see evidence of this in the child, in the parents, and in their interaction. If the system is not functioning well, one often sees that there is little pleasure, and the range of emotional expression is restricted; instead of interest, there may be evidence of a "turning off" or apathy. In more extreme circumstances, there may be sadness and depression. Other maladaptive patterns, such as fearfulness and vigilance or sustained anger and hostility, may also be apparent.

In one sense, this kind of assessment is obvious. Clinicians have long found emotions to be at the center of everyday work. Discomfort is the basis for consultation; patients want to "feel better." Further, in treatment, whether with children or adults, emotional expressions allow for ongoing assessment; both patient (through feeling) and clinician (through observation and empathy) monitor therapeutic progress. In another sense, however, this kind of obvious assessment is often overlooked or avoided. This is due not only to busy scheduling and the press of technical aspects of health care but also to a seeming paradox that emerges from the relational nature of emotional availability; namely, in order to assess emotional availability, *the clinician must also be emotionally available*. The clinician must use his or her own feelings. This is not easy and may take considerable effort, for expressions of sadness and depression are painful to acknowledge when they are experienced as resonant responses. It is probably because of similar discomforts among clinicians that depression in childhood went unacknowledged in psychiatry until quite recently (Emde, Harmon, & Good, in press), and that painful observations of child abuse went unappreciated for decades (Radbill, 1980).

Thus far we have discussed emotional availability in terms of features that exist throughout development. We now turn to some age-related, developmental aspects, beginning with emotional assessment on the child's side and then considering the parent's side.

The newborn not only has the capacity to take in and process information but also has the capacity to turn off stimulation by regulating behavioral state, as Brazelton and his co-workers have shown and as the Neonatal Behavioral Assessment Scale demonstrates so vividly (Brazelton, 1973). When development is progresing well, the newborn seeks out stimulation (particularly when in the "quiet alert" state) and actively engages in coping behaviors to regulate arousal and stimulation. When things are not going well because of illness or a continually stressful environment, the newborn can become lethargic, excessively sleepy, or irritable and difficult to engage in wakeful attentiveness. This may alert the sensitive clinician to a problem in need of intervention. Whatever its cause, we might say there is a likely deficit in emotional availability from the infant's perspective.

After 2 postnatal months, one normally expects to see the infant's pleasure system blossoming with social smiling, enhanced eye-to-eye contact, motoric activation in social encounters, and social cooing. There is less fussiness and more sustained daytime wakefulness, which is characterized by enhanced exploration with objects and people (Emde, Gaensbauer, & Harmon, 1976). With time, more is sought, more is enjoyed, and more is learned. If development is not going well, however, or if there is no emotionally available caregiver, there is apt to be less pleasure and less engagement with the world, and there may even be lethargy and social avoidance.

By 7 to 9 months, the infant increasingly shows preference for one or more primary caregivers. This is the age when the infant begins to manifest specific or focused attachments. Not only is there obvious pleasure in greeting the attachment figure, but there is apt to be specific displeasure when she or he leaves (separation distress) or when a stranger initially approaches (stranger distress). Toward the end of the first year and throughout the second year, the infant increasingly uses the attachment figure as a secure base from which to explore the environment (Ainsworth, Blehar, Waters, & Wall, 1978). With the onset of walking, there is a surge of exploratory activity, which frequently includes a mood of elation described by some as "the child's love affair with the world" (Greenacre, 1971). Mahler and her colleagues have described the periodic returns to mother for "emotional refueling" at this age (Mahler, Pine, & Bergman, 1975), as well as the importance of the mother's emotional availability for this process. If development is not going well, one may see manifestations of what Ainsworth and her colleagues have referred to as "insecure attachment" of the infant to its mother or father. This may be manifested by a lack of positive greeting and avoidance of the attachment figure or by resistance to interaction with mother or father during a reunion after a brief separation. One might also see evidence of a turning off, in which the child restricts both exploration and emotional expressiveness, as well as of a defensive use of play that looks stereotypic and less than joyful (Harmon, Suwalsky, & Klein, 1979).

On the parents' side of emotional assessment, the clinician expects to see evidence of pride and pleasure with renewed excitement following the child's developmental accomplishments (e.g., the social smile, walking, language). Such is the case when development is on track. Research has indicated that negative parental perceptions and attitudes about their children's development (including the absence of the above) are important risk indicators for emotional problems (Broussard & Hartner, 1971; Gray, Cutler, Dean, & Kempe, 1977; Thomas & Chess, 1977).

Elsewhere, we have stated our belief that the health care professional should be aggressive in finding out how parents feel about their children's development and in assessing the ratio of pleasure to distress in parental activities (Emde *et al.*, 1982). In addition to asking about this directly, we have found responses to questions about the baby's personality to be revealing. (For example, does your baby have a personality yet? If so, what's it like?) We have also found it helpful to ask how the mother perceives her infant's emotions. Reports of a lot of anger, fearfulness, or guilt during the first year may indicate problems that are worth pursuing. Our research is currently documenting normal and deviant maternal perceptions of infant emotions at different ages in order to gain useful information for the clinician.

One final point about practical guidelines. The term *emotional availability* emphasizes an important fact about emotions, namely, their social relatedness. Some believe emotions may have evolved primarily for social signaling and social bonding (Emde, 1980; Hamburg, 1963; Myers, 1976), and, in practice, the fundamental emotions are assessed through their relational features. Emotions reveal internalized, sustained aspects of interpersonal relationships, even in infancy. On the side of the positive emotions, the relational aspect of pleasure is affection. The relational aspect of interest is sociability, with the parent and child able to look outward, to engage other social partners. Surprise and mock surprise are emotions that lead to favorite games, which many parents and infants construct in unique ways during the first year. We find it useful to ask about games the baby plays with the mother. Toward the end of the first year, can the baby demonstrate peek-a-boo and reciprocal games? Is there evidence of anticipatory pleasure in these games?

Negative emotions, also important in everyday life, have problematic relational aspects if they are predominant, sustained, and internalized. Fear and anxiety can lead to insecurity, vigilance, and turning away from the social partner. Anger can lead to hostility and rejection. Sadness can have its relational aspects in turning off and depression, as has been noted. In all of this, it is important for the clinician to be aware of the fact that affective relationships, within a family, can be quite specific such that an infant can show vigilance, turning off, or anger with one parent and not another (Gaensbauer & Sands, 1980).

## THEORETICAL BACKGROUND: RECENT EMOTIONS RESEARCH AND THE AFFECTIVE SELF

A theoretical background for the above guidelines emerges from recent emotions research. Increasingly, emotions have become appreciated as biologically adaptive—as active, ongoing, and useful processes rather than reactive, intermittent, and disruptive states. Although peak emotions can be disruptive, these are unusual in everyday life, and sustained maladaptive disturbances in emotional regulation are a cause for concern.

How are emotions adaptive? From a psychological standpoint, emotions serve an evaluative function. They provide signals and incentives for learning, for new plans, and for new actions according to what is pleasant or unpleasant. Further, emotions have a monitoring function: At any given moment, they allow us to monitor ourselves, our states of being, and our engagement with the world. As the previous discussion illustrates, they also allow us to monitor others, their intentions, their needs, and their states of well-being and engagement. Emotions thus have a crucial set of adaptive functions for caregiving and for social life in general.

Another set of adaptive functions of our emotions may be equally important in providing a theoretical background for assessment of emotional availability. These concern an *affective self*, a construct (Emde, 1983) that rests on research showing that emotions are biologically patterned with a similar organization throughout the lifespan. Because of this organization, our emotions provide us with a core of continuity for our self-experience across development. This is adaptive in two ways. First, because we are able to access our own consistent feelings, we know we are the same in spite of the many ways we change over the years. Second, because of the biological consistency of our human "affective core," we are also able to appreciate the feelings of others and be empathic. Thus, it is the affective self and its human core which allow for emotional availability. A review of some lines of evidence for an affective self, therefore, seems appropriate.

**Evidence for the Affective Self**

The first line of evidence, quite simply, comes from everyday experience as well as clinical practice. We are aware of how much we rely on knowing other people by understanding their feelings. In clinical work, we go beyond monitoring distress; once we are in touch with another's emotional life, we are in touch with his or her humanity. This can become the basis for going further in appreciating that individual as a unique human being.

A second line of evidence for affective continuity concerns research that has documented the similar organization of emotional expression in infants, children, and adults. A variety of scaling studies of the facial expressions of emotions over the life span have revealed a strikingly similar dimensional organization, with hedonic tone (*pleasant* to *unpleasant*) consistently the most predominant dimension, and with activation the second most prominent dimension. (A third dimension is more variable and is sometimes labeled "control," "acceptance/rejection," or "internally oriented/externally oriented.") Our infancy studies, in which this pattern is found regularly after 3 months, are consistent with a host of experimental investigations in adults, and similar organization has been found in school children from Grades 3 through 7. (For a review of these studies, see Ekman, Friesen, & Ellsworth, 1972; Emde, 1980; and Russell & Ridgeway, 1983.)

Another line of evidence for affective continuity comes from cross-cultural studies of discrete emotions. Following on Darwin's (1877) postulation of species-wide discrete emotional expressions and Tomkins' (1962–1963) more recent theoretical elaboration, two separate teams of investigators (Izard, 1971; and Ekman *et al.*, 1972),using photographs of posed facial expressions of adults, found remarkable agreement concerning specific emotions. This agreement was found among adults in non-Western as well as Western cultures and in nonliterate as well as literate cultures for the emotions of joy, surprise, anger, fear, sadness, disgust, and, to a lesser extent, interest. These findings implied a universal human basis for both emotional recognition and expression. Subsequently, the facial movements involved in each of these discrete emotions have been specified (for a review of the latter, see Izard, 1982; and Ekman, 1982).

### Evidence for the Affective Self in Infancy

More evidence for affective continuity comes from infancy, where recent research has indicated a preadapted readiness to express discrete emotions. Data show that infant facial expressions of emotion can be judged reliably, and such expressions fit the patterning suggested from research on adult discrete emotions. This has thus far been found true for happiness, fear, surprise, sadness, anger, disgust, and pain (Emde, Kligman, Reich, & Wade, 1978; Hiatt, Campos, & Emde, 1979; Izard, Huebner, Risser, McGinnes, & Dougherty, 1980; Stenberg, Campos, & Emde, 1983; and Stenberg, 1982). Research on vocal expressions of emotion in infancy is just beginning, but there are already indications of a patterned signaling channel of major importance there, also.

Now we come more explicitly to the social domain in infancy. The very existence of an emotional signaling system, one that seems essential for caregiving and development, argues strongly for a prepatterned biological organization of emotions with some consistency over time. Again, some of this is obvious. As every parent knows, emotional expressions seem to be the "language of the baby." Not only are they prominent, but they guide caregiving by allowing the monitoring of the infant's current state of need or satisfaction. Some expressions are unequivocal and have clear survival value, such as crying, which communicates pain or distress and gives a peremptory universal message for change. Smiling communicates a universal message of pleasure and encourages approach and continuation. A current aspect of our research documents the rich array of infant emotional expressions and their caregiving consequences (see Johnson, Emde, Pannabecker, Stenberg, & Davis, 1982; and Klinnert, Sorce, Emde, Stenberg, & Gaensbauer, 1984). Indeed, when there is a dampening of infant signals, as in Down's syndrome, caregiving is more difficult (Cicchetti & Sroufe, 1978; Emde & Brown, 1978; Sorce & Emde, 1982).

Most recently, we have been absorbed in researching a phenomenon that has been termed "social referencing" (Campos & Stenberg, 1981; Klinnert, Campos, Sorce, Emde, & Svejda, 1982; Feinman & Lewis, 1981; Sorce, Emde, Campos, & Klinnert, 1985). In contrast to caregiver use of infant emotional signals, social referencing is concerned with the other side of the communication system; namely, the infant's appreciation and use of emotional signals in those around him or her, particularly the caregiver. *Social referencing* refers to a process in which the infant seeks out emotional information from a significant other in order to make sense of an event which is otherwise ambiguous. Toward the end of the first year and during the second year, this seems especially important.

For example, in a recent study (Sorce *et al.*, 1985) of 12-month-olds on the visual cliff, a glass-topped table was used in which one-half shows apparent depth (a checkerboard pattern 30 cm below the glass surface instead of directly under it). When infants appreciated the apparent drop-off, they looked to mother's face before exploring the cliff and reaching an interesting toy. If mothers (who were trained) displayed an expression of joy or interest, 75% of the infants explored and crossed the deep side to the toy; if mothers displayed an expression of fear or anger, less than 10% of the infants crossed the visual cliff. Other experimental paradigms of uncertainty (with unusual toys, for example) have also been used to elicit social referencing and consequent behavioral regulation on the part of infants. Clearly such an active form of emotional signaling, with the infant's searching for emotional information and using this information to regulate subsequent behavior, could not take place without a consistent pattern of organization.

Finally, we could add that research on emotional availability, although indirect, provides another indication of an adaptively patterned system. The importance of the emotional availability of the caregiver in infancy has been implicit in investigations of attachment (Bowlby, 1973; Matas, Arend, & Sroufe, 1978) and has been explicitly noted by Mahler and her colleagues (Mahler *et al.*, 1975). In one of our studies, we found striking evidence for the effects of mother's emotional availability on exploration and play in 15-month-olds (Sorce & Emde, 1982); the experimental effects depended on whether the mother was reading a newspaper or not.

Further propositions for a theory of an affective self have been stated elsewhere (Emde, 1983). Some features operate from the beginning of life. These include self-regulation, social fittedness, and affective monitoring. Other features develop during the course of infancy, reaching a nodal point in the middle of the second year with the acquisition of self-awareness and the emergence of prosocial inclinations and empathy (Zahn-Waxler & Radke-Yarrow, 1982). But, in all of this, the important point for our purposes is that emotional development cannot be viewed in isolation. We believe it must be assessed in the context of emotional availability, a concept that involves self-regulation and its social context.

## RESEARCH PARADIGMS FOR ASSESSMENT OF EMOTIONAL AVAILABILITY

With this general theoretical background, we now turn to research paradigms of promise. As was mentioned earlier, no screening device now exists to assess emotional availability, but future instruments are likely to be based on current research paradigms.

The social context of early emotional development is clearly apparent in existing research paradigms; most examine characteristics of emotional availability in interactions between young children and significant social partners (primarily caregivers, but also peers and unfamiliar adults). In addition, many focus on characteristics of the child-rearing environment in which emotional development unfolds (assessing family attitudes toward emotional expressiveness, for example).

Especially in infancy, before the development of sophisticated linguistic modes of communication, the child relies on emotional signaling to express his or her needs and wishes. Similarly, before the baby can understand the semantic context of an adult's verbal utterances, the baby encodes the emotional signals expressed through the vocal, facial, and tactile channels of adult caregivers. As these emotional experiences arise within the family, most assessment paradigms focus on infant–parent interaction, particularly interactions between infants and their mothers. Emotional availability within an infant–caregiver dyad is determined in part by the constitutional organization of the infant (the neural and physical organization necessary to encode and produce emotional signals clearly) and in part by characteristics of the caregiver. Few assessment paradigms, however, address the neural organization of the infant, and the focus of assessment is centered on the caregiving environment, particularly in early infancy. In order to have emotional availability in the dyad, caregivers must be able to *monitor* or perceive the emotional signals of the infant, to *interpret* their meaning accurately, to *select* an appropriate response from their behavioral repertoire, and to *execute* the response promptly or contingently. Many researchers call this sequence of events "parental sensitivity" (Ainsworth *et al.*, 1978; Lamb & Easterbrooks, 1981). According to Ainsworth, "highly sensitive mothers are usually accessible to their infants and are aware of even their more subtle communications, signals, wishes and moods . . . they accurately interpret their perceptions and show empathy with their infants (1985, p. 4).

A lack of sensitive empathy may result in the caregiver's distortion of the meaning or urgency of infant emotional signals (for instance, a distress cry may be interpreted as boredom or a sign of manipulation and may be responded to less promptly or with an inappropriate accompanying affect). Further, this inability on the part of the parent to be accessible to the affective content of the baby's communications may be manifest in the maintenance of physical proximity between the dyad, the manner of physical contact, or even denial of the signal value of infant emotional expressions. Emotional unavailability or lack of empathy on the part of a caregiver may also lead to interactions which, from the infant's perspective, are poorly timed or not well-resolved. In the empathic or sensitive interaction, the tempo of the interaction will be sensitive to the baby's cues and will be well-resolved, not ending before the affect modulation accompanying the interaction is completed.

The manner in which characteristics of maternal sensitivity during the first year of life relate to the development of infant–mother attachment bonds has been a research interest for the last decade. The assessment of emotional availability may provide information about the nature of these interpersonal relationships prior to the time at which attachment bonds are firmly established (the latter part of the first year of life). In fact, the caregiver's emotional availability in perceiving, interpreting, and empathizing with the infant's emotional signals probably plays an important role in establishing and maintaining attachment bonds and subsequent interpersonal relationships.

Given the transactional nature of the developing infant–caregiver system, it is important to keep in mind the developmental reorganization in biobehavioral systems during the first 2 years of life (Emde *et al.*, 1976; Sander, 1976; Spitz, 1959), for these shifts are marked by changes in the affective experience and expression of emotions. Through repeated experiences with the caregiver, the infant comes to understand the meaning and consequences of his/her own emotional signals and gains a sense of his/her efficacy. In effect, these experiences influence the child's developing sense of self and others in the environment. Infants with an emotionally available caregiver will learn the communicative value of emotional signaling between themselves and others. Without these experiences, infants may soon mask their own emotional expressiveness and reflect an inability to decode or empathize with the affective experiences of others.

### Assessment Paradigms

The nature of assessment tools for emotional availability varies greatly. Although the large majority involve observations of interactions between young children and their caregivers, others involve observations of interactions with unfamiliar social partners (adults and peers); nonobservational paradigms assess characteristics of the family environment (attitudes toward emotional expressiveness) or the ability of caregivers to accurately interpret emotional signals (using standardized materials). We will selectively review a variety of these methods.

## Observational Paradigms

The observational assessment of emotional availability encompasses a wide variety of techniques, including assessments of the caregiver's style of interaction with the child; the ability of the child to produce clear emotional signals; the emotional climate of the family (i.e., marital adjustment, emotional communication between parents); and assessment of the child's emotional reactions to strangers.

In addition to the social unit of analysis, assessment paradigms vary according to the observational context. Both structured assessments and observations of spontaneous interaction have strengths and weaknesses. Does one structure the interactional context in hopes of eliciting certain critical events, or is it best to observe unstructured interaction that may be more characteristic of spontaneous interchanges? Either of these types of observational assessments can be conducted in home or laboratory settings.

## Observations in the Home and Natural Environments

In one of the most widely known studies of early infant–mother interaction, Ainsworth and her colleagues (see Ainsworth *et al.*, 1978) observed mothers and infants at home over the course of the first year of life. To characterize maternal behavior, they devised a set of four qualitative rating scales based on observations of spontaneous interactions in a variety of contexts (e.g., feeding, emotional communication, physical contact). The assumptions underlying the ratings noted various components of sensitive responsiveness: monitoring, interpreting, selecting an appropriate response behavior, and responding promptly. The four 9-point scales assess dimensions of (a) sensitivity/insensitivity to the infant's signals, (b) cooperation/interference with the baby's desires, (c) acceptance/rejection of the baby, and (d) accessibility/ignoring. Together, these scales were found to differentiate interactions of caregivers of securely attached infants from those who later were assessed as insecurely attached (at the end of the first year of life—see below for further discussion of attachment). While these scales contain components other than emotional availability, the contribution of the affective component of the interaction was significant. Further, two additional rating scales developed by Main (see Ainsworth *et al.*, 1978) characterized a group of mothers of infants assessed as insecure/

avoidant. These mothers lacked emotional expressiveness (their range of expression was restricted), and they received high scores on a scale of maternal rigidity. Main suggested that these women were suppressing anger that was communicated to the infant in aversive experiences with physical contact. Interestingly, their infants were later themselves notable for their overt emotional blandness in the "Strange Situation" (Ainsworth & Wittig, 1969), although they expressed inappropriate modulation of anger at home and with others in later developmental periods. Although the scales were designed to be used in home observations of mother and infant in the first year of life, they can be modified for use with fathers or in nonhome settings, provided the observation period is extended.

For the clinical researcher, rating scales are probably the most useful technique for assessing emotional availability. A set of scales devised for the Chicago Mother's Project (Clark, Musick, Stott, & Klehr, 1980) provides a comprehensive assessment of individual and dyadic components of mother–child interaction in a variety of semistructured and unstructured situations (infant feeding, a mother–child task, and play). Although the scales were targeted for use with a population of diagnosed mentally ill mothers with their young children (newborn to 4 years), many are appropriate for capturing emotional availability in normal and at-risk populations. The set of fifty-three 5-point scales is noteworthy for the range of dimensions covered for both mother (e.g., tone of voice, involvement with child, appropriateness of behavior toward child) and child (e.g., facial affect, communicative competence, compliance). Similarly, they could be useful in observations of young children interacting with their fathers, siblings, or nonfamily members. Further, these ratings may be conducted on the basis of relatively short periods of observation (5–15 minutes).

The Infant Social Development Laboratory at the National Institute of Mental Health (which was under the direction of the late Leon Yarrow) has published the Infant Social Behavior Manual (Durfee, Klein, Fivel, Bennett, Morgan, & Blehar, 1977). This manual includes a set of rating scales designed to assess qualitative dimensions of spontaneous interaction and play behavior between infants and mothers either in the home or laboratory environments. One particular scale ("mutual accessibility between mother and baby") focuses on the social aspects of interaction, particularly the physical and psychological availability of the members of the dyad. The similarities between this scale and those developed by Ainsworth and colleagues are apparent, and both would require an extended period of observation in order to gain a sense of the dyad as an interactive system.

## Structured Observational Paradigms

### *The "Strange Situation"*

A classic and widely used and modified structured observation of the parent–infant (or toddler) relationship is the "Strange Situation" (Ainsworth & Wittig, 1969). Originally developed as a laboratory-based research tool to assess "security of attachment" in a manner that would reflect the historical patterns of mother–infant interaction in the home during the first year of life, the Strange Situation has yielded several variations that are employed for clinical purposes. Although this procedure was not designed for the specific evaluation of infant emotions, the patterning of emotional responses is a component in the assessment of the security of infant–parent attachment bonds. In contrast to the rating scales discussed previously, evaluation of security of attachment focuses on child behavior in this situation, not on parental behavior.

The 20-minute procedure is comprised of a series of successively more stressful episodes (exploration of a novel environment, interaction with an unfamiliar adult, separation from and reunion with the attachment figure) aimed at understanding the behavioral organization of the attachment, exploration, and affiliative systems. Six 7-point rating scales (based on behavioral frequency, intensity, duration, and latency) are used to assess the child's avoidance of and resistance to interaction with the caregiver, the achievement and maintenance of physical proximity and contact, and search behavior during separation and distal communication. The organization of these behaviors leads to the classification of infants and toddlers into three qualitative categories of attachment: secure, insecure/avoidant, and insecure/resistant (the three major classifications contain eight subgroups). Characteristics of emotional responses of the child are incorporated into these ratings and classifications (for example, securely attached infants typically engage in positive affect sharing with their parents, which requires emotional availability of both partners; insecure-avoidant infants may be characterized as emotionally bland in this situation; insecure-resistant infants may engage in positive affect sharing accompanied by negative emotional behavior, such as anger/tantrums, directed toward the caregiver). In variations of the Strange Situation paradigm (see Gaensbauer & Harmon, 1982; and Solyom, 1982), emotional expressiveness is assessed directly.

The laboratory-based Strange Situation design is appropriate for infants and toddlers approximately 11 to 24 months of age. Several investigators, recognizing that separations from and reunions with an attachment figure are salient thoroughout life, are presently attempting to develop extensions of the paradigm/notions of security of attachment to use with children in the third and fourth years of life (e.g., D. Cicchetti, personal communication, January, 1984; R. Marvin, personal communication, January, 1984; M. Greenberg, personal communication, January, 1984; Waters & Deane, in press). Although designed to assess infant–mother attachment, the Strange Situation is useful for assessing the quality of the child–father bond as well (Easterbrooks & Goldberg, 1984; Main & Weston, 1981). It is useful to bear in mind that quality of attachments to mother and father are independent, reflecting the dyadic nature behind the attachment bond.

### *The Gaensbauer and Harmon Paradigm*

A modified version of the Strange Situation assessment of attachment is incorporated into the Gaensbauer and Harmon paradigm (Gaensbauer & Harmon, 1982), with additional assessments arranged in order to provide a more complete picture of the child's functioning. The evaluation begins with observation of unstructured free-play between child and caregiver, followed by assessments of stranger sociability, separation from and reunion with the attachment figure, and developmental testing (the Bayley Mental Development Index) (Bayley, 1966). In addition to assessing security of attachment, specific ratings are conducted of the infant's affective responses across the situations. Ratings are conducted (every 30 seconds) of infant pleasure, interest (in mother, stranger, non-social environment), fear, anger, distress, and sadness. The patterning of these discrete emotions across the various interactive situations is used to construct an affect profile of the child, which may be used to forecast later coping mechanisms and modalities by which the developing child modulates affective arousal. To date, a variety of infant populations have been studied that evidence different affect profiles; these include full-term healthy infants, premature infants, and infants with a documented history of abuse or neglect. The abuse–neglect sample appeared particularly affectively withdrawn and depressed, avoided interaction with their mothers, and were indiscriminately responsive to the unfamiliar adult. These findings are supported by the work of George and Main (1979) with abused toddlers.

In order to conduct the above-detailed emotion ratings, one should conduct the paradigm in a laboratory setting equipped with videotape equipment. Although designed for infants and their mothers, the paradigm would be appropriate for assessing infants and fathers as well, and the assessments may be made from the end of the first year through the second year of life.

### *The Infant Clinical Assessment Procedure*

Closely related to the Gaensbauer and Harmon paradigm is the Infant Clinical Assessment Procedure (ICAP) and the accompanying Michigan Infant Affect Scales (MIAS) (Solyom, 1982). This set of procedures is formulated directly from the Ainsworth and the Gaensbauer and Harmon paradigms. The clinical observation, which is used with a wide age range (3–30 months), may be conducted in a laboratory playroom or home setting and entails detailed coding of the expression and regulation of affect in a variety of situations, most of which involve interaction with a caregiver. The assessment of affect is central, because the paradigm is based on the assumption that affect serves an organizing role in the motivation and regulation of social and nonsocial behavior.

The procedure includes the Gaensbauer and Harmon modified Strange Situation for assessing quality of attachment to the caregiver and responsiveness to an unfamiliar adult, as well as developmental testing (the Bayley MDI). An age-appropriate child–mother task and assessment of neuromuscular functioning complete the paradigm. The inclusion of the neuromuscular evaluation as a screening device for problems in the ability to produce or encode emotional signals or to regulate affect is noteworthy.

In contrast to the Gaensbauer and Harmon ratings of affect every 30 seconds, this procedure calls for 10-second ratings throughout the session (also making videotape analysis a necessity). Observations and ratings of discrete emotions are conducted (range, intensity, duration) for the emotions of pleasure, interest (in mother, toys, examiner), anger, sadness, distress. The unique aspect of the scales is the attempt to tease apart the modalities of affect expression; separate ratings are conducted for the facial, vocal, and motoric channels. From these ratings, affect profiles (similar to Gaensbauer & Harmon, 1982 and Lewis & Michalson, 1983, discussed below) are developed, based on (a) the organization of affect across the situations; (b) affect differentiation (context specificity, range of expression); (c) mechanisms of affect regulation (for example, whether the infant or toddler uses avoidance of the social partner, self-soothing, verbal mediation or various defense mechanisms to maintain or reduce affective arousal); and (d) the facilitative nature of the surrounding social environment (or how the child uses interpersonal relationships to regulate emotional expressiveness).

### *Scales of Socioemotional Development*

Also targeted for the assessment of children from 3 to 30 months are the Scales of Socioemotional Development (Lewis & Michalson,

1983). The scales were developed to assess the behavior of children in daycare settings and to reflect general response tendencies in a variety of social and nonsocial settings (not behavioral tendencies that may be specific to a particular relationship). In so doing, this paradigm focuses on characteristics of interactive behavior other than with the parental attachment figures (for instance, with peers and nonparental caregivers). In this manner it differs from most of the other assessment schemes that assume that the best index of emotional development of very young children can be made by observing interactions with their primary caregivers or attachment figures. The scales evaluate functioning in five discrete realms: fear, anger, happiness, affiliation, and competence (the latter two are considered social emotions in this scheme). The scales of affiliation and competence and assessment of peer interaction are not equivalently useful over the entire age range of 3 to 30 months and would be least appropriate with the youngest children. An array of naturally occurring situations are sampled, and many interactions may be observed as well in home or laboratory settings (such as responses to the approach of a stranger, game-playing with the caregiver, separation and reunion sequence, violations of social rules). The composite scores of responses for each of the five emotions averaged across the different observations are used to construct emotional profiles (similar to those discussed earlier). From their research study in the daycare setting, Lewis and Michalson developed profiles of five "types" of children: "happy," "competent," "excitable," "depressed," and "dependent."

### *Affect Attunement*

Another alternative assessment of emotional availability that does not entail observation of the Strange Situation or its modifications is observation of "affect attunement" (Stern, 1984). This concept reflects a belief that humans possess a biological propensity for affect matching, or affect resonance, which serves important functions for the human infant. Assessment of affect attunement in infancy places responsibility on the parent to monitor, interpret, and appropriately respond to infant emotional signals in an empathic manner (similar to Ainsworth's concept of sensitivity). Although there is no standardized measurement system, affect attunement may be observed at home, in the laboratory, or other environments in which brief periods of unstructured child–parent interaction are possible. According to Stern, the critical feature of the interaction is the proportion of time that the parent can empathize with the baby's internal state and will attune his or her own behavior accordingly. The concept of affect attunement is similar to Mahler's (Mahler *et al.*, 1975) notions of mirroring or echoing, with the parent attuning to the child's subjective state, not necessarily the overt behavior. One hallmark of successful affect attunement on the part of the parent is the facilitation of longer interactional bouts and the development of shared meanings or intersubjectivity between the social partners. Infant distress, avoidance, and withdrawal from the interaction present evidence that affect attunement is not met.

Finally, researchers have begun to assess the effects of emotional availability more directly by introducing simple perturbations in the usual mother–infant interactive system. Tronick, Als, Adamson, Wise, and Brazelton (1978) have shown the dramatic effects, in early infancy, of mothers' facial unresponsiveness. Mothers are asked to be "stoney-faced" for a minute or two, and, typically, infants attempt to engage interaction, then avert their gaze and become distressed. Tronick, who believes this sequence may be similar to what happens with infants of depressed caregivers, is developing standard measurement situations. For later infancy, Sorce and Emde (1982) have developed a paradigm in which there is a perturbation in emotional availability introduced by the mother's reading a newspaper. Fifteen-month-olds explore less and are less playful in playroom situations when the mother is thus occupied as compared with times when the mother is not reading. As in the case for the Tronick work, individual difference assessments are not yet available. Most recently, however, the work of Zahn-Waxler, Cummings, McKnew, and Radke-Yarrow (1984) has indicated considerable promise in this area. Eighteen- and 20-month-olds of depressed and nondepressed mothers showed marked individual differences in their responses to mothers who were facially unresponsive for 2 minutes. The significance of different infant responses (degree of upset, apathy, engagement behaviors) remains to be clarified, but the possibility of a standardized assessment procedure emerging from more research seems likely.

## Nonobservational Methods for Assessing Emotional Availability

This chapter has reviewed a selected sample of observational procedures for assessing emotional availability, primarily between young children and their caregivers. Useful information about emotional availability may be derived through nonobservational methods of assessment as well. We have focused on the social nature of emotional availability (the relationship and interactions between 2 or more persons, primarily the child and parental caregiver). Important information regarding the caregiving or familial context of emotional availability or affect expressiveness may be obtained using interviews or questionnaires investigating parental attitudes, practices, and perceptions about emotional expression. As indicated earlier, interviews may alert the clinician to the possible existence of problems that may be observed in actual interactions; identification of infants or dyads at risk may be facilitated.

### *Questionnaires*

Data from questionnaires may provide an additional or complementary format for assessing the degree to which parents may demonstrate the propensity to be emotionally available to their children or, to use Stern's (1984) term, their affect attunement. The Differential Emotions Scale (Izard, 1972) can be used as a caregiver report instrument (Johnson *et al.*, 1982) that captures perceptions of their infant's emotional experience. The caregiver notes the frequency (on a 5-point scale) with which the child has experienced 30 feeling terms (representing a variety of discrete emotions, including fear, anger, happiness, interest, disgust, shame) during the course of the past week. Highly aberrant parental perceptions can then be identified.

### *Photographs*

Similar in some respects to assessment with questionnaires is the use of photographs depicting facial expressions of emotion that parents are asked to interpret (Emde *et al.*, 1978; and Emde, Izard, Huebner, Sorce, & Klinnert, in press). A standard series of photographs of infants with various facial expressions of emotion is presented to the adult, whose task it is to define the most clearly expressed emotion. The procedure is brief (approximately 10–15 minutes are needed for responses to 40 pictures) and uses a standard lexicon for categorizing parental responses and comparing them with a reference sample. The instrument is aimed at detecting variations in the perception of infants' facial expressions of emotion and has been useful in differentiating risk and nonrisk populations of mothers.

### *Emotion Lexicon*

A recent development in the domain of linguistic communication is research designed to assess the child's developmental acquisition of an emotion lexicon (Bretherton & Beeghly, 1982). Using a questionnaire format, parents record the occurrence of their child's use of words depicting emotions or emotion labels (e.g., happy, scared, love). Although the measure has been used to identify the normative development of the use of emotion terms, it may be possible to use these norms (and other developmental data) to identify whether children are on track in the acquisition of emotion labels. Thus, this procedure might serve as an early screening device from which further investigation may be deemed warranted (for example, if a child uses certain types of emotion terms such as shame, sad, or bad to the exclusion of others such as interest, pride, and joy). Unlike most of the paradigms reviewed, the linguistic nature of this procedure makes it especially appropriate toward the end of the second year and into the third year of life.

## IMPLICATIONS FOR YOUNG CHILDREN'S DEVELOPMENT

For the clinician and researcher interested in early identification of children at risk and the developmental sequelae of emotional availability (or emotional unavailability) during infancy, there is some promise in longitudinal research on the security of attachment. At later ages, securely attached infants are more sociable with unfamiliar adults and peers, more effective in problem-solving settings, demonstrate more empathic behavior, and are better able to regulate their affective behavior appropriately. For example, toddlers who were assessed as securely attached during infancy demonstrate the ability to inhibit frustration behavior and negative affect in a problem-solving setting. Similarly, preschoolers who, as infants, were securely attached to their mothers were rated by their teachers as more ego-resilient, which includes components of affective flexibility (neither over- nor undercontrolled) (e.g., George & Main, 1979; Main & Weston, 1981; Matas *et al.*, 1978; and Waters, Wippman, & Sroufe, 1979). It appears, then, that secure attachment—with the concomitant ability to regulate positive and negative affect appropriately—provides a foundation for future positive interpersonal relations. Those infants with rejecting, emotionally unavailable mothers (insecure/avoidant) most often manifest the poorest developmental outcome (particularly in interpersonal relations and affect regulation) (Sroufe & Fleeson, 1984). Typically, environmental and caregiving conditions that foster either secure or insecure attachment remain relatively stable, facilitating developmental continuity (Vaughn, Egeland, Sroufe, & Waters, 1979) and highlighting the need for early identification of children at risk.

Further evidence for the critical nature of emotional availability during childhood comes from a recent study in which insecurely attached infants had mothers who reported that their own mothers were emotionally unavailable to them during childhood (Main, Kaplan, & Cassidy, 1984). These findings are reminiscent of clinical reports and, in particular, of the powerful cross-generational patterns of child abuse and neglect (Steele & Pollock, 1974). They lead us once again to a central idea: Emotional availability and self-regulation are intimately related. What begins in the caregiving dyad becomes internalized and added to the affective self of the young child, influencing the range of experienced emotions and the capacity for empathy. Then, as self interacts with others, emotional availability and its variations are apt to be transmitted. Perhaps the most dramatic instance of such transmission is when child becomes parent and the patterns recur. In any case, research directed toward early screening for problems in emotional availability should now occupy a high priority for our time.

## REFERENCES

Ainsworth, M. D. S. (1985). *Sensitivity vs. insensitivity to the baby's communications.* Unpublished manuscript.

Ainsworth, M. D. S., Blehar, M., Waters, E., & Wall, S. (1978). *Patterns of attachment.* Hillsdale, NJ: Lawrence Erlbaum.

Ainsworth, M. D. S., & Wittig, B. (1969). Attachment and exploratory behavior of one-year-olds in a strange situation. In B. M. Foss (Ed.), *Determinants of infant behaviour* (Vol. 4, pp. 111–136). New York: Wiley.

Bayley, N. (1966). *Bayley Scales of Infant Development.* New York: Psychological Corp.

Bowlby, J. (1973). *Attachment and loss: Vol. 2. Separation, anxiety and anger.* New York: Basic Books.

Brazelton, T. B. (1973). *Neonatal behavioral assessment scale.* Philadelphia: J. B. Lippincott.

Bretherton, I., & Beeghly, M. (1982). Talking about internal states. The acquisition of an explicit theory of mind. *Developmental Psychology, 18,* 906–921.

Broussard, E. R., & Hartner, M. S. (1971). Further considerations regarding maternal perception of the first born. In J. Hellmuth (Ed.), *Exceptional infant: Studies in abnormalities* (Vol. 2). New York: Bruner/Mazel.

Campos, J. J., & Stenberg, C. (1981). Perception, appraisal and emotion: The onset of social referencing. In M. E. Lamb & L. R. Sherrod (Eds.), *Infant social cognition* (pp. 273–314). Hillsdale, NJ: Lawrence Erlbaum.

Cicchetti, D., & Sroufe, L. A. (1978). An organizational view of affect: Illustration from the study of Down's syndrome infants. In M. Lewis & L. Rosenblum (Eds.), *The development of affect.* New York: Plenum.

Clark, R., Musick, J., Stott, F., & Klehr, K. (1980). *The mother's project: Rating scales of mother–child interaction.* Unpublished manuscript.

Darwin, C. (1877). A biological sketch of an infant. *Mind, 2,* 285–294.

Durfee, J. T., Klein, R. P., Fivel, M. W., Bennett, C. A., Morgan, G. A., & Blehar, M. C. (1977). Infant social behavior manual. *JSAS Catalog of Selected Documents in Psychology, 7,* 38, MS 1467.

Easterbrooks, M. A., & Goldberg, W. A. (1984). Toddler development in the family: Impact of father involvement and parenting characteristics. *Child Development, 55,* 740–752.

Ekman, P. (Ed.). (1982). *Emotion in the human face* (2nd ed.). Cambridge: Cambridge Univ. Press.

Ekman, P., Friesen, W., & Ellsworth, P. (1972). *Emotion in the human face: Guidelines for research and an integration of findings.* New York: Pergamon Press.

Emde, R. N. (1980). Levels of meaning for infant emotions: A biosocial view. In W. A. Collins (Ed.), *Development of cognition, affect and social relations: Vol 13. Minnesota symposia on child psychology* (pp. 1-37). Hillsdale, NJ: Lawrence Erlbaum.

Emde, R. N. (1983). The prerepresentational self and its affective core. *The Psychoanalytic Study of the Child, 38*, 165-192.

Emde, R. N., & Brown, C. (1978). Adaption to the birth of a Down's Syndrome infant: Grieving and maternal attachment. *Journal of the American Academy of Child Psychiatry, 17*, 299-323.

Emde, R. N., Gaensbauer, T., & Harmon, R. J. (1976). Emotional expression in infancy: A biobehavioral study. *Psychological Issues, A Monograph Series, Inc., 10*(37). New York: International Universities Press.

Emde, R. N., Gaensbauer, T., & Harmon, R. J. (1982). Using our emotions: Principles for appraising emotional development and intervention. In M. Lewis & L. Taft (Eds.), *Developmental disabilities: Theory assessment and intervention*. New York: S. P. Medical and Scientific Books.

Emde, R. N., Harmon, R. J., & Good, W. V. (in press). Depressive feeling in children: A transactional model for research. In M. Rutter, C. Izard, & P. Read (Eds.), *Depression in childhood: Developmental perspectives*. New York: Guilford Press.

Emde, R. N., Izard, C., Huebner, R., Sorce, J., & Klinnert, M. D. (1985). Adult judgments of infant emotions: Replication studies within and across laboratories. *Infant Behavior & Development, 8*(1), 79-88.

Emde, R. N., Kligman, D. H., Reich, J. H., & Wade, T. (1978). Emotional expression in infancy: I. Initial studies of social signaling and an emergent model. In M. Lewis & L. Rosenblum (Eds.), *The development of affect*. New York: Plenum.

Feinman, S., & Lewis, M. (1981, April). *Social referencing and second order effects in ten-month-old infants*. Paper presented at the meeting of the Society for Research in Child Development, Boston, MA.

Gaensbauer, T. J., & Harmon, R. J. (1982). Attachment behavior in abused/neglected and premature infants: Implications for the concept of attachment. In R. N. Emde & R. J. Harmon (Eds.), *The development of attachment and affiliative systems* (pp. 263-279). New York: Plenum.

Gaensbauer, T. J., & Sands, K. (1980). Distorted affective communications in abused/neglected infants and their potential impact on caretakers. *Journal of the American Academy of Child Psychiatry, 18*, 236-250.

George, C., & Main, M. (1979). Social interactions of young abused children: Approach, avoidance, and aggression. *Child Development, 50*, 306-318.

Gray, J. D., Cutler, C. A., Dean, J. G., & Kempe, C. H. (1977). Prediction and prevention of child abuse and neglect. *Child Abuse & Neglect, 1*, 45-58.

Greenacre, P. (1971). *Emotional growth*. New York: International Universities Press.

Hamburg, D. A. (1963). Emotions in the perspective of human evolution. In P. H. Knapp (Ed.), *Expression of the emotion in man* (pp. 300-315). New York: International Universities Press.

Harmon, R. J., Suwalsky, J. D., & Klein, R. P. (1979). Infants' preferential response for mother versus an unfamiliar adult: Relationship to attachment. *Journal of the American Academy of Child Psychiatry, 18*(3), 437-449.

Hiatt, S., Campos, J., & Emde, R. N. (1979). Facial patterning and infant emotional expression: Happiness, surprise, fear. *Child Development, 50*(4), 1020-1035.

Izard, C. (1971). *The face of emotion*. New York: Meredith & Appleton-Century Crofts.

Izard, C. (1972). *Patterns of emotion. A new analysis of anxiety and depression*. New York: Academic Press.

Izard, C. (1982). Measuring emotions in human development. In C. Izard (Ed.), *Measuring emotions in infants and children*. New York: Cambridge Univ. Press.

Izard, C., Huebner, R., Risser, D., McGinnes, G. C., & Dougherty, L. (1980). The young infant's ability to produce discrete emotional expressions. *Developmental Psychology, 16*(2), 132–140.

Johnson, W. F., Emde, R. N., Pannabecker, B. J., Stenberg, C., & Davis, M. (1982). Maternal perception of infant emotion from birth through 18 months. *Infant Behavior and Development, 5*, 313–322.

Klinnert, M. D., Campos, J., Sorce, J., Emde, R. N., & Svejda, M. (1982). The development of social referencing in infancy. In R. Plutchik & H. Kellerman (Eds.), *Emotion in early development. Vol. 2 of Emotion: Theory, research and experience*. New York: Academic Press.

Klinnert, M. D., Sorce, J. F., Emde, R. N., Stenberg, C., & Gaensbauer, T. J. (1984). Continuities and change in early emotional life: Maternal perceptions of surprise, fear, and anger. In R. N. Emde & R. J. Harmon (Eds.), *Continuities and discontinuities in development*. New York: Plenum.

Lamb, M. E., & Easterbrooks, M. A. (1981). Individual differences in parental sensitivity: Origins, components, and consequences. In M. E. Lamb & L. R. Sherrod (Eds.), *Infant social cognition: Empirical and theoretical considerations*. Hillsdale, NJ: Lawrence Erlbaum.

Lewis, M., & Michalson, L. (1983). *Children's emotions and moods*. New York: Plenum.

Mahler, M. S., Pine, E., & Bergman, A. (1975). *The psychological birth of the human infant*. New York: Basic Books.

Main, M., Kaplan, N., & Cassidy, J. (1984). *Security in infancy, childhood, and adulthood: A move to the level of representation*. Unpublished manuscript.

Main, M., & Weston, R. (1981). The quality of the toddler's relationship to mother and father: Related to conflict behavior and the readiness to establish new relationships. *Child Development, 52*(3), 932–940.

Matas, L., Arend, R., & Sroufe, L. (1978). Continuity of adaptation in the second year: The relationship between quality of attachment and later competence. *Child Development, 49*, 547–556.

Myers, R. E. (1976, September). *Cortical localization of emotion control*. Invited lecture presented at the American Psychological Association, Washington.

Radbill, S. X. (1980). Children in a world of violence: A history of child abuse. In C. H. Kempe & R. E. Helfer (Eds.), *The battered child* (3rd ed.) (pp. 3–20). Chicago: The Univ. of Chicago Press.

Russell, J. A., & Ridgeway, D. (1983). Dimensions underlying children's emotional concepts. *Developmental Psychology, 19*(6), 795–804.

Sander, L. W. (1976). Issues in early mother–child interaction. In E. Rexford, L. Sander, & T. Shapiro (Eds.), *Infant psychiatry: A new synthesis* (pp. 127–147). New Haven: Yale Univ. Press.

Solyom, A. E. (1982). Affect development and its assessment in infancy. *Infant Mental Health Journal, 3*, 276–277.

Sorce, J. F., & Emde, R. N. (1982). The meaning of infant emotional expressions: Regularities in caregiving responses in normal and Down's syndrome infants. *Journal of Child Psychology and Psychiatry, 23*(2), 145–158.

Sorce, J. F., Emde, R. N., Campos, J., & Klinnert, M. D. (1985). Maternal emotional signaling—its effect on the visual cliff behavior of one-year-olds. *Developmental Psychology, 21*(1), 195–200.

Spitz, R. (1959). *A genetic field theory of ego formation*. New York: International Universities Press.

Sroufe, L. A., & Fleeson, J. (1984). *Attachment and the construction of relationships*. Unpublished manuscript.

Steele, B. F., & Pollock, C. B. (1974). A psychiatric study of parents who abuse infants and small children. In C. H. Kempe & R. E. Helfer (Eds.), *The battered child* (2nd ed.). Chicago: Univ. of Chicago Press.

Stenberg, C. (1982). *The development of anger expressions in infancy*. Unpublished doctoral dissertation, University of Denver.

Stenberg, C., Campos, J., & Emde, R. N. (1983). The facial expression of anger in seven-month-old infants. *Child Development, 54*, 178–184.

Stern, D. M. (1984). Affect attunement. In J. Call, E. Galenson, & R. Tyson (Eds.), *Frontiers of infant psychiatry, Vol. II*. New York: Basic Books.

Thomas, A., & Chess, S. (1977). *Temperament and development*. New York: Bruner/Mazel.

Tomkins, S. S. (1962–1963). *Affect, imagery, consciousness* (Vols. 1–2). New York: Springer.

Tronick, E., Als, H., Adamson, L., Wise, S., & Brazelton, T. B. (1978). The infant's response to entrapment between contradictory messages in face-to-face interaction. *Journal of the American Academy of Child Psychiatry, 17*, 1–13.

Vaughn, B., Egeland, B., Sroufe, L. A., & Waters, E. (1979). Individual differences in infant–mother attachment at twelve and eighteen months. Stability and change in families under stress. *Child Development, 50*, 971–975.

Waters, E., & Deane, E. K. (in press). Defining and assessing individual differences in infant attachment relationships: Q-methodology and the organization of behavior. In I. Bretherton & E. Waters (Eds.), *Growing points in attachment theory and research. Monographs of the Society for Research in Child Development.*

Waters, E., Wippman, J., & Sroufe, L. A. (1979). Attachment, positive affect, and competence in the peer group: Two studies in construct validation. *Child Development, 50*(3), 821–829.

Zahn-Waxler, C., Cummings, E. M., McKnew, D. H., & Radke-Yarrow, M. (1984). Altruism, aggression and social interactions in young children with a manic-depressive parent. *Child Development, 55*, 112–122.

Zahn-Waxler, C., & Radke-Yarrow, M. (1982). The development of altruism: Alternative research strategies. In N. Eisenberg (Ed.), *The development of prosocial behavior*. New York: Academic Press.

CHAPTER 6

# Dyadic Interchanges in Families with At-Risk Children

## AN INDIVIDUAL DIFFERENCE APPROACH

*Jeanne Brooks-Gunn*

The study of between-group differences has a long history. In the search for explanations of behavioral differences, the emphasis has been on aggregates rather than on individuals. The focus has been on what is special about one group as compared to another, rather than on change and continuity over time within groups. Typically, the groups differ in that one represents a normative and the other a nonnormative condition. The nonnormative condition is usually one that may be characterized as "different" and/or "deficient" vis-à-vis the comparison group.

## THE STUDY OF SPECIAL POPULATIONS

The study of at-risk young children and their families is illustrative. Because *specialness* typically connotes different or deviant, underlying developmental processes and continuities may not be explored. Much dyadic research with delayed infants is driven by a deficit model. An exception involves the transactional model (Sameroff & Chandler, 1975), which has been eagerly accepted by most developmentalists. Surprisingly, however, little research has directly tested this model, especially for children with biological risk indicators.

***Jeanne Brooks-Gunn*** • Institute for the Study of Exceptional Children, Educational Testing Service, Rosedale Road, Princeton, New Jersey 08541. The research reported in this chapter was supported by a grant from the Bureau of Education of the Handicapped (now Office of Special Education, U.S. Department of Education).

In this chapter, the effects of using between-group difference approaches to the approach are discussed and alternatives presented. Parent and child characteristics that may contribute to interaction patterns in risk dyads are discussed, with emphasis on what may be special about such characteristics. Examples from research involving 143 handicapped young children and their mothers are presented. The children ranged in age from 3 to 26 months of age and had Down's syndrome, cerebral palsy, developmental delay, or multiple handicaps. Mothers and children were observed in a free-play setting for 15 minutes; the observational system is described in Brooks-Gunn & Lewis (1982a, 1984).

## The Meaning of Between-Group Differences

When a difference is found between groups, it is linked to what is thought to be the most salient difference between the groups. In this way, the difference rapidly becomes imbued with meaning. Knowing that two groups differ, however, does not allow us to assume that these differences are due to the specific attributes of one or the other group (Lewis & Brooks-Gunn, 1982a; Brooks-Gunn & Lewis, 1983). At least one or the other group must be assessed before this claim has any validity. If a third group is chosen carefully, on the basis of the possession of certain attributes that may have resulted in the original difference, then at least some possible explanations for that original difference may be tested. For example, when maternal responsivity as a proportion of total maternal behavior is examined, mothers of normal infants are found to be more responsive than mothers of handicapped children (Brooks-Gunn & Lewis, 1984). However, whether this is due to being handicapped *per se* or to some more specific attribute of handicapped infants is not known. Mothers of normal infants differ from mothers of infants with Down's syndrome, but not from mothers of developmentally delayed infants, which suggests that developmental maturation plays a role.

An often overlooked problem with normal-handicapped comparisons has to do with the ages chosen to study. Research on age changes is rare in the handicapped infant literature. Knowing that infants or mothers differ at a specific age point provides a static snapshot that may or may not reflect the process of growth during the first 3 years of life. To circumvent this criticism, researchers have chosen their target ages based on normal infancy research. In addition, those researchers who discuss critical age periods often discuss them vis-à-vis major cognitive, linguistic, or symbolic reorganizations, or at the very least vis-à-vis spurts in growth (Bee, Bernard, Eyres, Gray, Hammond, Spietz, Synder, & Clark, 1982; Ramey & Haskins, 1981; Wachs & Gruen, 1982).

Given the facts that the majority of handicapped infants are delayed in many skills and that the interindividual variability within such samples is large, concentration on chronological age markers may be misleading.

Concentration on one age point obscures rate changes, catch-up effects, or diverging capacities in between-group comparisons. For example, maternal smiles that are responses to an infant behavior (as a proportion of all maternal smiles) increased in our normal and handicapped samples with age, being similar at 3 months of age, but diverging at 12 and 24 months of age. This divergence was due to the steeper increase in the proportion of responsive smiles mothers of normal infants receive between 3 and 12 months; this is an example of a rate difference (Brooks-Gunn & Lewis, 1982a).

## Alternatives to the Study of Between-Group Differences

### *Differences among Handicapped Groups*

An obvious alternative to normal-handicapped comparison research is to explore differences among handicapped groups rather than to compare children in these groups with groups of normal children. An even more finely tuned approach might involve comparing infants with a similar diagnostic classification who differ with respect to some specific competency. For example, cerebral palsied infants with intact informational processing skills and those with delays might be compared. Zelazo (1979) and Kearsley (1979) adopted such an approach with developmentally delayed infants, finding that those with intact attentional abilities responded to an intervention program more favorably than infants with attentional deficits. Even groups considered to be relatively homogeneous, at least from an etiologic viewpoint, are quite heterogeneous with respect to cognitive and social skills. Thus, infants with Down's syndrome can be divided into different subgroups on the basis of general intellectual functioning, linguistic ability, or degree of motor impairment.

### *Change and Continuity*

Another approach is to conduct longitudinal studies of change and continuity within samples of at-risk infants. Short-term follow-ups may be conducted in order to examine how early deficits may lead to certain interaction patterns and how interaction patterns are altered by a child's status (growth and/or delay). Not only may child status be changed by the environment, but environmental stimulation or deprivation may alter child behavioral characteristics that are possibly related to biological structures. An example is the research on the interaction of nutrition and environmental stimulation and their effect on brain functioning (Winick, Meyer, & Harris, 1975; Winick & Morgan, 1980). Prospective studies do not exist from early to later childhood in handicapped samples. Even short-term longitudinal studies are scarce, except those linked to intervention (Karnes, Schwedel, Lewis, Ratts, & Esray, 1981; Ludlow & Allen, 1979; Moore, Fredericks, & Baldwin, 1981; Piper & Pless, 1980). Even in these studies, data on environment-child outcome links are not provided over and above the treatment dimension.

## CONTINUUM OF DELAY OR SPECIFIC DYSFUNCTION

One of the most intriguing problems in the field, and one that has special relevance for interaction research, is whether to attribute a between-group difference to specific dysfunctions or characteristics of one group as opposed to another, or whether to attribute the difference to general retardation in the acquisition of abilities. Do differences reflect delays in an underlying process, or different processes? Whereas both explanations imply that handicapped children (and/or risk dyads) are different, they would be characterized as unique in the former but not unique in the latter. Both might describe the child as deficient, however.

The strong form of the special characteristics explanation states that parents are unable to interpret their handicapped children's signals, which in normal infants are easily seen and understood. This is in direct contradistinction to the argument that signals are delayed, and therefore unreadable because they are not present or are less sophisticated or differentiated than the parent expects (based on the progression of most normal infants). In addition, it is implied—through reference to the transactional model—that these effects are cumulative, and that interactions in the first few months set the stage for subsequent ones. Parents are seen as unable to adjust to their child's special characteristics; or, if they try to adjust, they are seen as overresponding. Thus, there is an interesting shift from the child's unreadable signals (special characteristics) to the parent's inability to adjust to these unique signals, which emphasizes their special characteristics. This research, although building on the early work of Stern (1974) and others who emphasize interchanges in terms of turn-taking and fine tuning, suggests not only that mutuality is disrupted (Thoman, 1980) but that parents are unable to respond effectively without direct intervention. The lack of longitudinal interaction research, information on the continuity of maternal interaction pattern over time, and studies of interventions centered on altering instructions make it difficult to evaluate these hypotheses.

## Research on Cognitive Delay versus Dysfunction

Several approaches to studying the delay versus dysfunction issue have been developed. First, the relative contribution of mental age (or some proxy) and chronological age on aspects of maternal behavior within samples may be examined. This technique especially favors handicapped samples, because mental and chronological age are not tightly linked and because great variability in mental age functioning exists in handicapped infants. In our large cross-sectional sample of handicapped infants ranging from 3 to 36 months of age, responsivity was found to increase with both. Partial correlational analyses indicated that the relationship between responsivity and chronological age disappeared when controlling for mental age. In contrast, when controlling for chronological age, responsivity and mental age were still significantly and positively related (Brooks-Gunn & Lewis, 1984).

Second, several investigators have defined development in terms of specific abilities (in particular sensorimotor functioning or linguistic competence), matching groups with respect to a particular competency. For example, Dunst (1980) divided mentally retarded and normal infants into those functioning at Uzgiris and Hunt's (1975) sensorimotor Stage IV and those at Stage V. Mothers of Stage V infants were more responsive than those with Stage IV infants. Matching of infants with Down's syndrome with a normal sample on chronological age and mean length of utterance, Leifer and Lewis (1983) found that maternal vocalization patterns were related to the child's linguistic ability, rather than to chronological age (see also Rondal, 1978; Vietze, Abernathy, Ashe, & Faulstich, 1977). Buckhalt, Rutherford, and Goldberg (1979) report a similar finding for complexity of maternal language. Mothers of normal infants have been shown to adjust their speech to reflect their child's linguistic competence (Moerk, 1974; Shatz & Gleitman, 1973; Snow, 1972).

## Research on Special Characteristics

Whether or not handicapped infants have special characteristics rather than general delays has been studied with regard to social and emotional competencies. A necessary assumption of this research is that affective and cognitive systems are not perfectly related; how tightly emotion and cognition are linked is a major (and as yet unanswered) issue in the normal infancy literature (Emde, Katz, & Thorpe, 1978; Izard, 1977; Kagan, Kearsley, & Zelazo, 1978; Lewis & Michalson, 1983). However, the strength of the possible links has not been studied as systematically in handicapped samples (Cicchetti & Sroufe, 1978; Emde &

Brown, 1978). Given this limitation, the literature points to some possible special handicapped characteristics, or at the very least, delays that are not totally accounted for by cognitive delays. Four examples will be mentioned.

### *Smiling*

Handicapped infants have been found to smile less and to smile later than normal infants (Emde, Katz, & Thorpe, 1978; Gallagher, 1979). These differences are not totally accounted for by developmental age (Brooks-Gunn & Lewis, 1982a). In addition, handicapped group differences have been reported; in our work, infants with Down's syndrome smiled less than physically impaired and developmentally delayed infants, even when controlling for mental age (Brooks-Gunn & Lewis, 1982a). This counters the stereotype of the Down's syndrome infant as typically exhibiting high positive affect (Baron, 1972).

In addition, the actual quality of the handicapped infant's smile may be different in terms of intensity, type of stimulation needed to elicit it, latency of onset, and its configuration. Whereas the first two dimensions have been studied in infants with handicaps, (Cicchetti & Sroufe, 1976), others have not, although several investigations are underway.

Given these possible special characteristics of the smiles of infants with handicaps, it comes as no surprise that maternal affective responses are reported to be dampened. Not only do handicapped infants smile less frequently in free-play settings than normal infants from 12 months on (even when taking mental age into account), but so do their mothers, whose responses are also dampened from the time their children are 12 months of age (Brooks-Gunn & Lewis, 1982a). (Also see suggested lowering of threshold of response by mothers of Down's syndrome infants in Sorce, Emde, & Frank, 1981.) In addition, after 3 months of age, mothers of handicapped infants are less likely to respond to any infant behavior with a smile than are mothers of normal infants; and at 24 months of age, the mothers are less likely to respond to an infant smile, even after taking mental age into account.

### *Irritability*

Irritability, as reflected in fretting, crying, and fussing, also has been hypothesized to be characteristic of handicapped infants. Again, little systematic work on the intensity and frequency of crying behavior has been conducted in risk samples (an exception is Thoman, 1980). Maternal responsivity to distress is of particular interest, because being more responsive to a young normal infant's cries has been shown to be related to a decrease in crying by the end of the first year (Bell & Ainsworth, 1972), because the infant's cry seems to hold great signal value for the mother (Lewis, 1972; Yarrow, Rubenstein, & Pedersen, 1975) and because mothers differentiate among their infant's cries in the first months of life (Wolff, 1969). In our study, maternal responsivity to fretting decreased dramatically as the child grew older in all samples (Brooks-Gunn & Lewis, 1982a). Mothers of handicapped infants were more responsive to this behavior than mothers of normal infants in the first few months of life, but not thereafter. If handicapped infants continue to be irritable, responsivity may become attenuated, as mothers believe the behavior to be inappropriate or have discovered that their attempts to alter it are not successful (see Moss, 1967, for a similar argument as it relates to the greater irritability of male than female infants).

Finally, the acoustic features of the handicapped infant's cry may be unique, as has been found for biologically at-risk newborns (Zeskind & Lester, 1978). These qualitative differences may result in adults and parents both perceiving the at-risk child's cues quite differently (Frodi & Lamb, 1980; Zeskind & Lester, 1978).

### *Physical Care and Feeding*

Another special characteristic that may influence subsequent interaction involves the extra and sometimes specialized physical care that the handicapped infant requires. Although little systematic information is available, mothers of handicapped infants list physical care demands as a problem, and the number of care demands relate to the amount of stress reported by mothers (Bell, 1980). Feeding problems, one of the physical problems often noted, have been studied vis-à-vis maternal reactions in premature infants, whose mothers sometimes have to work harder than mothers of normal infants to get their babies to feed (Beckwith & Cohen, 1980; Field, 1980; Bakeman & Brown, 1980).

### *Temperament*

The last example of a possible special characteristic of handicapped infants to be discussed is temperament. In general, variability in temperament is similar across infants and young children who are normal, or who have Down's syndrome, physical impairment, or rubella (Baron, 1972; Bridges & Cicchetti, 1982; Chess & Korn, 1970a, 1970b; Thomas & Chess, 1977). However, handicapped infants are more likely to have a low threshold for stimulation than normal infants (Baron, 1972; Bridges & Cicchetti, 1982; Brooks-Gunn & Lewis, 1982b).

Across handicapped infants, those with Down's syndrome have been rated by their mothers as more positive in mood, less active, and having a lower threshold than developmentally delayed or physically impaired infants (Brooks-Gunn & Lewis, 1982b). It is interesting that Down's syndrome infants were rated as more positive in mood even though they smiled less overall in our free-play setting. This raises issues of across-situation generalizability, information-processing biases on the part of mothers, and the meaning that mothers attach to certain behaviors, such as smiles.

Of interest from an individual difference approach is how temperament characteristics influence maternal interactions within a sample of handicapped. Mothers of difficult infants did not exhibit less positive affect than those with easy infants, nor were they less responsive. Thus, our mothers do not find the infants so difficult that they altered affective or responsive exchanges.[1] Another approach to the question of difficulty is to pinpoint the behaviors that do diminish responsivity, such as in research on premature cries (Frodi & Lamb, 1980). Examining our data in this way, we found that maternal language interaction was attenuated when infants were distractible, not persistent, very active, and intense (even when controlling for mental age differences); maternal affective interaction was not affected by these temperament characteristics.

## SUMMARY

Research on the at-risk dyad has implicitly relied on a deficit model, even while espousing a more interactive approach. In this chapter, several approaches were suggested to remedy this incongruence. First, when using between-group approaches, more than two groups of at-risk infants may be studied in order to generate partial explanations for observed differences between dyads. Second, more consideration may be given to within-group designs. Either children from a number of diagnostic categories or children with different competencies within diagnostic categories may be studied. Third, developmental change in interaction patterns, both cross-sectionally and longitudinally, may be explored.

With regard to interaction research, research needs to focus on the issue of general retardation or cognitive delay versus different abilities.

[1]Classification of an infant as difficult is based on the system described by Carey (1970). Five of the nine temperament categories are used: "irregular," "low in adaptability, "initial withdrawal," "intense," and "predominantly negative mood." Temperamentally difficult infants were not less likely to smile in the free-play setting than were temperamentally easy children. That a relationship was found between maternal affect and infant smiling while no corresponding relationship was found for difficult temperament suggests that maternal affect may be related to very specific infant characteristics (Carey, 1972).

It is clear that general mental functioning of the handicapped child does affect maternal responsivity, just as does the child's level of language, at least in handicapped infants. At the same time, infants' affective expression, which is not totally accounted for by the mental age of the child, also affects mothers' interaction styles. Thus, both mental delays and specific child characteristics may contribute to the mother's interaction patterns.

## ACKNOWLEDGMENTS

Special thanks go to Lorraine Luciano, Alice Kass, Rosemary Deibler, Richard Brinker, and Michael Lewis.

## REFERENCES

Bakeman, R., & Brown, J. (1980). Early intervention: Consequence for social and mental development at three years. *Child Development, 51,* 437–447.

Baron, J. (1972). Temperament profile of children with Down's Syndrome. *Development and Child Neurology, 14,* 640–643.

Beckwith, L., & Cohen, S. (1980). Interactions of preterm infants with their caregivers and test performance at age 2. In T. Field, S. Goldberg, D. Stern, & A. Sostek (Eds.), *High-risk infant and children: Adult and peer interactions.* New York: Academic Press.

Bee, H. L., Barnard, K. E., Eyres, S. J., Gray, C. A., Hammond, M. A., Spietz, A. L., Snyder, C., & Clark, B. (1982). Prediction of IQ and language skill from perinatal status, child performance, family characteristics,and mother-infant interaction. *Child Development, 53*(5), 1134–1156.

Bell, P. B. (1980). *Characteristics of handicapped infants: A study of the relationship between child characteristics and stress as reported by mothers.* Unpublished doctoral dissertation, University of North Carolina at Chapel Hill.

Bell, S., & Ainsworth, M. (1972). Infant crying and maternal responsiveness. *Child Development, 43,* 1171–1190.

Bridges, F. A., & Cicchetti, D. (1982). Mothers' ratings of the temperament characteristics of Downs syndrome infants. *Developmental Psychology, 18*(2), 238–244.

Brooks-Gunn, J., & Lewis, M. (1982a). Affective exchanges between normal and handicapped infants and their mothers. In T. Field & A. Fogel (Eds.), *Emotion and interaction: Normal and high-risk infants.* Hillsdale, NJ: Earlbaum.

Brooks-Gunn, J., & Lewis, M. (1982b). Temperament and affective interaction in handicapped infants. *Journal of the Division of Early Childhood, 5,* 31–41.

Brooks-Gunn, J., & Lewis, M. (1983). Screening and diagnosing handicapped infants. *Topics in Early Childhood Special Education, 3*(1), 14–28.

Brooks-Gunn, J., & Lewis, M. (1984). Maternal responsivity in interactions with handicapped infants. *Child Development, 55*(3), 782–793.

Buckhalt, J. A., Rutherford, R. B., & Goldberg, K. E. (1978). Verbal and nonverbal interaction of mothers with their Down's syndrome and nonretarded infants. *American Journal of Mental Deficiency, 82*(4), 337–343.

Carey, W. B. (1970). A simplified method for measuring infant temperament. *Journal of Pediatrics, 77,* 188–194.

Carey, W. B. (1972). Measuring infant temperament. *Journal of Pediatrics, 81*(4), 823–828.

Chess, S., & Korn, S. (1970a). The influence of temperament of education of mentally retarded children. *Journal of Special Education, 4*(1), 13–27.

Chess, S., & Korn, S. (1970b). Temperament and behavior disorders in mentally retarded children. *Archives of General Psychiatry, 23,* 122–130.

Cicchetti, D., & Sroufe, L. A. (1976). The relationship between affective and cognitive development in Down's syndrome infants. *Child Development, 47,* 920–929.

Cicchetti, D., & Sroufe, L. A. (1978). An organization view of affect: Illustration from the study of Down's syndrome infants. In M. Lewis & L. Rosenblum (Eds.), *The development of affect.* New York: Plenum.

Dunst, C. (1980, April). *Developmental characteristics of communicative acts among Down's syndrome infants and nonretarded infants.* Paper presented at the biennial meeting of the Southeastern Conference on Human Development, Alexandria, Virginia.

Emde, R. N., & Brown, C. (1978). Adaptation to the birth of a Down's syndrome infant: Grieving and maternal attachment. *Journal of American Academy Child Psychiatry, 17,* 299–323.

Emde, R., Katz, E. L., & Thorpe, J. K. (1978). Emotional expression in infancy: Early deviations in Down's syndrome. In M. Lewis & L. Rosenblum (Eds.), *The development of affect: Genesis of behavior* (Vol. 1). New York: Plenum.

Field, T. (1980). Supplemental stimulation of preterm neonates. *Early Human Development, 4,* 301–314.

Frodi, A., & Lamb, M. (1980). Child abusers' responses to infant smiles and cries. *Child Development, 51*(1), 238–241.

Gallagher, R. (1979). *Positive affect in multiply handicapped infants: Its relationship to developmental age, temperament, physical status, and setting.* Unpublished doctoral dissertation, University of North Carolina at Chapel Hill.

Izard, C. E. (1977). *Human emotions.* New York: Plenum.

Kagan, J., Kearsley, R., & Zelazo, P. (1978). *Infancy: Its place in human development.* Cambridge: Harvard Univ. Press.

Karnes, M., Schwedel, A., Lewis, G., Ratts, D., & Esray, D. (1981). Impact of early programming for the handicapped: A follow-up study into the elementary school. *Journal of the Division for Early Childhood, 4,* 62–79.

Kearsley, R. B. (1979). Iatrogenic retardation: A syndrome of learned incompetence. In R. Kearsley & I. Sigel (Eds.), *Infants at risk: Assessment of cognitive functioning.* New York: Wiley.

Leifer, J., & Lewis, M. (1983). Maternal speech to normal and handicapped children: A look at question-asking behavior. *Infant Behavior and Development, 6*(2), 175–187.

Lewis, M. (1972). State as an infant-environment interaction: An analysis of mother-infant interaction as a function of sex. *Merrill-Palmer Quarterly, 18,* 95–121.

Lewis, M., & Brooks-Gunn, J. (1982). Developmental models and assessment issues. In N. Anastasiow, W. Frankenburg, & A. Fandal (Eds.), *Identifying the developmentally delayed child.* Maryland: University Park Press.

Lewis, M., & Michalson, L. (1983). *Children's emotions and moods: Development, theory, and measurement.* New York: Plenum.

Ludlow, J., & Allen, L. (1979). The effect of early intervention and preschool stimulus on the development of the Down's syndrome child. *Journal of Mental Deficiency Research, 23,* 29–44.

Moerk, E. (1974). Changes in verbal mother–child interaction with increasing language skills of the child. *Journal of Psycholinguistic Research, 3,* 101–116.

Moore, M., Fredericks, H., & Baldwin, V. (1981). The long-range effects of early childhood education on a trainable mentally retarded population. *Journal of the Division for Early Childhood, 4,* 92–110.

Moss, H. (1967). Sex, age, and state as determinants of mother–infant interaction. *Merrill-Palmer Quarterly, 13,* 19–36.

Piper, M., & Pless, I. (1980). Early intervention for infants with Down's syndrome: A controlled trial. *Pediatrics, 65,* 463–468.

Ramey, C. T., & Haskins, R. (1981). The causes and treatment of school failure: Insights from the Carolina Abecedarian Project. In M. Begab, H. Garber, & H. C. Haywood (Eds.), *Causes and prevention of retarded development in psychosocially disadvantaged children*. Baltimore: University Park Press.

Rondal, J. (1978). Maternal speech to Down's syndrome and normal children matched for mean-length of utterance. In E. Myers (Ed.), *Quality of life in severely and profoundly retarded people: Research foundations for improvement*. Washington, DC: American Association on Mental Deficiency.

Sameroff, A. J., & Chandler, M. J. (1975). Reproductive risk and the continuum of caretaking casualty. In F. D. Horowitz, M. Hetherington, S. Scarr-Salapatek, & G. Siegel (Eds.), *Review of child development research* (Vol. 4). Chicago, IL: Univ. of Chicago Press.

Shatz, M., & Gleitman, R. (1973). The development of communication skills: Modifications in speech of young children as a function of the listener. *Monographs of the Society for Research in Child Development, 38*(5, Serial No. 152).

Snow, C. (1972). Mother's speech to children learning language. *Child Development, 43*, 549–565.

Sorce, J. F., Emde, R. N., & Frank, M. (1981). Maternal referencing in normal and Down's syndrome infants: A longitudinal analysis. In R. N. Emde & R. Harmon (Eds.), *The development of attachment and affiliative systems* (pp. 281–292). New York: Plenum.

Stern, D. (1974). Mother and infant at play: The dyadic interaction involving facial, vocal, and gaze behaviors. In M. Lewis & L. Rosenblum (Eds.), *The effect of the infant on its caregiver: The origins of behavior* (Vol. 1). New York: Wiley.

Thoman, E. B. (1980). Disruption and asynchrony in early parent–infant interaction. In D. B. Sawin, R. C. Hawkins, L. O. Walker, & J. H. Penticuff (Eds.), *Exceptional infant: Psychosocial risks in infant–environment transactions* (Vol. 4). New York: Brunner/Mazel.

Thomas, A., & Chess, S. (1977). *Temperament and development*. New York: Brunner/Mazel.

Uzgiris, I. C., & Hunt, J. (1975). *Assessment in infancy: Ordinal scales of psychological development*. Urbana, IL: Univ. of Illinois Press.

Vietze, P., Abernathy, S., Ashe, M., & Faulstich, G. (1977). Contingent interaction between mothers and their developmentally delayed infants. In G. Sackett (Ed.), *Observing behavior: Theory and application in mental retardation* (Vol. 1). Baltimore: University Park Press.

Wachs, T. D., & Gruen, G. E. (1982). *Early experience in human development*. New York: Plenum.

Winick, M., & Morgan, B. (1980). Effects of administration of N-Aceylnew-raminic acid (NANA) on brain NANA content and behavior. *Journal of Nutrition, 110*(3), 416–424.

Winick, M., Meyer, K. K., & Harris, R. C. (1975). Malnutrition and environmental enrichment by early adoption. *Science, 190*, 1173–1175.

Wolff, P. H. (1969). The natural history of crying and other vocalizations in early infancy. In B. M. Foss (Ed.), *Determinants of infant behavior* (Vol. 4). London: Metheun.

Yarrow, L. J., Rubenstein, J. L., & Pedersen, F. A. (1975). *Infant and environment: Early cognitive and motivational development*. New York: Wiley.

Zelazo, P. R. (1979). Reactivity to perceptual-cognitive events: Application for infant assessment. In R. Kearsley & I. Sigel (Eds.), *Infants at risk: Assessment of cognitive functioning*. New York: Wiley.

Zeskind, P. S., & Lester, B. M. (1978). Acoustic features and auditory perceptions of the cries of newborns with prenatal and perinatal complications. *Child Development, 49*, 580–589.

PART III

# New and Updated Approaches to Screening

CHAPTER 7

# Prediction of School and Behavior Problems in Children Followed from Birth to Age Eight

*Sandra K. Mitchell, Helen L. Bee, Mary A. Hammond, and Kathryn E. Barnard*

For a number of years in the late 1960s and early 1970s there was astonishing agreement among those interested in child welfare that the best way to serve children's interests was through the early detection of learning and behavior problems. This belief was due in part to the outcomes of two major longitudinal studies—the Kauai study (Werner, Bierman, & French, 1971; Werner & Smith, 1977) and the National Collaborative Perinatal Study (Broman, Nichols, & Kennedy, 1975). Both of these had demonstrated that perinatal status variables had significant, although modest, relationships with later cognitive and motor development (Smith, Flick, Ferris, & Sellman, 1972; Werner *et al.*, 1971). Moreover, it appeared that the effects of these perinatal status variables were mediated by the quality of the environment in which the child was raised.

At about the same time, other investigators were directly studying these environmental variables. For example, Yarrow and his colleagues (Yarrow, Rubenstein, Pedersen, & Jankowski, 1972) showed that the variety and amount of animate and inanimate stimulation provided in the home were important predictors of the child's cognitive development.

***Sandra K. Mitchell, Helen L. Bee, Mary A. Hammond, and Kathryn E. Barnard*** • School of Nursing and Child Development and Mental Retardation Center, University of Washington, Seattle, Washington 98195. The research reported here was supported by the Division of Nursing, Department of Health & Human Services, Contract No. 1-NU-14174 and Grants NU-00559 and NU-00816.

Other research pointed to the importance of the contingent nature of stimulation (Lewis & Goldberg, 1969), the style of parent–child communication (Bee, Van Egeren, Streissguth, Nyman, & Leckie, 1969; Hess & Shipman, 1967), the mother's perception of whether her baby was better or worse than the average baby (Broussard & Hartner, 1970), and the overall level of life change and stress in the family (Wyler, Masuda, & Holmes, 1971).

Although several programs of early screening and detection were undertaken about this time, it soon became clear that two kinds of research would be needed to establish a strong scientific base for the undertaking. First, there was a need for practical ways of assessing the infant and relevant aspects of the environment. Second, prospective, longitudinal studies were needed to validate the predictive usefulness of these assessments.

The methods chosen for these endeavors were generally those of traditional developmental psychology: Fairly large samples of families were selected, repeatedly assessed, and then followed longitudinally until the child was old enough for reliable measures of developmental progress to be made. Although the original question asked which children would show poor outcomes, the data analyses of most of these studies reflected the extent to which the *whole range* of outcomes (good as well as bad) could be predicted from early assessments. In the present report, categorical outcomes (problem vs. no problem) have been chosen instead of continuous variables (like school acheivement scores), and the analyses reflect the extent to which a child's status in second grade can be predicted (albeit in retrospect) from data collected earlier in life.

## METHOD

The longitudinal study to be discussed here has been described in detail elsewhere (Barnard & Douglas, 1974; Barnard & Eyres, 1979; Bee, Barnard, Eyres, Gray, Hammond, Spietz, Snyder, & Clark, 1982), so only a brief explanation of the procedures up to age 4 will be provided here.

### Subjects

The subjects in the study were 193 primiparous mothers and their infants, selected from among births during 1973 and 1974 at a large health maintenance organization hospital in Seattle, Washington. The sample was largely well-educated and economically well off: Most parents had some college education, and the median family income was between $11,000 and $12,000 (in 1973 dollars). Consequently, analyses of data from these subjects is an attempt to see what would have predicted developmental problems in a basically low-risk group of families.

## Earlier Data-Collection Procedures

Mothers were first interviewed during the eighth prenatal month, and then again when the child was 1, 4, 8, 12, 24, 36, and 48 months of age. Mother–infant interaction was observed at 4, 8, 12, 24, 36, and 48 months, and the children were tested or assessed extensively at birth and at 12, 24, 36, and 48 months. A home visit was completed at each point after birth except 24 months, when all testing and interviewing was done in the laboratory. Data collected at 1 and 8 months are not included with the present analysis. For the purposes of analyses, the assessments have been grouped into four clusters.

### *Perinatal and Infant Status*

These measures included the Dubowitz estimate of gestational age (Dubowitz, Dubowitz, & Goldberg, 1970); Apgar score at 1 and 5 minutes; weight, length, and head circumference at birth; and sex. Minor congenital anomalies (Smith, 1970; Waldrop, Pedersen, & Bell, 1968) were assessed by the home visitor at 4 and 8 months of age, and the Brazelton Neonatal Behavioral Assessment Scale (Brazelton, 1973) was used on the second post-partum day, yielding seven cluster scores (Lester, 1978). In addition, mothers reported on the children's sleep–wake patterns during the first year in a series of 1-week diaries, collected at 1, 4, 8, and 12 months. Finally, a summary perinatal risk score was constructed by counting the total number of individual prenatal, perinatal, and postnatal complications observed in the mother and infant (out of a list of 36).

### *Child Outcomes*

Measures of mental development included the Bayley Scales of Infant Development (Bayley, 1969) at 12 and 24 months, and the Stanford-Binet Intelligence Scale (Terman & Merrill, 1973) at 48 months. Motor development was measured with the Bayley, the Denver Developmental Screening Test (Frankenburg & Dodds, 1967) at 36 months, and the motor section of the McCarthy Scales of Children's Abilities (McCarthy, 1972) at 48 months. Receptive and expressive language skills were assessed using the Sequenced Inventory of Communication Development

(Hedrick, Prather, & Tobin, 1975) at 12 and 36 months. At 24 months, 10 items from the Bayley scales that assess aspects of language skill were used to generate language scores, and at 48 months the Fluharty Speech and Language Screening Test (Fluharty, 1974) was used.

The measure of social and emotional development in this cluster was the Preschool Behavior Questionaire (Behar & Stringfield, 1974), which was completed at 36 and 48 months by the mother. Mothers also reported the illnesses and accidents experienced by their child at yearly intervals.

### *Family Ecology and Parent Perceptions*

Along with standard demographic variables, mothers completed the Schedule of Recent Events (Holmes & Rahe, 1967) at most interviews and the Neonatal Perception Inventory (Broussard & Hartner, 1970) at 2 days and at 1 month. Information from the prenatal interview was used to construct an index of the mother's "developmental expectations" (Snyder, Eyres, & Barnard, 1979) and an index of social support.

To this cluster were added certain variables obtained in the 8-year-old interview that reflected life circumstances during the child's earlier life. These included years spent with only one parent, years spent with one parent full time at home, number of partnerships by the parent, number of different child care arrangements experienced by the child, and the Hollingshead Four-Factor Index of Social Status (Hollingshead, 1975).

### *Family Environment and Parent–Child Interaction*

This final cluster includes measures of both family environment and of special interaction patterns. The Home Observation for Measurement of the Environment (HOME) Inventory (Caldwell & Bradley, 1978) was administered at 4, 8, 12, 24, 36, and 48 months. Scores of the HOME can be taken as reflective of a variety of family environmental characteristics. Each mother–infant pair was observed in two different tasks, feeding (at 1, 4, 8, and 12 months) and teaching (at every contact point). These interactions were scored by a project staff member on a series of rating scales, and the scales were then combined to yield two summary scores, one for the parent and one for the child.

## Data Collection at Age Eight

Assessment of the families and children occurred during the middle third of second grade. Most children were tested at a university laboratory in a session that lasted about 2 hours and included a rest break with a snack. At the visit the parent accompanying the child was interviewed by another staff member, and was asked to complete a questionnaire about the child's self-help development and the Schedule of Recent Events (Holmes & Rahe, 1967).

Academic achievement was assessed using the Peabody Individual Achievement Test (PIAT) (Dunn & Markwardt, 1970), and general intelligence was measured with the Wechsler Intelligence Scale for Children-Revised (WISC-R) (Wechsler, 1974). Because of time constraints, we followed the procedure suggested by Wechsler of omitting two subtests.

Classroom behavior characteristics were assessed by the children's teachers using the Pupil Rating Scale (PRS) (Myklebust, 1981). Although the 24 PRS items are grouped in five behavioral areas, only the total score was used in the data analyses. Teachers were also asked to report whether the child had been a behavioral problem in the class or had participated in any special programs in school (for gifted children, for children with specific learning disabilities, etc.).

The data collection at this point also included certain family ecology variables mentioned earlier, and the McDaniels-Piers Young Children's Self-Concept Scale (McDaniel & Piers, 1973). Parents were also asked to provide information about the health and development of the child, including reports about health habits, accidents, illnesses, and growth measures. Reports on these characteristics of the children are reported elsewhere.

### Defining Problem Groups

Twenty-one children were classified as having *learning problems* using one of two criteria: (a) those identified by their teachers as being in remedial or special classes for a learning disability, or (b) those identified by testing with the PIAT as performing three-quarters of a school year or more below their expected grade. Children whose records were missing either of these pieces of information were not classified. It is important to note that a low IQ score or a low PRS score by itself did *not* classify a child as having a learning problem, although most children with very low scores were included in the problem group by the criteria used.

The *behavior problem* definition, which classified 15 children as having problems, was based solely on the report of the child's teacher. Teachers were asked whether or not the child's classroom behavior had been a problem, and, if so, to describe the problem and what actions had been taken. Teachers reported problems including temper outbursts, fighting, stealing, lack of self-control, excessive talking, inattentiveness, and attention-seeking behavior. Seven children in the behavior problem group were also in the learning problem group.

Although formal validity data are not available for these problem classifications, there is some support for their reasonableness. For example, the learning problem group included 4 of the 5 children with the lowest WISC-R scores and 4 of the 5 children with the lowest PRS scores. Similarly, parent reports of the presence or absence of behavior problems were consistent with teacher reports about 84% of the time ($\chi^2$ = 10.18, p. < .01), although the teachers did identify 8 children not identified by the parents.

## RESULTS

The basic strategy for the data analysis was to use each of these two divisions of the sample (presence vs. absence of learning problems, and presence vs. absence of behavior problems) as an outcome for discriminant function analyses, using variables from the four clusters of predictors, variables from each age point, and the combined variables in a single analysis.

### Learning Problems

The results of the discriminant function analyses comparing children with learning problems ($N$ = 21) and those without learning problems ($N$ = 109) are shown in Table 1 (for the clusters of predictors) and Table 2 (for predictors from different age periods).

The canonical correlations shown in Table 1 indicate that variables from all four of the clusters significantly predict whether or not a child will be classified as having a learning problem in second grade, although the coefficient for the perinatal and infant status variables is not large (representing less than 10% of the variance). The significantly discriminating variables in the child outcome cluster were expressive language (poorer at 24 months), motor development (better at 36 months), IQ (lower at 48 months), and accidents (more reported at 48 months). In the interaction/environmental cluster, the significant discriminators reflect both interactive capacities and general environmental quality. Among those measures from the ecological cluster, family intactness and social status seem the most relevant to whether a child has problems.

The discriminant functions summarized in Table 2 show these relationships in a slightly different way, with variables entered according to the age at which they were collected, rather than according to their

**Table 1.** Discriminant Analyses for Four Clusters of Predictor Variables

| Cluster | Learning problems: Variables | Learning problems: Standard discriminant function coefficients | Behavior problems: Variables | Behavior problems: Standard discriminant function coefficients |
|---|---|---|---|---|
| Perinatal & infant status | Sex (1-girl, 2-boy) | .95 | No significant variables | |
| | Birth weight | −.78 | | |
| Canonical correlation | | .29 | | |
| Child outcomes | IQ (48 months) | −.47 | Expressive language (12 Mo.) | .74 |
| | | | IQ (48 mo.) | −.65 |
| | Expressive language (24 mo.) | −.66 | Receptive language (12 mo.) | .42 |
| | Motor development (36 mo.) | .45 | Psychomotor development (12 mo.) | −.45 |
| | Medically attended accidents (48 mo.) | .44 | Medically attended accidents (48 mo.) | .41 |
| Canonical correlation | | .50 | | .45 |
| Family ecology and and parent perceptions | Years with only one parent | .80 | Years with only one parent | .79 |
| | Social status | −.63 | Life change (24 mo.) | −.47 |
| | Number of partnerships | −.48 | Social support (prenatal) | −.39 |
| Canonical correlation | | .44 | | .48 |
| Interaction and environmental quality | HOME Inventory (48 mo.) | −.52 | Mother feeding (12 mo.) | −.72 |
| | Infant feeding (12 mo.) | −.56 | HOME Inventory (36 mo.) | −.56 |
| | HOME Inventory (24 mo.) | −.39 | Infant feeding (4 mo.) | .46 |
| Canonical correlation | | .54 | | .56 |

**Table 2.** Discriminant Analyses for Six Time Points

| Timepoint | Learning problems: Variables | Learning problems: Standard discriminant function coefficients | Behavior problems: Variables | Behavior problems: Standard discriminant function coefficients |
|---|---|---|---|---|
| Prenatal | Social status | −.70 | Social support | |
| | Sex (1-girl, 2-boy) | .51 | | |
| | Social support | −.56 | | −1.00 |
| Canoncial correlation | | .43 | | .30 |
| 4 months | HOME Inventory | | HOME Inventory | −.86 |
| | | −1.00 | Infant feeding | .79 |
| Canonical correlation | | .31 | | .35 |
| 12 months | Infant feeding | −.63 | Mother feeding | −.71 |
| | HOME Inventory | −.60 | Expressive language | .67 |
| | Total illnesses | .44 | HOME Inventory | −.42 |
| | | | Mental development | −.41 |
| Canonical correlation | | .52 | | .58 |
| 24 months | HOME Inventory | −.67 | HOME Inventory | .86 |
| | Expressive language | −.58 | Life change | −.57 |
| | Life change | −.37 | | |
| | Child teaching | .38 | | |
| Canonical correlation | | .52 | | .35 |
| 36 Months | Receptive language | −.53 | HOME Inventory | |
| | HOME Inventory | −.66 | | −1.00 |
| Canonical correlation | | .41 | | .38 |
| 48 Months | HOME Inventory | | HOME Inventory | −.82 |
| | Medically attended | −.73 | Medically attended | |
| | accidents | .41 | accidents | .67 |
| | IQ | −.41 | | |
| Canonical correlation | | .49 | | .33 |

content. From the results, it seems clear that the combination of variables that can be obtained during the perinatal period (including the family ecology measures of social status and social support) is a fairly potent predictor of learning problems.

One is also struck in Table 2 by the consistency with which scores on the HOME Inventory contribute to the prediction of learning problems. In addition, it is interesting that earlier measures of mental development (Bayley scores from 12 and 24 months) do not appear as significant discriminators.

Overall, it appears that later learning problems can be detected best by observing or testing the child and the ecological and stimulating qualities of his or her environment. The child's sex, birth weight, later motor development, language skill, and ability to enter effectively into an interactive activity all appear to be elements in the equation. This impression is confirmed when variables from all four clusters are combined in a single discriminant function analysis (shown in Table 3).

For this analysis only the significant variables from each cluster were entered, and a stepwise method was used that entered infant status variables first, then child outcome variables, then ecological variables, and finally interaction/environment variables. Because this analysis capitalizes heavily on chance, the results must be viewed with a particularly skeptical eye.

Table 3 shows that each cluster *does* add predictive information not found in the clusters which preceded it into the discriminant function. In our sample, the child outcome variables seem to have less relative importance in discriminating between the learning problem groups than do variables from other clusters. If we were to summarize the results from this analysis, we would say that a child with a learning problem at age 8 tends to have one or more of the following characteristics: male, lower birth weight, poor interactive skill in infancy (infant feeding at 12 months), a less rich preschool-age environment (HOME Inventory at 48 months), a single parent home, and more accidents (48 months).

When variables are combined in this way, we are able to identify 13 of the 21 children with learning problems while misclassifying 4 of the children with no learning problems. No single cluster of variables did as well, nor did scores from any one age (Table 4). This table also shows that there is a very low rate of children falsely identified but a rather high rate of children with problems who were missed. In other words, a "bad" combination of predictor variables very rarely occurs in a child who turns out to be problem-free. However, even with extensive testing and assessment, there are many children who will develop problems who could not have been identified ahead of time using this scheme.

**Table 3.** Overall Discriminant Analyses (Across Clusters)

| | Step/Variables | Standard and discriminant function coefficients |
|---|---|---|
| | Learning problems vs. no learning problems | |
| 1 | Sex | .39 |
| | Birth weight | −.25 |
| 2 | IQ (48 mo.) | −.23 |
| | Motor development (36 mo.) | .22 |
| | Expressive language (24 mo.) | −.23 |
| | Medically attended accidents (48 mo.) | .30 |
| 3 | Years with only one parent | .30 |
| 4 | Infant feeding (12 mo.) | −.43 |
| | HOME Inventory (48 mo.) | −.37 |
| | Canonical correlation = .64 | |
| | Behavior problems vs. no behavior problems | |
| 1 | (No perinatal status variables entered) | |
| 2 | Expressive language (12 mo.) | .47 |
| | IQ (48 mo.) | −.26 |
| | Receptive language (12 mo.) | .27 |
| | Psychomotor development (12 mo.) | −.36 |
| | Medically attended accidents (48 mo.) | .29 |
| 3 | Years with only one parent | .50 |
| | Social support (prenatal) | −.33 |
| | Life change (24 mo.) | −.20 |
| 4 | Mother feeding (12 mo.) | −.52 |
| | Infant feeding (4 mo.) | .35 |
| | Canonical correlation = .70 | |

## Behavior Problems

A parallel set of analyses was done to discriminate children rated by the teacher as having problem behavior problems in the classroom from those with no problems, and these are also reported in Tables 1 through 4.

The analysis of the four clusters of variables (Table 1) shows clearly that perinatal and infant status variables are not significant discriminators of these two groups of children. Behavior problems in second grade are associated with precocious language development combined with somewhat delayed motor development at the end of the first year of life. By the fourth year, these children have lower IQ scores and more

**Table 4.** Discriminant Analysis Classification Results

| | Learning problems | | | | Behavior problems | | | |
|---|---|---|---|---|---|---|---|---|
| | Problem ($N$ = 21) | | No problem ($N$ = 109) | | Problem ($N$ = 15) | | No problem ($N$ = 122) | |
| Variable set | True positive | False negative | True negative | False positive | True positive | False negative | True negative | False positive |
| Perinatal & infant status | 5% | 95% | 100% | 0% | NA | NA | NA | NA |
| Child outcomes | 43 | 57 | 97 | 3 | 27% | 73% | 98% | 2% |
| Ecological & perceptual | 29 | 71 | 97 | 3 | 33 | 67 | 98 | 2 |
| Interaction & environmental | 38 | 62 | 98 | 2 | 53 | 47 | 98 | 2 |
| Perinatal | 33 | 67 | 97 | 3 | 33 | 67 | 95 | 5 |
| 4 Month | 19 | 81 | 100 | 0 | 13 | 87 | 99 | 1 |
| 12 Month | 43 | 57 | 97 | 3 | 53 | 47 | 95 | 5 |
| 24 Month | 43 | 57 | 96 | 4 | 20 | 80 | 99 | 1 |
| 36 Month | 29 | 71 | 96 | 4 | 33 | 67 | 99 | 1 |
| 48 Month | 33 | 67 | 96 | 4 | 13 | 87 | 99 | 1 |
| Overall (across clusters) | 62% | 38% | 96% | 4% | 87% | 13% | 100% | 0% |

fairly serious accidents. In the ecological cluster, more years spent in a single parent home appears to be related to behavior problems (as it was to learning problems). And in the interaction/environmental cluster, behavior problems appear to be associated with poor maternal sensitivity during interaction (feeding at 12 months) and a less stimulating environment (HOME Inventory at 36 months).

The discriminant function results for each age point (Table 2) show that the interaction/environmental variables are predominent at each point in time. In contrast to the analysis of learning problems (where predictive accuracy was about the same at all age points), the age of 12 months appears to be one where behavior problems can be especially accurately predicted.

The overall discriminant function analyses (Table 3) are consonant with the individual ones. That is, variables from both the ecological and the interaction/environmental clusters add significant information to what is known from the child outcome cluster. The child with second grade behavior problems is one with some combination of the following characteristics and experiences: advanced early language development (expressive and receptive at 12 months), poor early motor development (12 months), relatively frequent accidents in the preschool years (48 months), a single parent household, and low maternal sensitivity during infancy feeding at 12 months.

The accuracy with which screening decisions could have been made from these data is shown in Table 4. As was the case with learning problems, our ability to detect behavior problems with a single cluster of variables or at a single time point is somewhat limited. However, one cluster (interaction/environmental) and one time point (12 months) appear to be notably better than the others for this purpose. And when all of our information is combined, we manage to correctly identify a creditable 87% of the children with later behavior problems.

### Traditional Prediction Equations

Because the analyses reported here (which focus on the variables that discriminate between problem and no-problem groups) were somewhat unusual, it may be helpful to briefly summarize more traditional analyses of these same data. Multiple regression analyses from this project (reported by Hammond & Bee, 1983) focused on the variables that *predict* individual outcomes, both good and bad. Of course in some sense, both kinds of analyses are really *post*-diction, because they were done after the fact, but the contrast between general prediction and early identification of problems is an important one.

First, the variables in the perinatal and infant status cluster do not *predict* either IQ or school achievement, even though they did *discriminate* between children who did and did not have learning problems in the present analysis. Second, the best predictors of the cognitive outcomes (in terms of the size of *R*) were the child outcome variables, with the 48-month Stanford-Binet IQ playing a central role. Nonetheless, the ecological cluster and the interaction/environmental cluster showed significant and interesting patterns of prediction. Third, the pattern of general prediction of school achievement (PIAT) was fairly similar to the pattern of discrimination for learning problems, especially for the ecological and interaction/environmental clusters. The pattern of discrimination for behavior problems, however, was not paralleled in these multiple regression results.

## DISCUSSION AND IMPLICATIONS

A single data set can yield somewhat different results, depending on how the research question is asked. The perinatal status variables in the present study, for example, are useful at discriminating between groups of children with and without learning problems, but they do not predict cognitive functioning in general (either IQ or school achievement).

Infant status indexes alone, however, were not very accurate at predicting later learning problems for these children. Still, the generally more vulnerable children (boys and somewhat low birth weights) who were reared in a less optimum cognitive environment had a greater probability of a later learning problems. Note that a poor environment alone was not associated with significant learning problems in this group of children; it was the combination of heightened physical risk and poor environment that mattered. This certainly replicates the basic findings from both the Kauai study and the National Collaborative Perinatal Project: really poor outcomes for a child most often arise when an initial vulnerability (low birth weight or some other difficulty) is combined with a less-than-optimally stimulating or supporting environment.

A quite different pattern appears when we attempt to predict later behavior problems. As was suggested earlier, this pattern appears to describe a group of children with good early language skills accompanied by slow motor development—a combination that might present a special challenge to parents. Once again, it is the *combination* of this pattern of child development with family disruption (a high number of years with only one parent) that is associated with teachers' ratings of behavior problems.

## Implications for Screening

A simple model of early detection is not supported by these data. On the contrary, it appears that some families function rather well at first, with good interaction and environment and a competent child, but then later run into difficulties (of many kinds) that are related to the child's later problems.

The current study found that children born into homes with stable and well-educated parents are at fairly low risk for further problems—certainly below the rate of risk that would make screening economically feasible. Children in high risk situations, however, those with physiological vulnerabilities and those whose families face high stress with low social support, probably require screening at repeated intervals through their lives. Children whose lives change markedly, through divorce or financial reverses or other family stresses, should probably be included in this latter group.

## A Methodological Note

We began by noting that research like ours, which was designed to provide a scientific basis for early screening, usually took a particular form—the multivariate longitudinal study. As much as these studies have taught us, they are not very well suited to the questions that they are meant to answer. The statistical procedures used in the current study answer questions about shared variance among different variables in the same sample of subjects. The sad methodological truth of the matter is that existing techniques of assessing children and families are at the stage where their psychometric shortcomings may seriously mislead us. The amount of shared variance that can be detected is strongly influenced by the distribution of scores on every variable that is entered into the equations. Uncertain range, wide (or narrow) variability, and lack of representativeness of the sample (to some real-world population of interest) can skew the results. These shortcomings make it nearly impossible to answer questions about the relative importance of different domains in predicting developmental outcomes.

Researchers must reevaluate ways of thinking about screening before new research designs and assessment methods can be developed that will serve our needs more exactly. In the meantime, practitioners involved in early screening programs should realize that not all results from longitudinal studies can be directly applied to screening. Only if the data analysis is specifically aimed at identifying children with specific problems—and not if it is aimed at prediction of the whole range of functioning—can the results be responsibly used to guide clinical applications.

# REFERENCES


Barnard, K. E., & Douglas, H. B. (1974). *Child health assessment, Part 1: A literature review* (DHEW Publication No. HRA 75-30). Bethesda, MD: U.S. Dept. of Health, Education, & Welfare, Public Health Service, HRA, Bureau of Health Resources Development, Division of Nursing.

Barnard, K. E., & Eyres, S. J. (1979). *Child health assessment, Part II: The first year of life* (DHEW Publication No. HRA 79-25). Hyattsville, MD: U.S. Dept. of Health, Education, & Welfare, Public Health Service, HRA, Bureau of Health Manpower, Division of Nursing.

Bayley, N. (1969). *Bayley scales of infant development: Birth to two years.* New York: Psychological Corp.

Bee, H. L., Barnard, K. E., Eyres, S. J., Gray, C. A., Hammond, M. A., Spietz, A. L., Snyder, C., & Clark, B. (1982). Prediction of IQ and language skill from perinatal status, child performance, family characteristic, and mother-infant interaction. *Child Development, 53,* 1134–1156.

Bee, H. L., Van Egeren, L. F., Streissguth, A. P., Nyman, B. A., & Leckie, M. A. (1969). Social class differences in maternal teaching strategies and speech patterns. *Developmental Psychology, 1,* 726–734.

Behar, L., & Stringfield, S. (1974). A behavior rating scale for the preschool child. *Developmental Psychology, 10,* 601–610.

Brazelton, T. B. (1973). *Neonatal Behavioral Assessment Scale.* Philadelphia: Lippincott.

Broman, S. H., Nichols, P. L., & Kennedy, W. A. (1975). *Preschool IQ: Prenatal and early developmental correlates.* Hillsdale, NJ: Erlbaum.

Broussard, E. R., & Hartner, M. (1970). Maternal perception of the neonate as related to development. *Child Psychiatry and Human Development, 1,* 16–25.

Caldwell, B. M., & Bradley, R. H. (1978). *Manual for the Home Observation for Measurement of the Environment.* Unpublished manuscript, University of Arkansas, Little Rock, AR.

Dubowitz, L. M. S., Dubowitz, V., & Goldberg, C. (1970). Clinical assessment of gestational age in the newborn infant. *Pediatrics, 77,* 1-10.

Dunn, L. M., & Markwardt, F. C. (1970). *Manual for Peabody individual achievement test.* Circle Pines, MN: American Guidance Service.

Fluharty, N. B. (1974). The design and standardization of a speech and language screening test for use with preschool children. *Journal of Speech and Hearing Disorders, 39,* 75–88.

Frankenburg, W. K., & Dodds, J. B. (1967). The Denver Developmental Screening Test. *Journal of Pediatrics, 71,* 181–191.

Hammond, M. A., & Bee, H. L. (1983, April). *Prediction of IQ and achievement test scores at second grade from measures obtained in infancy and early childhood: An update on longitudinal data.* Paper presented at the biennial meeting of the Society for Research in Child Development, Detroit, MI.

Hedrick, D. L., Prather, E. M., & Tobin, A. R. (1975). *Sequenced inventory of communication development.* Seattle: Univ. of Washington Press.

Hess, R. D., & Shipman, V. C. (1967). Cognitive elements in maternal behavior. In J. P. Hill (Ed.), *Minnesota symposia on child psychology.* Minneapolis: Univ. of Minnesota Press.

Hollingshead, A. B. (1975). *Four factor index of social status.* Unpublished manual, Yale University, New Haven, CT.

Holmes, T. H., & Rahe, R. H. (1967). The social adjustment rating scale. *Journal of Psychomatic Research, 11,* 213–218.

Lester, B. M. (1978). *A priori clusters for the Brazelton neonatal behavioral assessment scale.* Mimeographed report.

Lewis, M., & Goldberg, S. (1969). Perceptual-cognitive development in infancy: A generalized expectancy model as a function of mother–infant interaction. *Merrill-Palmer Quarterly, 15,* 81–100.

McCarthy, D. (1972). *Manual for the McCarthy scales of children's abilities.* New York: Psychological Corp.

McDaniel, E. D., & Piers, E. V. (1973). *McDaniel-Piers young children's self-concept scale.* West Lafayetter, IN: Purdue Educational Research Center.

Myklebust, H. R. (1981). *The pupil rating scale revised: Screening for learning disabilities.* New York: Grune & Stratton.

Smith, A. C., Flick, G. L., Ferris, G. S., & Sellman, A. H. (1972). Prediction of developmental outcome at seven years from prenatal, perinatal, and postnatal events. *Child Development, 43,* 495–507.

Smith, D. W. (1970). *Recognizable patterns of human malformations.* Philadelphia: Saunders.

Snyder, C., Eyres, S. J., & Barnard, K. (1979). New findings about mothers' antenatal expectations and their relationship to infant development. *MCN, 4,* 354–357.

Terman, L. M., & Merrill, M. A. (1973). *Stanford-Binet intelligence scale: Manual for the third revision form L-M.* Boston: Houghton-Mifflin.

Waldrop, M. F., Pedersen, F. A., & Bell, R. Q. (1968). Minor physical anomalies and behavior in preschool children. *Child Development, 39,* 391–400.

Wechsler, D. (1974). *Manual for the Wechsler intelligence scale for children—revised.* New York: Psychological Corp.

Werner, E. E., Bierman, J. M., & French, F. E. (1971). *The children of Kauai.* Honolulu: Univ. of Hawaii Press.

Werner, E. E., & Smith, R. S. (1977). *Kauai's children come of age.* Honolulu: Univ. of Hawaii Press.

Wyler, A. R., Masuda, M., & Holmes, T. H. (1971). The magnitude of life events and seriousness of illness. *Psychosomatic Medicine, 33,* 115–122.

Yarrow, L. J., Rubenstein, J. L., Pedersen, F. A., & Jankowski, J. J. (1972). Dimensions of early stimulation and their differential effects on infant development. *Merrill-Palmer Quarterly, 18,* 205–219.

# PART III

## SCREENING INSTRUMENTS

*CHAPTER 8*

# The Denver Approach to Early Case Finding

## A REVIEW OF THE DENVER DEVELOPMENTAL SCREENING TEST AND A BRIEF TRAINING PROGRAM IN DEVELOPMENTAL DIAGNOSIS

*William K. Frankenburg*

The purpose of this chapter is to review the evolution of the Denver Developmental Screening Test (DDST) and the currently recommended process for developmental screening.

### ORIGINAL STANDARDIZATION OF THE DDST

The Denver Developmental Screening Test (DDST) (Frankenburg & Dodds, 1967) was devised to provide a simple method of screening the development of infants and preschool children. This test was designed to be a quick, simple procedure that would be applied to a presumptively asymptomatic population to identify children highly suspect of being delayed in development. In contrast to developmental psychological tests that are intended for use by psychologists, developmental screening tests are designed for use by a variety of professionals such as nurses, physicians, and day care teachers as well as by paraprofessionals who come into contact with young children.

The DDST consists of 105 test items arranged in one of four functional sectors: gross motor, fine motor-adaptive, language, and personal-social. Each test item is represented schematically by a distribu-

*William K. Frankenburg* • Rocky Mountain Child Development Center, University of Colorado School of Medicine, Denver, Colorado 80262.

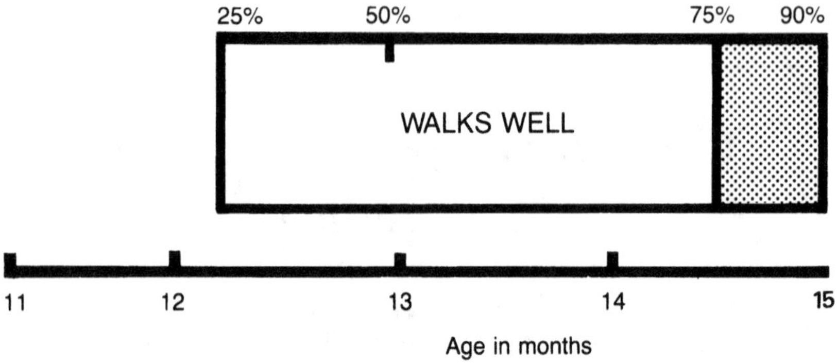


**Figure 1.** Age distribution of children performing a DDST test item.

tion bar so located in relation to a horizontal age line from birth to 6 years that it depicts at a glance the age at which 25%, 50%, 75%, and 90% of children could perform the task. Figure 1 illustrates the item Walks Well. To depict the bars accurately, the Denver group standardized the test on 1,036 presumably normal children whose families reflect the occupational and ethnic characteristics of the Denver population. Norms were calculated for boys, girls, and children whose fathers were laborers, managers, and professionals. Few marked differences were found between ages at which boys and girls performed the individual test items. The authors initially had the notion that through the derivation of accurate norms and comparison of a child's development to those norms, potential developmental delays could be identified. This expectation, however, turned out not to be the case. What was required was to determine a method of scoring the entire test in a simple yet accurate manner.

## SCORING THE DDST

### Reliability Studies

Following the calculation of norms, two reliability studies were undertaken: a study of tester–observer reliability and a study of test–retest stability. On individual test items, tester–observer agreement was 97.7% ($N$ = 76), and for items passable by report, the agreement rate was 96.1%. Test–retest stability was determined by evaluating 186 subjects divided into 13 age groups (1.5–72 months) twice, at a week interval. Each child was evaluated by a different examiner at the time of the second evaluation to avoid tester bias. For this study, mental ages were calculated. The coefficients for the subjects varied from .66 to .93, with no age trend displayed (Frankenburg & Dodds, 1967). The overall analysis of the results indicates that the test–retest stability of the DDST is not only satisfactory for a screening test but compares favorably with test–retest stability of diagnostic tests, such as the Revised Bayley Scale of Mental and Motor Development (Frankenburg, Fandal, Sciarillo, & Burgess, 1981) at comparable ages.

### Concurrent Validity Studies

To determine the concurrent validity of the DDST, the Denver group evaluated 236 subjects (Frankenburg, Camp, Van Natta, Demersseman, & Voorhees, 1971) with the DDST and one of the following criterion tests: Stanford-Binet, Revised Yale Developmental Schedules (Provence, 1964), Cattell (1940), and the Revised Bayley Infant Scales (Bayley, 1969). Because each of the criterion tests generate mental ages, a DDST mental age was determined and the test was also scored as normal, questionable, or abnormal (Frankenburg, Dodds, Fandal, Kazuk, & Cohrs, 1975). Correlation coefficients based on an average of DDST sector mental ages was .85 with the Stanford-Binet, .95 with the Revised Yale Developmental Schedule, .97 with the Cattell, .89 with the Mental Scale of the Bayley, and .84 with the Psychomotor Scale of the Bayley.

The DDST results and results of the criterion tests were compared in terms of co-positivity, co-negativity, and overall agreement (Buck & Gart, 1966). (*Co-positivity* is the probability that the screening and criterion tests will call a subject abnormal, and *co-negativity* is the probability that the screening and criterion test will call a subject negative or normal. *Overall agreement* is the percentage of tested individuals who had identical results on the two tests.) For this analysis, criterion test results were considered normal if the DQ or IQ were 70 or above and abnormal if the DQ or IQ were below 70. Subjects classified as questionables on the DDST were grouped with those classified as normals. The highest correlations between the DDST and the criterion were with the Cattell and the Revised Yale Developmental Schedule; and correlations with the Stanford-Binet and the Bayley Mental and Motor scales were still above .83. The foregoing reliability and concurrent validity studies lend strong support to the use of the DDST as a screening test for identifying developmental deviations.

### Revision of the DDST Scoring Method

Because there was concern that a sizable proportion of children classified as *questionable* and *abnormal* by the DDST were found to have no problems on a criterion test, the DDST's scoring criteria of abnormal and questionable were modified to yield greater agreement with the criterion measures. The revised scoring method was then further evaluated for reliability. One medical student and one college student were trained to administer the DDST according to the manual and the revised scoring method. One-hundred-and-eighty-six children between the ages of 1.5 and 76 months were each evaluated at 7-day intervals by each examiner. Use of the old and revised scoring method yielded 76% and 97% agreement, respectively (Frankenburg, Goldstein, & Camp, 1971).

To further evaluate the validity of the revised scoring method, four health aides were trained to administer the DDST until each achieved 95% interobserver reliability with a pediatrician on 10 consecutive examinations. Subsequently, the aides screened 2,000 children who came to Denver's neighborhood health program. DDST results were scored by the original and the revised scoring method. Of the 2,000 children screened, 237 children were brought back for validation 1 to 3 weeks after screening. Each child was evaluated by a psychologist or a psychometrician utilizing the Revised Bayley Infant Scale for children under 2 years of age or the Stanford-Binet for children above 2 years.

In the sample of 237 children evaluated with the original and revised scoring methods, the co-positivity and the co-negativity, as well as the rate of overreferrals and underreferrals were compared. Through use of a revised scoring method, the overreferrals were reduced from 21% to 11%. Cross-validation of this new scoring method, utilizing 9 screening aides who had 95% interobserver reliability, with a sample of 1,292 children yielded a co-positivity of .92 and a co-negativity of .97.

The results of the foregoing three studies indicate that the revised scoring method increased test–retest stability and validity. No doubt the higher rate of agreement in the cross-validation study is in a great part due to retraining of the screeners. It therefore is recommended that screeners be periodically retrained to minimize screening errors.

## PREDICTIVE VALIDITY OF THE DDST

Because the purpose of screening is to move up the time of diagnosis to an earlier stage in the disease or handicapping process, subsequent to studies of concurrent validation, studies were undertaken to evaluate the predictive validity of the DDST. If screening tests lack predictive validity, then they will have little use in moving up the time of diagnosis. As this became more obvious to the developers of the test, new criteria for screening test validity had to be selected. It was with this in mind that the validation emphasis shifted from concurrent validation against criterion tests to the prediction of subsequent school failure.

School failure is a condition meeting most of the criteria in the selection of diseases or conditions for screening. For example, school failure is serious; it can be diagnosed with certainty and it can be prevented or mitigated if identified prior to school age; it has an adequate lead time; it is treatable or controllable; it is relatively prevalent; screening does not harm the individual being screened; facilities are available to diagnose and treat the condition, and—last but most important—the cost of screening, diagnosis, and treatment is reasonable when compared to the human misery and cost of treatment after the usual time of treatment. Drawbacks in screening for school failure are that school failure is not a clear-cut entity but instead may be due to factors within the child (such as mental retardation or hearing loss), factors in the child's home environment (which can result in lack of cognitive stimulation or lack of motivation), and factors in the school environment (such as a teacher who is unable to discern a child's problem and therefore meet his or her educational needs). Furthermore, since expectations may vary from one school district to another, a failure in one district may not constitute a failure in another.

Despite these shortcomings, school failure nevertheless constitutes an entity that meets most of the criteria in the selection of conditions for screening and, therefore, two studies were undertaken to establish the predictive validity of the DDST in predicting later school failure. The first was a study reported by Camp, van Doorninck, Frankenburg, and Lampe (1977), which compared DDST results for 65 children from low socioeconomic status (SES) families. The subjects were evaluated with the DDST and the Stanford-Binet when they were 4 to 6 years of age and were followed up 3 years later to determine school status. For purposes of this study, school failure was operationally defined as one or more of the following: repetition of a grade, enrollment in a program for the educationally handicapped, enrollment in a program for the educable or trainable mentally retarded, third grade achievement test grade equivalent scores more than 1.5 years below grade level, teacher checklist scores indicating significant behavior problems interfering with school performance, health records citing referral for evaluation of hyperactivity, or behavior and learning problems. Results of the study indicated that 88% ($N$ = 17) of the 4- to 6-year-old children with abnormal DDST scores, 66% ($N$ = 23) with questionable DDST scores and 32% ($N$ = 25) with normal scores met the above criteria for school failure when reevaluated 3 years later (Frankenburg, Goldstein, & Camp, 1971).

Combining DDST with IQ scores in this study did not lessen the total number of children who were misclassified. This failure to increase screening accuracy by the addition of an IQ score was of concern, because it had always been recommended that individuals with deviant DDST results should be referred to a psychologist for diagnostic evaluation.

The second study of predictive validity was of children who had been screened with the DDST between 3 months and 6 years of age and were reevaluated after a time span of 5 to 6 years to determine school status. School failure was operationally defined by the same criteria as utilized by Camp *et al*. (1977). The study population was 3,000 children of low SES families. A total of 169 children (40 abnormal, 69 questionable, and 60 normal) were later located for reevaluation.

On follow-up, 89% ($N$ = 31) of the abnormals, 63% ($N$ = 41) of the questionables, and 38% ($N$ = 19) of those with normal results had later school problems. In comparing the predictive accuracy for 3 age groups (less than 24 months, 24–47 months, and 48–72 months) at the time of initial screening, predictive accuracy was found to increase with age. One reason for the lower predictive accuracy of the DDST abnormals for children screened below 24 months of age may be due to the fact that 5 to 6 years later the children were only in first or second grade and therefore had not had time to meet all of the school failure criteria.

The findings in these two studies should be viewed with the realization that school failure among this low SES population may run as high as 30%, which is far higher than the prevalence in children from high SES populations. Thus, the predictive accuracy of the DDST for a cross-section of the population would be lower than that presented above.

## SELECTING SCREENING CUTOFF SCORES THROUGH DECISION ANALYSIS

As use of the DDST gained widespread implementation (it is estimated that about 30 million children have been screened with the DDST since its first publication), the authors turned their attention to the cutoff separating suspect from nonsuspect children. In setting the cutoff point, a major consideration involved weighing the relative costs of over- and underreferrals. Because society bears both the benefits and burdens of test results, the authors felt it was most appropriate that society should be involved in the decision-making process of setting the screening cutoff point.

Decision analysis (described earlier in this volume, see Frankenburg, "The Concept of Screening Revisited") seemed ideally suited in selecting a cutoff point even though, to the knowledge of the DDST authors, it had not previously been employed in selecting a screening test's cutoff point (Coons, Gay, Frankenburg, McClelland, & Krieger, 1978). The decision analysis technique indicates the most desirable ratio of overreferrals to underreferrals that can be obtained with a screening instrument. Use of the optimum cutoff score should produce results (in terms of correct identifications, overreferrals, and underreferrals) that approximate this ratio. Thus, the results are reflective of current abilities to follow up and intervene with children found to be positive on screening. They are also consistent with current values regarding the detrimental effects of missed cases, and the problems associated with overreferrals (Coons *et al.*, 1978).

Implementation of the decision-analysis procedure includes the following steps:

1. Determination of specific facts and values that are pertinent to decisions regarding developmental screening;
2. Obtaining the best possible information regarding the specific, needed facts;
3. Obtaining the best possible information regarding the public's values as they relate to screening issues;
4. For each possible screening cutoff score, integrating both values and facts with outcome probabilities obtained for that score so as to get a total value for the score. The highest total value indicates the optimum cutoff score.

These relationships may be illustrated as follows. Table 1 reviews the four possibilities that occur when screening results are compared with a diagnosis. Costs and benefits are generated for each subject falling into any of the four quadrants (A, B, C, and D). Through a series of steps involving a review of the literature, the development of a con-

**Table 1.** Relationship between Diagnostic and Screening Test Findings

| | | Diagnostic findings | | |
|---|---|---|---|---|
| | | + | − | |
| Screening Test Findings | + | A<br>Agreement | B<br>Overreferral | A + B |
| | − | C<br>Underreferal | D<br>Agreement | C + D |
| | | A + C | B + D | |

Sensitivity = × 100     Overreferral rate = × 100

Specificity = × 100     Underreferral rate = × 100

Predictive validity of a positive test = × 100

Predictive validity of a negative test = × 100

sensus among experts in the field utilizing the Delphi process, and interviews with the lay public, positive and negative values (in terms of dollars) were obtained for each factor and for each of the four quadrants in Table 2. For example, for each subject falling into Quadrant A, there would be the following costs: screening, diagnostic evaluation, and treatment. Similarly, there would be the following benefits: economic gain (increase in lifetime earnings) and intrinsic gain (increased feeling of self-worth). Conversely, for each subject falling into Quadrant B, there would be the costs of screening, diagnosis, and undue parental anxiety (false concern); there would be no benefits.

Summing the factors for each quadrant made it possible to derive one number for each quadrant. The final step involved summing the four quadrants for possible cutoff points. For each cutoff point the number of individuals expected to fall in each cell was multiplied by the sum of the positive and negative values. Table 3 illustrates two cutoff points and the values derived.

Having obtained an optimum cutoff point, one must determine if there are possible constraining or compromising factors. In our initial study, my colleagues and I found that the economic benefits of Quadrant A far outweighed all the other values so that no case should be missed regardless of the number of overreferrals. However, actual field

**Table 2.** Costs and Benefits for Screening Outcomes, 4 Quadrants

| | | True developmental status | |
|---|---|---|---|
| | | Delayed | Normal |
| Screening result | + | A<br>Abnormal outcome<br>– Cost of screen<br>– Cost of diagnosis<br>– Cost of treatment<br>+ Economic impact of intervention<br>+ Intrinsic value of IQ increment | B<br>Overreferral outcome<br>– Cost of screen<br>– Cost of diagnosis<br>– Parental anxiety |
| | – | C<br>Underreferral outcome<br>– Cost of screen<br>– Economic impact of intervention<br>– Intrinsic value of IQ increment<br>– Parental anxiety | D<br>Normal outcome<br>– Cost of screen<br>(0) + Value of documenting Child's normal status |

*Note.* From *A decision analysis approach to the selection of screening test cutoff scores* by C. E. Coons, E. C. Gay, & W. K. Frankenburg (1978, April 24). Paper presented at the Ambulatory Pediatrics Association meeting, New York.

**Table 3.** Results of High versus Low Cutoff Score

| High cutoff | |
|---|---|
| Correct ID delay<br>10% | Overreferral<br>40% |
| Underreferral<br>.0% | Correct ID normal<br>50% |

.10(8,797) + .40(−221) + 0(−309) + .50(0) = +870.86

| Low cutoff | |
|---|---|
| Correct ID delay<br>5% | Overreferral<br>20% |
| Underreferral<br>5% | Correct ID normal<br>70% |

.05(8,797) + .20(−221) + .05(−309) + .70(0) = +380.20

experience suggested that diagnosticians performing follow-ups of children who were suspect on screening would only tolerate a limited number of false positives (Quadrant B). Thus, it was necessary to derive a cutoff point that was a compromise between the ideal (derived from decision analysis) and limiting factors determined largely by the diagnosticians in the community.

Although some observers may not agree with the values obtained through use of this Delphi process, it has value as a method that avoids test developer bias in selection of screening cutoff points. To our knowledge, this attempt at bringing the public into the process of deciding screening definition of suspects is unique. It is our opinion that selection of the cutoff points should be made by various sectors of society if society has to bear the burden of "paying" for screening errors and will reap the benefits of screening. All too often it is not realized that society at large bears the benefits and costs of screening, not the developers of the screening test in question.

## USE OF THE DDST IN SCREENING DIFFERENT POPULATIONS

One criterion in the selection of a screening test is selection of a test that is appropriate to the population being screened. This is particularly true for tests that require the cooperation of the child. The age of the child is an important factor. Whether a developmental screening test should be restandardized for various subgroups of the population is often discussed. Some observers feel that it is unfair to compare disadvantaged children with advantaged children, as children's culture and past experiences are major determinants of future development. It is this reasoning that has led to suggestions that the DDST be restandardized on low SES children, such as children enrolled in Head Start. On the basis of past studies one could predict that Head Start norms would lower expectations and therefore lead to fewer low SES children being classified as abnormal or questionable on the DDST. In deciding whether to restandardize the DDST or any other developmental screening test on various populations, one might begin by defining what is being attempted. In the case of the DDST, the purpose is to predict school failure, which is far more common among children in the low SES population. The reason that school failure is more common among children in these groups is that expectations of school performance are rather homogeneous across most SES groups, but low SES children often have not had the environmental advantages common among high SES homes. Standardization in the colloquial sense means gathering data on central tendencies. These data differentiate what is common from what is uncommon but they do not tell who needs treatment. Restandardizing the DDST among Head Start children and using such norms for low SES children would be a disservice because it would fail to identify children in need of extra help if they are to be successful in school.

A number of years go, there arose the question of whether or not the DDST is racially biased and therefore should be banned from use in so-called "spring kindergarten roundups" in which prekindergarten-aged children are evaluated to determine school readiness. Prior to the time that this question arose, a cross-sectional study involving 2,230 children had previously been conducted to determine the developmental status (as portrayed by the DDST) of preschool-aged children of different social and ethnic groups (Frankenburg, Dick, & Carland, 1975). In this study the developmental status of 1,180 children representing a cross-section of Denver's ethnic and parental occupation groups was compared with that of 1,055 children (349 Anglo, 354 Spanish surname, and 352 Afro) whose parents were unskilled workers. In both groups the children varied in age from 2 weeks to 6.4 years and were evaluated with the DDST. The first analysis compared 910 Anglo children from the cross-sectional sample (primarily middle SES) with 349 Anglo children from the unskilled families; it demonstrated significant differences ($p < .05$) for 39 of the 105 DDST items. Below 20 months of age, children in the unskilled sample were advanced in all sectors, whereas after 20 months of age, the children of the middle SES sample were advanced in all test items except those in the personal-social sector. One might speculate that this difference in development is due to environmental factors, and that there is a lapse between the time the environment begins to influence the child's development and the time the child's development appears to be delayed—a so-called "sleeper" effect. If one accepts this reasoning, one may conclude that the ideal time to provide low SES children with supplementary environmental experiences is at 1 year of age, and that Head Start may actually be a "Hind Start." Comparisons of Anglo, Afro, and Spanish surname children from unskilled families showed few differences in rates of development. The failure of the present study to show marked differences in development between the 3 ethnic groups when SES was held constant suggests that the DDST is not racially biased. The answer to the question of whether the DDST should be used without restandardization must be answered locally by considering what developmental screening is expected to accomplish, and deciding whether the DDST is the most appropriate test to accomplish that end.

## SIMPLIFYING THE DDST

Though the DDST is taught at most of this nation's medical and nursing schools, its use by health professionals is limited by its cost in terms of space, trained personnel, and time required. In addition, health practitioners are generally not paid to perform the test. Thus, there is little financial incentive to routinely perform the test. These reasons explain the findings of Smith (1978), who demonstrated that physicians, even when taught the test, used it primarily to confirm their clinical impression that a child's development was delayed.

To encourage routine test application, the Denver group devised several approaches, all of which involve the use of a two-stage screen. This process is illustrated in Figure 2. In such a two-stage process, the first stage is quick and simple, making it economical; it is also valid and accurate in identifying all of the developmentally handicapped children screened. Use of such a two-stage process requires that the first stage not miss any children (few underreferrals or false negatives), and that errors be in the direction of overreferrals (false positives). This is important because underreferrals would not be identified until a later screening, a time when treatment may not be as efficacious.

In a two-stage process, all children who are suspect on the first-stage screen require a more costly and lengthy second-stage screen. A second-stage screen is generally more time-consuming, may require special training in administration and interpretation, and may require a special space for testing, each of which will tend to increase the cost.

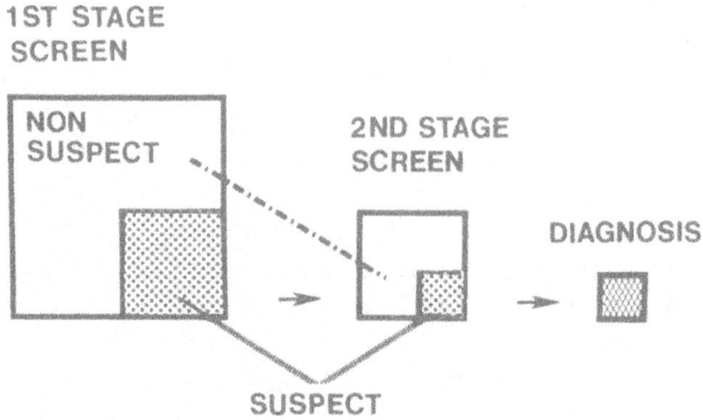


**Figure 2.** Two-stage screening process.

A recent application of the two-stage screening process has been in airport screening for hijackers. Such screening consists of Stage one (walking through a metal detector) and Stage two (body "combing" of individuals found to be suspect on stage one to determine the location of the metal).

The first two-stage process developed by the Denver group appeared in 1976. At that time, the authors recommended use of the Prescreening Developmental Questionnaire (PDQ) which consisted of 97 of the 105 standard DDST items formulated into questions designed to be answered by the parent. To validate the PDQ, 1,155 parents answered 10 age-appropriate questions. Next, each child in the study was evaluated blindly by a DDST examiner to determine agreement between parental report and DDST evaluation. The agreement rate varied for specific items from 68% to 100% with a mean of 93.3% (Frankenburg, van Doorninck, Liddell, & Dick, 1976).

Subsequently, in another study (Frankenburg, 1983), 10,000 children (5,000 from low SES and 5,000 from high SES families) were evaluated blindly in the following sequence: (a) PDQ followed by a second PDQ 1 week later, (b) DDST, and (c) psychological validation with the Revised Bayley Infant Scale or the Stanford-Binet. This study of concurrent validity demonstrated that the most cost-efficient screening approach for high SES families consisted of use of the PDQ; suspect children would be rescreened with the PDQ 1 week later and all individuals suspect on the second PDQ would be referred for diagnosis. For low SES families the PDQ answered by a parent without assistance generated too many errors; as a result, the PDQ is not recommended for families in which both parents have not completed high school. (However, it is possible that the PDQ, with the assistance of office personnel, may generate accurate results among low SES families.)

A recent attempt to further simplify and shorten screening time and to involve parents in child development has resulted in a book for parents called, *Your Child's Development: Charting the First Six Years* (Frankenburg, 1984).This book is to be given to parents at the time of the first health maintenance visit by the child's physician, who explains that the parents are being enlisted to help monitor their child's development. All of the developmental items in the book are taken from the PDQ, and so have been validated. The parent records the child's age at the time of attainment of the various developmental milestones. If the physician chooses, the parents can be asked to take a further step, which is to chart the child's development on the developmental chart (which is a revised DDST form, illustrated as Figure 3). Use of this book for parents is currently being explored in a number of physicians' offices in the Denver area.

A second two-stage approach developed by the Denver group consists of use of the abbreviated DDST, which requires administration of only 12 of the usual 20 to 25 DDST items (Frankenburg *et al.*, 1981). The 12 items administered are the 3 items in each of the four sectors that are immediately to the left of, but not touching, the age line (see Figure 4). Children who receive suspect scores on the abbreviated DDST (failure to pass all 12 items) then undergo the second stage, which is given as an expansion of the first stage screen and consists of administering the rest of the DDST (or about 12 additional items). The reason for immediately administering the balance of the DDST to children who are suspect on the abbreviated version is to check the findings with a more comprehensive screen and thus to decrease the number of false positives. Because 10,000 actual DDST profiles were entered on computer cards, it was possible to use the computer to try various scoring methods to determine the method that would yield the least number of false negatives. This computer simulation revealed that the previously described abbreviated DDST will identify 100% of suspect children on the full screen, and that only 25% of the children undergoing the abbreviated DDST will be suspect and will therefore require the full DDST. The time shown to be saved is 10 to 15 minutes per test on 75% of children who are nonsuspect on the abbreviated DDST. It is noteworthy that in the People's Republic of China, where the DDST has been restandardized, only 21% of children undergoing the abbreviated DDST require the full DDST. The Denver group's computer simulation findings seem therefore to hold up across continents.

Another approach to simplifying the administration of the DDST has been through use of a revised test form (Frankenburg *et al.*, 1981). To develop the new form, the Denver group arranged the 105 DDST items in a chronological stepwise order within each of the four sectors

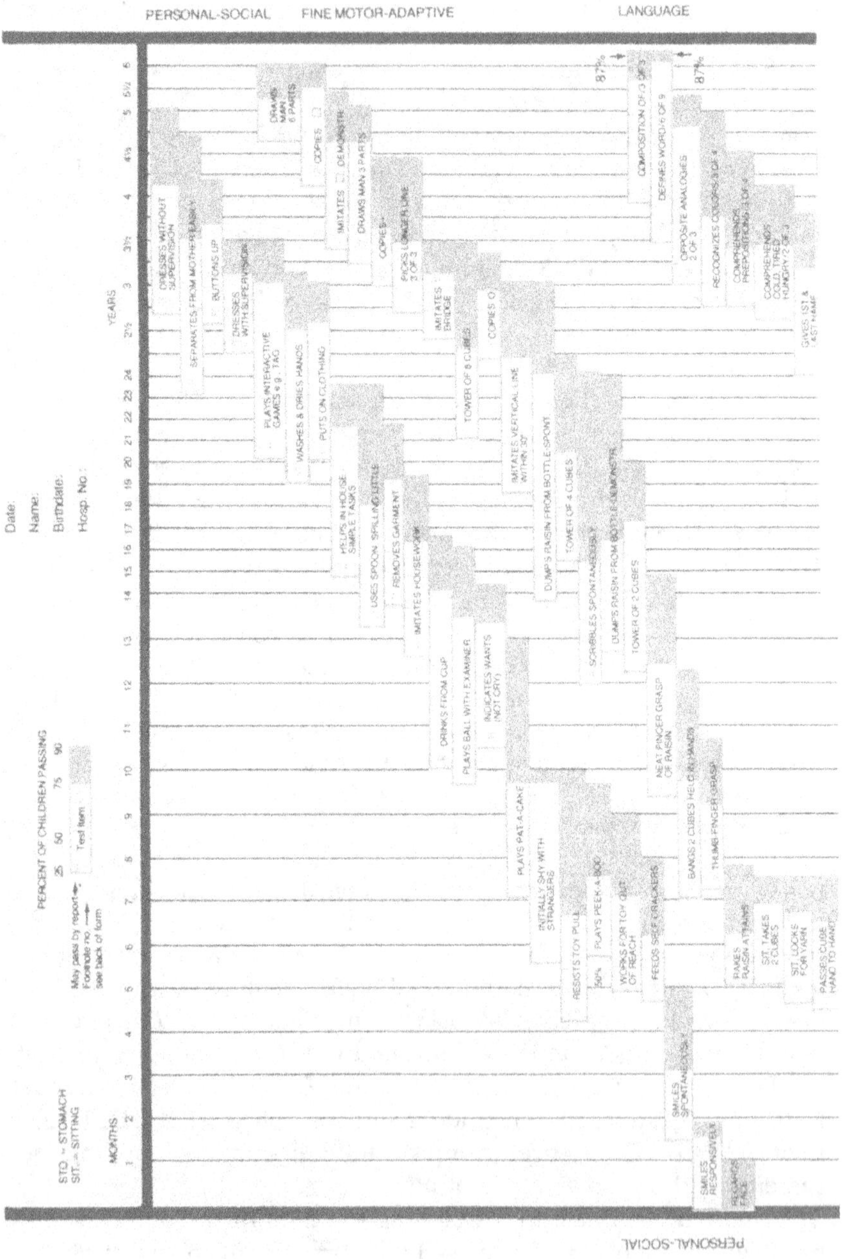
PERSONAL-SOCIAL
FINE MOTOR-ADAPTIVE
LANGUAGE

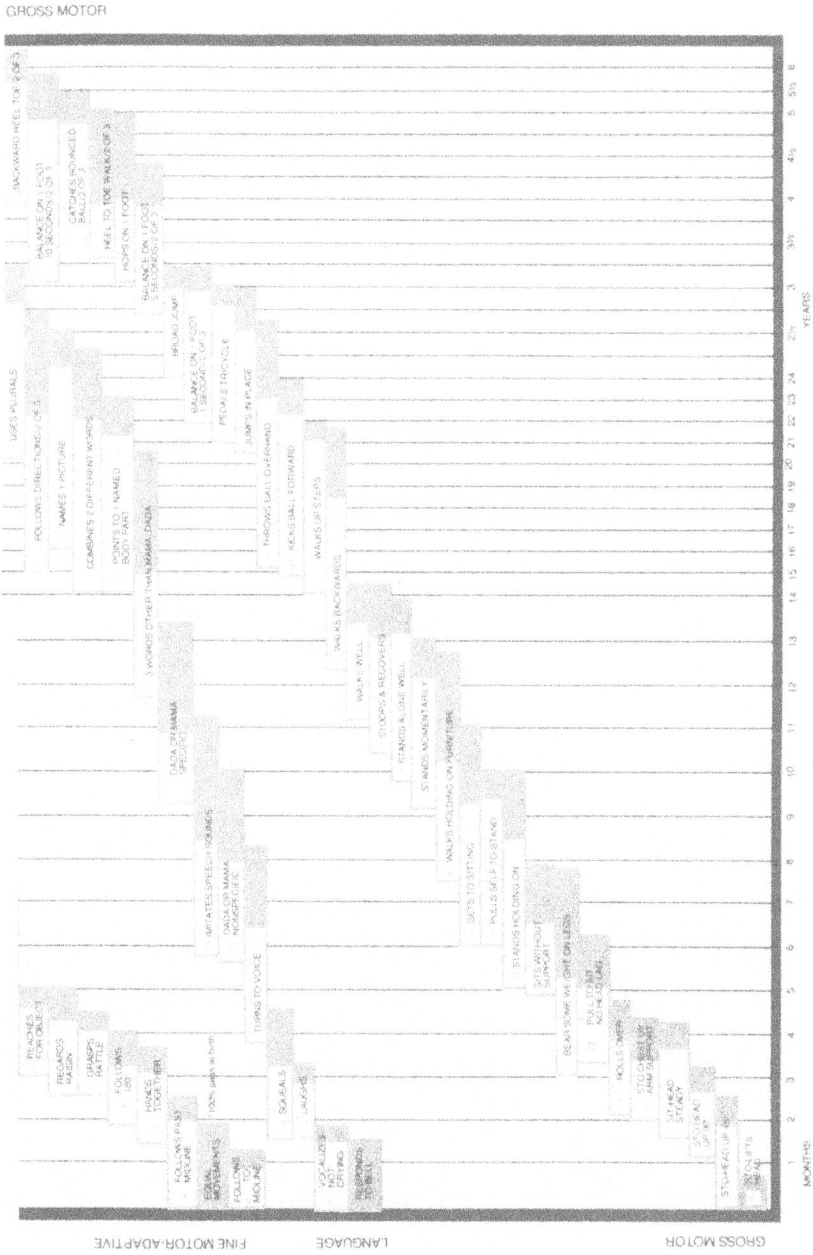


**Figure 3.** Revised Denver Developmental Screening Test form (DDST-R).

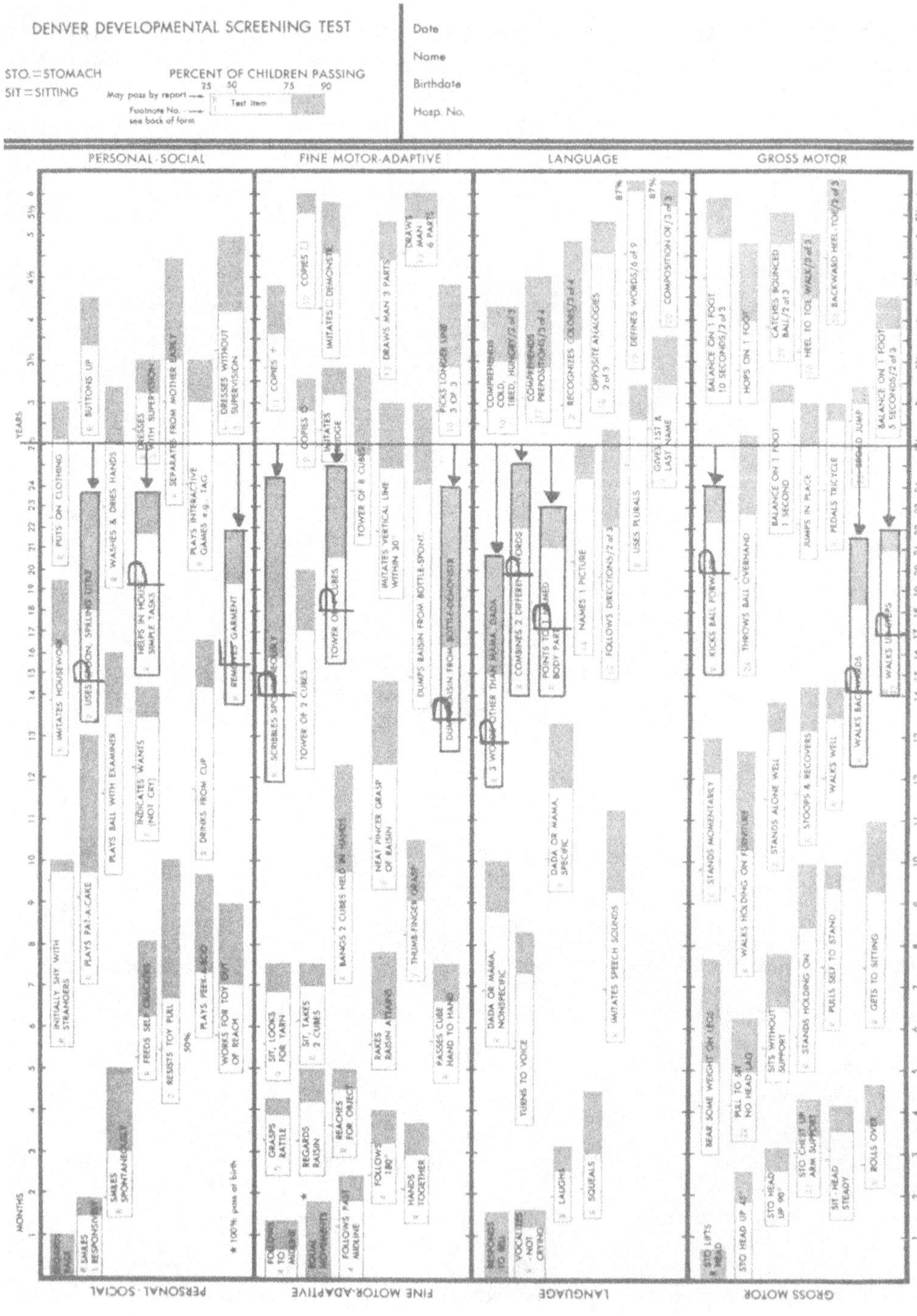


**Figure 4.** Abbreviated scoring of original Denver Developmental Screening Test form.

of the test. This order is based on the age at which 90% of the children in the original normative study passed the item. The result is a more condensed DDST form that resembles a growth curve, in that items at the lowest age level start at the bottom left side of the form and progress upward to the right with increasing age (Figure 3). This revised form, referred to as the DDST-R, has two basic advantages over the original form. First, it is far easier to administer the abbreviated DDST because it is easier to identify the 12 age-appropriate items than it had been using the original DDST form. The second advantage is that use of the form makes it easier to visualize a given child's rate of development much as one looks at rates of growth on growth curves.

A study comparing the accuracy of DDST scores for the original form and the DDST-R revealed the agreement to be 98% for the abbreviated DDST administered on the two forms, and 100% for the full DDST when evaluating 200 children varying in age from birth to 6 years (Frankenburg *et al.*, 1981). These findings suggest that use of the abbreviated manner of administration and the revised form will yield the same accurate results as the parent DDST. Although there are advantages to using the DDST-R over the original test form, some people who are used to the older form prefer to continue to use it rather than change to the DDST-R. Because accuracy is not affected appreciably by one form or the other, the form used is a matter of screener preference.

## INTERNATIONAL APPLICATION OF THE DDST

To date, the DDST has been utilized in more than 54 countries and has been restandardized in more than 15 countries. Each restandardization has involved more than 1,000 children. (The most recent restandardization, in Beijing, China, involved more than 6,000 children.) Although the restandardization procedures (primarily the selection of subjects) regrettably have varied from country to country, the similarity in rates of development found across countries and cultures has been striking. To be sure, minor variations have been noted, especially in the language sector. In addition, the results suggest that children in northern climates develop motorically slower than their southern counterparts (Ueda, Litt, & Yokozawa, 1980). This difference has been hypothesized to be related to the amount of restrictive clothing children wear in colder climates. Another difference suggested is that Asiatic children are slower than their American and European counterparts in concept formation (Sung, Chu, & Koo, 1980). Whether this finding will be confirmed by further studies remains to be seen.

One regrettable lack is that although a number of countries have restandardized the DDST, to the author's knowledge no new scoring criteria have been developed in these (or other) countries. As a result, the DDST may not be optimally effective in identifying children with delayed development in countries other than the United States. As countries operationally define what constitutes a developmental status of concern, it is to be hoped that they will determine how to score their version of the DDST to maximize agreement with their criteria of a "developmental problem." It is hoped that countries using the DDST will begin to develop their own scoring criteria in the near future.

## EVALUATION OF THE HOME ENVIRONMENT

Because the child's home environment is a major determinant of later development (Bradley & Caldwell, 1981), it is appropriate to combine developmental with environmental screening. Previous work by Sameroff (1975) popularized the transactional model of development. This model, as applied to developmental screening, proposes that a child's future development is best predicted through a measure of the child's current developmental status, combined with a measure of the child's environment. This is because environmental factors may potentially depress a child's development (or if conducive, may promote a child's development). Thus, a child receiving an abnormal score on the DDST (and therefore having an 89% probability of later school failure) and also receiving a low environmental score is at double risk. The interrelation between the DDST and the home environment is illustrated in Table 4.

Evaluation of the home environment is a relatively new and still evolving field. One of the best known instruments is the Home Observation for Measurement of the Environment (HOME) Inventory (Bradley & Caldwell, 1981). The HOME is composed of two scales: One covers birth to 3 years, and the other 3 to 6 years. To complete the HOME Inventory, a trained evaluator schedules a home visit when the child is awake and the primary caretaker is present. The evaluator interviews the parent and observes interactions in the home, a process that takes

**Table 4.** Relationship between Denver Developmental Screening Test Scores and Home Environment

| DDST scores | Low score | High score |
|---|---|---|
| Abnormal | Very high risk | High risk |
| Questionable | High risk | Moderate risk |
| Normal | Moderate risk | Low risk |

6. How many books do you own?
   ____ 0-9
   ____ 10-20
   ____ or more than 20
   *And*, where do you keep them?
   ____ in boxes
   ____ on a bookcase
   ____ or other — explain

7. How often does someone take your child into a grocery store:
   ____ hardly ever; prefer to go alone
   ____ at least once a month
   ____ at least twice a month
   ____ at least once a week

8. How many different babysitters or day care centers have you used in the past three months? ____

**Figure 5.** Sample questions from the Home Screening Questionnaire.

about 1 hour (plus travel time). From a screening standpoint, the two main drawbacks of the HOME are the requirement that a trained evaluator be involved and the time required to conduct the home visit. This latter point precludes use of the HOME to routinely and periodically screen the home environments of large numbers of children.

To develop a first-stage environmental screening instrument, the Denver group—with the assistance of Caldwell and Bradley—revised the HOME Inventory into a parent-answered questionnaire called the Home Screening Questionnaire (HSQ). Two HSQ scales (birth to age 3 and 3 to 6 years) correspond to the two ages on the HOME. Sample HSQ questions are depicted in Figure 5. For a parent to complete the HSQ requires only about 15 minutes. The questions are written at a sixth-grade reading level; the HSQ is designed for use by parents who have not completed high school, because these parents are the ones whose HSQ and HOME scores show the greatest diversity (Frankenburg, Coons, van Doorninck, Goldstein, Berrenberg, & Moriarty, 1977). Furthermore, it is this population that has a relatively high percentage of school failure (van Doorninck, Caldwell, Wright, & Frankenburg, 1976). If a home is suspect on the HSQ, follow-up should be by a trained professional using an instrument like the HOME Inventory.

## CURRENT DEVELOPMENTAL SCREENING RECOMMENDATIONS

On the basis of these past experiences, the Denver group makes developmental screening recommendations for 2 separate populations based on level of parental education (which is generally related to SES). The reason for separate recommendations is that the most cost-efficient approach for high SES families is not the same as far as low SES families. Both recommended approaches make use of a two-stage process to increase their economic efficiency.

### Screening When Parents Have Less Than a High School Education

When screening children from homes in which either parent has less than a high school education, it is recommended that the first-stage screen consist of the abbreviated DDST. Children who do not pass all 12 items (about 25% of children screened) then receive the second-stage screen consisting of the remainder of the DDST, or about 12 to 15 more items. Children who receive nonnormal scores on the full DDST should be rescreened about a week later. If they again receive nonnormal scores, they should receive a diagnostic evaluation.

It is recommended that children be screened with the abbreviated DDST at 3 to 6 months, 9 to 12 months, and 3, 4, and 5 years of age to facilitate early detection and to identify children who develop delays after the initial screening. The revised DDST form (Figure 3) is ideally suited for such screening because its graphic presentation simplifies identification of the 12 items and is well suited for noting trends in development.

All children coming from families in which either parent has not graduated from high school should also be screened with the HSQ. If they are suspect on the HSQ, a home visit and administration of the full HOME Inventory (or similar instrument) are indicated. If the full HOME Inventory yields a low score, it can be used to develop a strategy for helping the families.

### Screening When Both Parents Have at Least a High School Education

The most economical method of screening children from more educated families is with the PDQ. If the child passes at least 9 out of 10 age-appropriate items, the results are nonsuspect. If the child passes fewer than 9 items, the results are considered to be suspect, and the child should be rescreened with the PDQ 1 week later. If the child passes 8 or fewer items on rescreening, the child should receive a diagnostic evaluation.

A new screening approach (described previously in this chapter) has been developed to further speed up the screening process and encourage parent involvement in child development. This approach involves use of the parents' book, *Your Child's Development: Charting the*

*First Six Years*. The book is to be given to parents by their child's physician; the parents record their child's development, possibly also chart the child's development, and bring the book to the physician's office whenever the child comes for a health maintenance visit. The health provider reviews the parents' reports in the book and may elect to perform a few of the 12 items of the abbreviated DDST at the visit. Children who seem to be falling behind in development on the basis of the chart should be screened with the abbreviated-full DDST to substantiate the delay. Studies are currently underway to answer such questions as the following: Will parents fill out the book? Will parents' reports be accurate? Will parents remember to bring the book to periodic health maintenance visits?

### Screening Families Having Varied Educational Levels

Because it may be best to utilize one approach to screening a population in which education levels vary, it is suggested by the Denver group that the abbreviated-full DDST be employed.

## TRAINING IN DEVELOPMENTAL DIAGNOSIS

Because case finding is not only presumptive identification, but also diagnosis or confirmation of screening results, it is logical to discuss training in developmental diagnosis under the broader topic of "Early Case Finding."

If all children were to be screened as mandated by such legislation as Medicaid-EPSDT, Child-Find, and Head Start, and as recommended by various professional groups, virtually every child in this country would undergo developmental screening. As a result of such screening 5% to 15% of this nation's children would require diagnostic follow-up to determine if they actually have a problem, the cause of the problem, and what might be done about it. Multidisciplinary team evaluations, which are quite expensive and time-consuming, are not readily available to children in all communities, and there are simply not enough centers offering this type of evaluation to meet the expected needs of the population. Thus, it becomes clear that existing diagnostic facilities are gravely inadequate. It is therefore of the utmost urgency that massive nationwide efforts be undertaken to train professionals in diagnostic evaluation.

Follow-up of many children screened with the DDST has led the Denver group to speculate that not every child who is suspect on screening or whose parents are concerned about the child's development needs a complete multidisciplinary evaluation. Instead, approximately 80% of the children who are suspect on screening could be satisfactorily evaluated by a pediatrician or family practitioner who has received special training in diagnostic evaluation. The remaining 20% of suspect children who have more complex and/or time-consuming psychosocial problems, or who are severely multiply handicapped, would require a more exhaustive evaluation by a multidisciplinary team.

On the basis of the above assumptions, the Denver group has developed a concise pre- and in-service training program for primary care physicians. In this training program the four functions of the primary care physician are the following:

1. To make a categorical diagnosis and thereby establish a cause for the problem
2. To determine whether or not a child should be referred to another physician or to allied health workers for further evaluation
3. To assemble diverse test results into a comprehensive and coherent treatment plan
4. To counsel families on the meaning of evaluation findings

To facilitate widespread dissemination at a minimum cost, the Denver group assembled a relatively structured training program consisting of a tutor, videotaped demonstrations, a tutor's guide, and a student text. Eleven diagnostic lessons, together with lessons on screening and use of community resources, are generally taught in 20 hours. Lessons are presented by a tutor who trains small groups of 8 to 15 persons. Videotapes are frequently interrupted by the tutor to facilitate group discussions, to review local resources, and to offer practicum time to the trainees. At this writing, more than 200 instructors have taught the lessons to more than 1,000 primary health care providers. The first 120 professionals taking the course demonstrated gains in knowledge and increases in perceived self-competence. More than 95% of them stated that they would recommend this course and form of teaching to other physicians.

## CONCLUSION

Seventeen years ago, the Denver group started out to develop a developmental screening test; at that time it was not recognized how widely the test would be applied nor was there much consideration given to reliability and cost efficiency. As the test was applied to ever larger populations (about 30 million children to date), further consideration was given to simplifying the test to facilitate its applicability in mass screening efforts. To yield maximum efficiency, the authors proposed a two-stage process that differs depending on the population to be screened. With the aim of increasing the predictive accuracy of children likely to fail in school, the HSQ has been developed to screen the home environments of children from poverty families. Most recently the authors have turned their attention to developing diagnostic follow-up training programs for psychologists, speech pathologists, social workers, educators, and foster parents, as well as physicians. The goal of these programs is to train professionals to follow up on suspect screening results, because screening by itself does little to improve the health and welfare of the child. Instead, screening followed by categorical diagnosis, educational assessment, and treatment is actually just the first step in the prevention of developmental disabilities.

## REFERENCES

Bayley, N. (1969). *Bayley Scales of Infant Development-Manual.* New York: Psychological Corp.

Buck, A. A., & Gart, J. J. (1966). Comparison of a screening test and a reference test in epidemiologic studies. *American Journal of Epidemiology, 83,* 586–592.

Bradley, R. B., & Caldwell, B. M. (1981). Pediatric usefulness of home assessment. *Behavioral Pediatrics, 2,* 61–80.

Camp, B. W., van Doorninck, W. J., Frankenburg, W. K., & Lampe, J. M. (1977). Preschool developmental testing as a predictor of school problems. *Clinical Pediatrics, 16*(3), 257–263.

Cattell, P. (1940). *The measurement of intelligence of infants and young children.* New York: Psychological Corp.

Coons, C. E., Gay, E. C., Frankenburg, W. K., McClelland, G., & Krieger, M. (1978, April 24). *A decision analysis approach to the selection of screening test cutoff scores.* Presented at the Ambulatory Pediatric Association meeting, New York.

Frankenburg, W. K. (1983). Infant and preschool developmental screening. In M.D. Levine, W. B. Carey, A. C. Crocker, & R. T. Gross (Eds.), *Developmental-behavioral pediatrics* (pp. 927–937). Philadelphia, PA: W.B. Saunders.

Frankenburg, W. K. (1984). *Your child's development: Charting the first six years.* Denver, CO: Preliminary manuscript published privately.

Frankenburg, W. K., Camp, B. W., Van Natta, P. A., Demersseman, J. A., & Voorhees, S. F. (1971). Reliability and stability of the Denver Developmental Screening Test. *Child Development, 42,* 1315–1325.

Frankenburg, W. K., Coons, M. A., van Doorninck, W. J., Goldstein, E. A., Berrenberg, J., & Moriarty, K. R. (1977, March 18). *Evaluation of the home environment using a self-administered questionnaire.* Paper presented at the Society for Research in Child Development, New Orleans, LA.

Frankenburg, W. K., Dick, N. P., & Carland, J. (1975). Behavioral pediatrics. *The Journal of Pediatrics, 87*(1), 125–132.

Frankenburg, W. K., & Dodds, J. B. (1967). The Denver Developmental Screening Test. *The Journal of Pediatrics, 71*(2), 181–191.

Frankenburg, W. K., Dodds, J. B., Fandal, A. W., Kazuk, E., & Cohrs, M. (1975). *The Denver Developmental Screening Test: Reference manual.* Denver: Univ. of Colorado Medical Center.

Frankenburg, W. K., Fandal, A., Sciarillo, W., & Burgess, D. (1981). The newly abbreviated and revised Denver Developmental Screening Test. *The Journal of Pediatrics, 99*(3), 995–999.

Frankenburg, W. K., Goldstein, A. D., & Camp, B. W. (1971). The Revised Denver Developmental Screening Test: Its accuracy as a screening instrument. *The Journal of Pediatrics, 79*(6), 988–995.

Frankenburg, W. K., van Doorninck, W. J., Liddell, T. N., & Dick, N. P. (1976). The Denver Prescreening Developmental Questionnaire (PDQ). *Pediatrics, 57*, 744–753.

Provence, S. (1964). *Revised Yale Developmental Schedule: A composite of Gesell examiniation with selected items from Merrill-Palmer, Stanford-Binet and Hetzer Woolf.* Unpublished manuscript, Yale Child Study Center.

Sameroff, A. J. (1975). Early influences on development: Fact or fancy? *Merrill-Palmer Quarterly, 21*, 267–294.

Smith, R. D. (1978). The use of developmental screening tests by primary-care physicians. *Journal of Pediatrics, 93*, 524.

Sung, C., Chu Y., & Koo X. (1980). The standardization of the Denver Developmental Screening Test on Chinese children. In A. W. Fandal, N. J. Anastasiow, & W. K. Frankenburg (Eds.), *Early identification of at-risk children: 3rd International Conference Proceedings.* Denver, CO: John F. Kennedy Child Development Center, Univ. of Colorado Health Sciences Center.

Ueda, R., Litt, M., & Yokozawa, S. (1980). Child development in Iwate as compared with Tokyo and Okinawa: Its implications for developmental screening. In A. W. Fandal, N. J. Anastasiow, & W. K. Frankenburg (Eds.), *Early identification of at-risk children: 3rd International Conference Proceedings.* Denver, CO: John F. Kennedy Child Development Center, Univ. of Colorado Health Sciences Center.

van Doorninck, W. J., Caldwell, B. M., Wright, C., & Frankenburg, W. K. (1976). *The relationship between the 12-month inventory of stimulation and school competence.* Unpublished manuscript.

CHAPTER 9

# The HOME Inventory

## ITS RELATION TO SCHOOL FAILURE AND DEVELOPMENT OF AN ELEMENTARY-AGE VERSION

*Robert H. Bradley and Stephen L. Rock*

---

The United States Commission on Excellence in Education recently reiterated concerns about the high percentage of school-age children who demonstrate poor academic performance and who show adjustment problems in school. Underachievement, classroom behavior problems, and other indicators of school failures have been of major concern to federal policymakers for quite some time.

Because of the high cost of school failure to the child, to the family, and to society at large, a number of attempts have been made to identify children who are at high risk for school failure. The risk factor most commonly identified is lower social class. However, although children from the lower social classes are represented in higher proportion among students who show school adjustment and school achievement problems, current measures of social class (i.e., socioeconomic status indexes) have generally provided too gross a screen to make them really valuable as predictors (Deutsch, 1973). As Bloom (1964) stated almost two decades ago, the experiences of children at every class level varies widely. It is unfair to characterize all low-income homes as not being stimulating. It is also inaccurate to assume that all middle-class homes are warm and stimulating for children.

Over the past 2 decades, there have been a number of efforts directed at developing more sensitive measures of children's developmental environments (Bradley & Caldwell, 1978). Rather than utilizing

---

***Robert H. Bradley and Stephen L. Rock.*** • Center for Child Development and Education, University of Arkansas at Little Rock, Little Rock, Arkansas 72204.

structural and status indexes such as parental occupation, parental education, size of family, and type of dwelling, the newer types of environmental measures assess processes within a child's environment, processes that are assumed to play a more direct and immediate role in children's development. The types of processes most commonly contained in the newer environmental measures include specific transactions between parent and child, the types and quantity of objects available in the environment, specific events that occur in the home environment, experiences designed to stimulate some aspect of a child's development, and the general quality of the physical environment in a home. These measures of more specific aspects of a child's developmental environment appear to be more strongly related to school achievement than socioeconomic status (SES) indexes (Bradley, Caldwell, & Elardo, 1977; Marjoribanks, 1972; Moore, 1968). The discrepancy may be particularly evident among minority populations where ethnicity and social status are often confounded (Bradley, Caldwell, & Elardo, 1977; Havighurst, 1976; White & Watts, 1973).

The use of environmental process measures appear to offer promise for increasing the efficiency of batteries used in screening for developmental risk (Bradley & Caldwell, 1978; Frankenburg, 1977). For example, van Doorninck (1977) conducted a 5-year longitudinal study of homes of 286 infants who were part of an early learning project in Syracuse, New York. The environments of the infants were all assessed using the Home Observation for Measurement of the Environment (HOME). Years later, 94 of these children were found still to be enrolled in elementary schools within the Syracuse area. About 60% of the participants were from lower SES groups, and 75% were white. The scores that families had made on the HOME Inventory when the participating child was 12 months old were correlated to school failure (defined in terms of repetiton of grade, referral for a learning problem, grades of D or F in reading and math). The overall correlation was .47. When the HOME score was below 16 (out of a possible 45), 71% later developed some type of school problem. Correspondingly, 81% of those with high scores on the HOME (at least 30 out of 45) were achieving at grade level. In this latter group, the HOME Inventory was a more accurate predictor of later school success than were SES variables.

The HOME Inventory used by van Doorninck *et al.* (1975) has become one of the most widely used environmental process measures. A series of investigations reported by Bradley, Caldwell, and Elardo has revealed a substantial relation between aspects of the home environments measured with the HOME inventory and children's intellectual and language development during the preschool years (Bradley & Caldwell, 1976, 1979, 1980, 1981; Bradley, Caldwell, & Elardo, 1979; Elardo,

Bradley, & Caldwell, 1975, 1977). Other investigators employing the HOME Inventory have also found substantial relationships with various measures of children's development during the first 3 years of life (Ramey, Mills, Campbell, & O'Brien, 1975; Siegel, 1981; Wulbert, Inglis, Kriegsmann, & Mills, 1975). A recent study by Bradley and Caldwell (1984b) reveals a similarly strong relationship between HOME scores taken when children were in the first 2 years of life and achievement test scores in the first grade.

This chapter addresses two main themes: (a) to describe the ability of the HOME Inventory by itself (preschool version) to predict children's later school failure, and (b) to describe development of an elementary-age version of the HOME.

## THE HOME INVENTORY AND SCHOOL FAILURE

The purpose of the current study is to examine the ability of the HOME Inventory by itself to predict poor achievement and poor school adjustment in children ages 10, 11, and 12. In addition, it is designed to examine the extent to which these school outcomes are, in theory, predictable from a battery of environmental measures; these measures include both the early HOME scores, the HOME scores obtained at elementary school age, and a variety of other status and structural measures (e.g., presence of father, mother's age, mother's education, SES).

### Method

#### *Sample*

Data from 56 normal fifth and sixth grade children and their families were used in the study. The children were obtained from a larger group of some 105 children who participated in a longitudinal observation and intervention study (Caldwell, Elardo, & Elardo, 1972). All of the participants originally resided in a catchment area in Little Rock, Arkansas, which contained a heterogeneous mixture of both black and white families. The black families were predominantly lower income and working class, but also included some middle class. The white families were predominantly working class and middle class. The current sample is 50% black and 50% white. The mean 3-year Stanford-Binet IQ scores for the participants in the current study was 99.4. The number of cases varied somewhat from analysis to analysis depending on the data that were available.

### *Instruments*

The HOME Inventory (infant version) was administered to all participating families when the children were 12 months of age. The HOME Inventory is an observation/interview technique that assesses the quality of stimulation available to the child in the home. It is composed of six subscales:

1. Emotional and verbal responsitivity of the parent
2. Acceptance of the child
3. Organization of the environment
4. Provision of appropriate play materials
5. Maternal involvement with child
6. Variety in daily stimulation

When the children were ages 10 and 11, the elementary version of the HOME Inventory was administered to the families. This version was composed of eight subscales:

1. Emotional and verbal responsivity
2. Encouragement of maturity
3. Emotional climate
4. Growth-fostering materials and experiments
5. Provision for active stimulation
6. Family participation in developmentally stimulating experiences
7. Paternal involvement
8. Aspects of the physical environment

The children were given the Stanford-Binet (1960) intelligence test when they were 3 years of age and the Science Research Associates' (SRA) (1971) achievement battery in fifth and sixth grade. During the same year that the achievement battery was administered, the classroom behavior of each children was rated by his or her teacher using the Classroom Behavior Inventory (Schaefer & Aaronson, 1965). It is composed of three bipolar scales: task orientation/distractibility; introversion/extroversion; and consideration/hostility. Teachers were also asked to rate the overall classroom adjustment for each child on a 4-point scale (1 = very poorly adjusted; 2 = some adjustment problems; 3 = generally adjusted; 4 = well adjusted).

## Results

Bivariate correlations were obtained between home environment variables at the two ages (1 year and 10–11 years) and child development measures (SRA composite scores and teacher ratings of student adjustment). Modest correlations ($N$ = 56 children) were obtained between SRA composite scores and the following variables: (a) total score of the Infant HOME; (b) play materials subscale of the Infant HOME; (c) materials and experiences subscale of the Elementary HOME; (d) physical environment subscale of the Elementary HOME; (e) mother's age; and (f) Stanford-Binet at 36 months. None of these correlations was above .38. For teacher ratings of student adjustment, significant correlations were found with the following variables: (a) play materials subscale of the Infant HOME; (b) total score for the Elementary HOME; (c) responsibility subscale of the Elementary HOME; (d) materials and experiences subscale of the Elementary HOME; and (e) SES. Again these correlations were modest, with none above .37.

Stepwise descriminant functions were computed for each variable to determine which combinations of variables would most efficiently predict performance on each child development criterion variable. For the discriminant analysis on SRA composite scores, students were classified as successful achievers if they recorded scores greater than the 33rd percentile or as poor achievers if they recorded scores less than or equal to the 33rd percentile. (The 33rd percentile was selected for two reasons, one statistical and one conceptual. First, to have selected a lower cutoff point would have resulted in too few students in one group. Second, the 33rd percentile includes many children who are having school achievement problems while not distorting the statistical results by including an excessive number of children who may have handicaps.) No significant relationships were identified by the discriminant analyses.

For teacher ratings of student adjustment, students were grouped into a well-adjusted group (rating of 3 or 4) and a poorly adjusted group (rating of 1 or 2). Table 1 shows the results of the stepwise discriminant analysis that was conducted. (The $N$ in Table 1 was 48 instead of 56 because CBI scores were available on only 48 subjects.) Five variables were found to significantly relate to teacher ratings of adjustment, entering into the equation in the following order: (a) SES; (b) parental responsivity subscale of the Elementary HOME; (c) mother's age; (d) the parental responsivity subscale of the Infant Home; and (e) Infant HOME total scores. With these five variables, a canonical correlation of .49 was obtained, accounting for approximately 24% of the total variance. Of the five variables that contributed significantly to the relationship with student adjustment, the responsivity subscale of the Infant HOME and the total score of the Infant HOME contributed the most to the relationship, as shown by the standardized discriminant function coefficients (Table 2). As shown in Table 3, this set of variables accurately predicted 83.3% of group membership.

**Table 1.** Stepwise Discriminant Functions with Groups Defined by Teacher's Rating of Adjustment ($N = 48$)

| Step | Variable entered | Significance |
|---|---|---|
| 1 | SES | .01 |
| 2 | Elementary HOME subscale 1—responsivity | .02 |
| 3 | Mother's age | .02 |
| 4 | Infant HOME subscale 1—responsivity | .03 |
| 5 | Infant HOME—total score | .03 |
| 6 | Stanford-Binet | .05 |
| 7 | Elementary HOME subscale 4—materials & experiences | .08 |
| 8 | Elementary HOME subscale 8—physical environment | .11 |
| 9 | Presence of father | .13 |
| 10 | Infant HOME subscale 4—toys | .18 |
| 11 | Elementary HOME—total score | .25 |

## Discussion

The relation between the early HOME scores and teachers' judgments about student adjustment were generally in line with what was hypothesized. Although no attempt was made to determine optimal cutoff scores for school adjustment, the overall hit-rate was reasonably good at 83%. The sensitivity to poor adjustment was also reasonably good at 71%.

The ability of the HOME scale to predict poor achievement test

**Table 2.** Standard Canonical Discriminant Function Coefficients for Significant Variables

| | Function 1 |
|---|---|
| Mother's age | .56 |
| SES | .37 |
| Infant HOME-total | .64 |
| Infant HOME—subscale 1—responsivity | −.83 |
| Elementary HOME—subscale 1—responsivity | .55 |
| Canonical correlation = .49 | |

**Table 3.** Classification of Cases by Discriminant Function

| | | Predicted | |
|---|---|---|---|
| Actual group | *n* | Group 1 | Group 2 |
| Group 1—poorly adjusted | 7 | 5 (71.4%) | 2 (28.6%) |
| Group 2—well adjusted | 41 | 6 (14.6%) | 35 (85.4%) |
| 83.8% classified correctly | | | |

scores was less than expected, given previous research showing strong relations with IQ scores during the preschool years. Part of the reason may lie in the inconsistency with which SRA tests were administered across schools. In addition to some informal information about test administration received from school personnel, there were several indications in the data that cast suspicion on the validity of the SRA scores. These were (a) the generally flat or platakurtic distribution of scores, (b) the higher-than-expected mean (61st percentile), (c) the low correlation with IQ (.38), and (d) the negligible correlation with SES (.16). For this reason, we are attempting to secure additional information about the participants' school performance, so that more meaningful analyses can be run.

## DEVELOPMENT OF THE HOME INVENTORY-ELEMENTARY VERSION

As part of our continuing efforts to examine the relation between home environment and children's development, we have begun work on a new version of the HOME Inventory. It is designed for use with families of elementary-age children (6–10 years of age). As with the infant and preschool versions of the HOME Inventory, the elementary version was designed to be a measure of the quality and quantity of support for cognitive, social, and emotional development available to a child in the home environment. Our intention in designing the instrument was that it not only be a sensitive barometer of the kinds of experiences typically available to children in the home but that it also be relatively easy to use. The instrument is constructed so that it requires approximately one hour to give; thus, it is not truly a screening measure. Nonetheless, it provides information on a broad array of environmental transactions, events, and objects in a relatively short span of time. It provides an array of information about a child's typical experiences in the home that can be useful in helping to make decisions regarding the need for or type of intervention for children who are at risk for developmental delays.

The elementary version of the HOME Inventory was developed in essentially the same fashion that the infant and preschool versions were developed. Specifically, an extensive review of the available empirical and theoretical literature in child development was conducted (Bradley & Tedesco, 1982; Caldwell, 1968). Based on these reviews, more than 100 items were constructed. Each item was designed to assess some aspect of a child's environment that seemed salient for the elementary school period. The items index such things as transactions between parent and child, varieties of enriching materials and experiences, the amount of contact with various adults in the family, physical conditions within the home and neighborhood, availability of certain intellectual and language experiences, the quality of nurturance and discipline, and maturing activities required of the children. As with the other versions of the HOME Inventory, scoring of items was based on observation and on interview questions obtained during a semistructured interview in the home with the child's primary caregiver. In all instances the child was also present during the interview. Preliminary field tests were conducted with 28 families, resulting in some modifications of administrative and scoring criteria for items. At that point, the number of items was reduced to 91.

The 91-item HOME was administered to 141 families rearing elementary-age children in Little Rock, Arkansas. Families were selected on the basis of the child's race and gender; approximately 50% were white, 50% were black, with equal proportions of each gender. The SES range in both racial groups was considerable, with the black group showing a greater percentage of low-income families and the white group showing a greater percentage of middle-income families. These demographic characteristics correspond to the demographic characteristics for the area.

### Results

During the process of scale construction, several data analytic studies were done: factor analysis, item analysis, and a variety of correlation analyses using various environmental and developmental measures. Factor analysis was used as a basis of determining which of the 91 items to retain and to help cluster items. The result was a 59-item scale.

The items are clustered into eight subscales. The names of the subscales are listed in previous sections, but will be referred to by more abbreviated titles:

1. Parental responsivity

2. Physical environment
3. Materials and experience
4. Active stimulation
5. Encouraging maturity
6. Emotional climate
7. Parental involvement
8. Family participation

### *Means, Standard Deviations, and Reliability Coefficients*

The means, standard deviations, interobserver agreement, and alpha coefficients were computed for each of the eight subscales and the total HOME score. Based on a sample of 55 cases across four home observers, the average level of interobserver agreement was 95%. The means, standard deviations, and alpha coefficients are displayed in Table 4. The mean for the total HOME score was 44.2 (*SD* 9.6). Alpha coefficients for the subscales ranged from .50 for emotional climate to .87 for emotional and verbal responsivity of parents. The alpha coefficient for the total score was .92. These findings are generally in line with those reported for the infant and preschool versions of the HOME Inventory (Caldwell & Bradley, 1979). In sum, the test seems to record a range of responses from home environments and appears to be reasonably reliable. It shows substantial reliability at the level of the total HOME score.

### *Socioeconomic Status, Family Structure, and Family History*

Among the validity studies conducted on the HOME for families of elementary-age children were those examining the relation between the HOME and other measures of the child's environment. Specifically,

**Table 4.** Means, Standard Deviations, and Reliability Coefficients for Elementary HOME

| HOME scales | No. of items | *M* | *SD* | Reliability coefficient |
|---|---|---|---|---|
| Parental responsivity | 10 | 8.9 | 2.3 | .87 |
| Physical environment | 8 | 7.1 | 1.6 | .82 |
| Materials & experiences | 8 | 5.5 | 2.0 | .70 |
| Active stimulation | 8 | 3.8 | 2.5 | .77 |
| Encouraging maturity | 7 | 4.8 | 1.8 | .70 |
| Emotional climate | 8 | 6.3 | 1.4 | .50 |
| Parental involvement | 4 | 2.5 | 1.5 | .71 |
| Family participation | 6 | 4.9 | 1.4 | .54 |
| Total score | 59 | 44.2 | 9.6 | .92 |

**Table 5.** Correlations between Elementary HOME Scores, Socioeconomic Status, Family Structure, and Family History ($N = 141$)

| HOME scales | Mother's education | Mother's occupation | Father's occupation | SES[a] | Father's presence | Life events |
|---|---|---|---|---|---|---|
| Parental responsivity | .32** | .38** | .30* | .23* | .25* | .08 |
| Physical environment | .30** | .35** | .26** | .28** | .14 | .04 |
| Materials & experience | .39** | .30** | .37** | .30** | .16 | .06 |
| Active stimulation | .43** | .28** | .42** | .25* | .25* | .01 |
| Encouraging maturity | .17 | .26** | .20* | .22* | .05 | .02 |
| Emotional climate | .08 | .24* | .09 | .22* | .01 | −.05 |
| Paternal involvement | .08 | .13 | .26** | .11 | .02 | .09 |
| Family participation | .40** | .37** | .36** | .32** | .25* | .13 |
| Total score | .34** | .46** | .46** | .36** | .25* | .07 |

[a]Based on Hollingshead's (1975) 4-Factor Index of Social Position.
*$p < .05$. **$p < .01$.

scores on the HOME were correlated with measures of SES, family structure, and family history. Previous research suggests that the infant and preschool versions of the HOME are moderately related to various SES and family structure characteristics (Bradley, & Caldwell, 1979, 1984a; Bradley, Caldwell, & Elardo, 1977; Elardo, Bradley, & Caldwell, 1975; Hollenbeck, 1978; Nihira, Meyers, & Mink, 1980).

Table 5 displays the correlations between the HOME and three specific SES indexes (maternal education, maternal occupation, paternal occupation), a composite SES index (Hollingshead's 4-factor Index) (Hollingshead, 1975), one family structure measure (father's presence), and one family history measure (Coddington's Life Events Record) (Coddington, 1972). In general, moderate correlations were obtained between the HOME and the four SES measures (.2 to .5). Marginally significant relations ($N = 141$) were observed between the HOME and the father's presence ($r = .25$). No significant relations were observed between the HOME and the Coddington Life Events Record.

As expected, the correlations were in the same general range as were obtained with the other two versions of the Inventory (Caldwell & Bradley, 1979). Relations are significant but modest. Any higher correlations might mean that the HOME was essentially redundant of these more global measures. Any lower correlations would mean that the HOME was not tapping some of the real differences in parenting practices, events, and materials that one typically finds in families from different social strata and family backgrounds.

The specific pattern of relations between HOME subscale scores and the various SES indexes followed predictable lines. To wit, parental education, occupational status, and overall SES were more strongly related to the general physical environment in the home, the richness of language used, the types of material and experiences provided for children, and the general experiences in which parents were involved. SES seemed less strongly associated with the general emotional climate of the home or the extent of the father's involvement, and the father's presence showed little relation to most HOME scores. A small but significant relation was obtained for the degree of family participation in developmentally stimulating activities, the amount of active stimulation provided to the child, and the level of emotional and verbal responsivity provided the child. This last relation is interesting in light of findings that mothers tend to be more responsive to their infants in the presence of the father than when no father is present (Pedersen, Yarrow, Anderson, & Coin, 1978).

### *Academic Achievement*

Because the HOME was designed to assess the quality of support for cognitive development available to a child in the home environment, examining the relation between the HOME and children's school achievement was an important facet of scale validation. It was anticipated that the correlation between the home environment and academic achievement of elementary children would not be as high as the correlation with cognitive development among preschool children. As expected, results indicated a moderate level of correlation between HOME and SRA scores. The strongest relation was between SRA scores and the provision for active stimulation subscale of the HOME ($r$ = .39). This subscale includes such things as judicious use of TV, encouragement of hobbies, provision for memberships in organizations, use of libraries, and arrangements for trips and visits to cultural events and facilities. Four other HOME subscales (parental responsivity, physical environment, materials and experiences, family participation) showed significant relations with SRA scores, with correlations ranging from .35 to .27 ($N$ = 141 children). The total HOME score was correlated .37 with SRA. Although correlation between elementary HOME and SRA were significant, they were not as high as those reported between the preschool HOME and first grade achievement scores (Bradley & Caldwell, 1984b); nonetheless, the correlations do indicate that the HOME may be valid in the sense that it is related to measures of cognitive performance.

### *California Q-Sort*

Because the HOME is also intended as a means of assessing the quality of the support for social and emotional development available to a child in the home environment, it was necessary to examine its relation to measures of socioemotional development in children. For this purpose, the California Q-Sort was administered to each child's parents. The responding parent was asked to describe his or her child using the 43 adjectives included in the scale. Items were sorted into seven categories from "most like" to "most unlike." A factor analysis was used to cluster the 43 items. The result was 13 brief scales that, on the basis of item content, were labeled as follows:

1. Mature
2. Considerate
3. Reflective
4. Feminine, task-oriented
5. Self-reliant, goal-directed
6. Optimistic
7. Competitive
8. Responsible
9. Masculine, noncompliant
10. Introverted
11. Extroverted
12. Creative
13. Easy-going

In general, the correlations are modest, with the highest being only around .4. Seven of the brief scales from the Q-sort showed little or no relation to HOME scores. These included mature, feminine, optimistic, competitive, introverted, extraverted, and easy-going. Still, other child characteristics had moderate relations to HOME scores. These included considerate, reflective, self-reliant, responsible, masculine, and creative.

For example, children rated as "considerate" by their parents came from homes with slightly higher scores in such areas as parental responsitivity, encouraging maturity, emotional climate, and paternal involvement. Children described as "self-reliant, goal-directed" came from homes with higher scores on such subscales as parental responsivity, materials and experiences, provision for active stimulation, encouraging maturity, emotional climate, and family participation. Children judged as "creative" came from homes with higher scores on parental responsivity, materials and experiences, provision for active stimulation, and family participation in developmentally enriching experiences.

In sum, the pattern of correlations obtained between HOME scores and scores on the California Q-sort may be taken as evidence that the HOME is tapping elements of the quality of support for socioemotional development available in the child's home environment. The observed correlations, although not strong, are basically in the direction one would predict.

## SUMMARY

The two studies reported in this chapter are related. They are part of a series of investigations that involve development of home environment measures and the use of those measures to delineate the relation between children's home environments and their behavioral development. Previous investigations in the series had established that the infant and the preschool versions of the HOME Inventory were reliable measures of the child's home environment and that they were significantly related to measures of cognitive and social development throughout the early childhood period (Bradley, 1982). In the first study reported in this chapter, 56 children who have been participating in a longitudinal study were assessed during fifth or sixth grade with the elementary version of the HOME, the SRA Achievement Battery, and the Classroom Behavior Inventory. Low to moderate correlations were observed between infant HOME, elementary HOME, 3-year IQ, 10-year SRA scores, and 10-year school adjustment scores (.3–.4). However, a discriminant function analysis using environmental variables and early developmental variables did not provide clear separation between poor achievers and adequate achievers.

The second study reported an attempt to develop and validate a version of the HOME Inventory of families of elementary-age children. Results indicated that the new elementary version was reliable. Data also suggested it was valid in terms of predicted associations with SES indexes and child development measures—albeit the correlations with developmental measures were not as high as for the infant and the preschool versions of HOME. Inconsistencies in the administration of the SRA achievement tests by local schools may have contributed to the lower-than-expected levels of correlation between HOME and SRA for both studies.

## REFERENCES

Bloom, B. (1964). *Stability and change in human characteristics.* New York: Wiley.

Bradley, R., & Caldwell, B. (1976). The relationship of infant's home environment to mental test performance at 54 months: A follow-up study. *Child Development, 47,* 1172–1174.

Bradley, R., & Caldwell, B. (1978). Screening the environment. *American Journal of Orthopsychiatry, 48,* 114–130.

Bradley, R., & Caldwell, B. (1979). Home observation for measurement of the environment: A revision of the preschool scale. *American Journal of Mental Deficiency, 84,* 235–244.

Bradley, R., & Caldwell, B. (1980). Home environment, cognitive competence, and IQ among males and females. *Child Development, 51,* 1140–1148.

Bradley, R., & Caldwell, B. (1981). The HOME Inventory: A validation of the preschool scale for black children. *Child Development, 52,* 708–710.

Bradley, R. 1982. The HOME Inventory: A review of the first fifteen years. In N. Anastasiow, W. Frankenburg, & A. Fandal (Eds.), *Identifying the developmentally delayed child.* Baltimore: Univ. Park Press.

Bradley, R., & Caldwell, B. (1984a). The HOME Inventory and family demographics. *Developmental Psychology, 20,* 315–320.

Bradley, R., & Caldwell, B. (1984b). The relation of infant's home environments to achievement test performance in first grade: A follow-up study. *Child Development, 55,* 516–524.

Bradley, R., Caldwell, B., & Elardo, R. (1977). Home environment, social status, and mental test performance. *Journal of Educational Psychology, 69,* 697–701.

Bradley, R., Caldwell, B., & Elardo, R. (1979). Home environment and cognitive development in the first two years of life: A cross-lagged panel analysis. *Developmental Psychology, 15,* 246–250.

Bradley, R., & Tedesco, L. (1982). Environmental correlates of mental retardation. In J. Lachenmeyer & McGibbs (Eds.), *Psychopathology in Childhood.* New York: Gardner Press.

Caldwell, B. (1968). On designing supplementary environments for early child development. *Boston Association for the Education of Young Children (BAEYC) Reports, 10,* 1–11.

Caldwell, B., & Bradley, R. (1979). *Home Observation for Measurement of the Environment.* Little Rock: Univ. of Arkansas at Little Rock.

Caldwell, B., Elardo, P., & Elardo, R. (1972). *The longitudinal observation and intervention study: A preliminary report.* Paper presented at the meeting of the Southeastern Conference on Research in Child Development, Williamsburg, Virginia.

Coddington, R. (1972). The significance of life events as etiologic factors in the diseases of children: II. A study of a normal population. *Journal of Psychosomatic Research, 16,* 205–213.

Deutsch, C. P. (1973). Social class and child development. In B. M. Caldwell & H. N. Ricciuti (Eds.), *Review of Child Development Research* (Vol. 3). Chicago: Univ. of Chicago Press.

Elardo, R., Bradley, R., & Caldwell, B. (1975). The relation of infants' home environments to mental test performance from 6 to 36 months: A longitudinal analysis. *Child Development, 46,* 71–76.

Elardo, R., Bradley, R., & Caldwell, B. (1977). A longitudinal study of the relation of infants' home environments to language development at age three. *Child Development, 48,* 595–603.

Hollenbeck, A. (1978). Early infant home environments: Validation of the Home Observation for Measurement of the Environment Inventory. *Developmental Psychology, 14,* 416–418.

Frankenburg, W. (1977). Increasing the lead time for the preschool-aged handicapped child. In M. Karnes (Ed.), *Not all little wagons are red.* Arlington, Virginia: Council for Exceptional Children.

Havighurst, R. (1976). The relative importance of social class and ethnicity in human development. *Human Development, 19,* 56–64.

Hollingshead, A. (1975). *Four-factor index of social status.* New Haven, CT: Privately printed.

Majoribanks, K. (1972). Environment, social class, and mental abilities. *Journal of Educational Psychology, 43,* 103–109.

Moore, T. (1968). Language and intelligence: A longitudinal study of the first eight years, Part II: Environmental correlates of mental growth. *Human Development, 11,* 1–24.

Nie, N., Hull, C., Jenkins, J., Steinbrenner, K., & Bent, C. (1975). *Statistical package for the social sciences.* New York: McGraw-Hill.

Nihira, K., Meyers, C., & Mink, I. (1980). Home environment, family adjustment, and the development of mentally retarded children. *Applied Research in Mental Retardation, 1,* 5–24.

Pedersen, F., Yarrow, L., Anderson, B., & Cain, R. (1978). Conceptualization of father influences in the infancy period. In M. Lewis & L. Rosenblum (Eds.), *The social network of the developing infant.* New York: Plenum.

Ramey, C., Mills, P., Campbell, R., & O'Brien, C. (1975). Infants' home environments: A comparison of high-risk families from general population. *American Journal of Mental Deficiency, 80,* 40–42.

*Science Research Associates Achievement Series.* (1971). Chicago, IL: Science Research Associates.

Schaefer, E., & Aaronson, M. (1965). *Classroom Behavior Inventory: Preschool to primary.* Chapel Hill, NC: Unpublished form.

Siegel, L. S. (1981). Infant tests as predictors of cognitive and language development at two years. *Child Development, 52,* 545–557.

*Stanford-Binet Intelligence Scales.* (1960). Boston: Houghton-Miflin.

van Doorninck, W. (1977). Families of children at risk for school problems. In M. Krajicek & A. Tearney (Eds.), *Detection of developmental problems in children.* Baltimore: University Park Press.

White, B., & Watts, J. (1973). *Experience and environment.* Englewood Cliffs, New Jersey: Prentice-Hall.

Wulbert, M., Inglis, S., Kriegsmann, E., & Mills, B. (1975). Language delay and associated mother–child interactions. *Developmental Psychology, 2,* 61–70.

*CHAPTER 10*

# Simultaneous Technique for Acuity and Readiness Testing

*Raymond A. Sturner, Sandra G. Funk, and James A. Green*

Almost all pediatricians feel that developmental screening should be a standard part of routine child health examinations (Smith, 1978). However, this belief is only rarely reflected in actual practice. The reason most often given by pediatricians for their failure to carry out the screening is that the tests are too time-consuming. Although pediatricians typically claim that they are able to accomplish developmental screening through informal observations of the child's responses to the usual health examination procedures, this approach to screening has been shown to be unreliable (Bierman, Connor, Vaage, & Honzik, 1964; Korsch, Cobb, & Ashe, 1961). On the theory that reliable, valid, and efficient developmental screening can be accomplished during the course of routine health examinations, providing simultaneous screening of health and development, the current study attempted to revitalize and systematize the observational process that pediatricians claim to do during health examinations. The research being reported here is an attempt to test the proposition that simultaneous screening can be both effective and efficient. Specifically, it uses the routine preschool vision acuity screening test to not only screen for visual acuity, but also as a means to detect children with educational handicaps.

The procedure used is designated Simultaneous Technique for Acuity and Readiness Testing (START). To date, approximately 3,000 preschool children (mostly between the ages of 4 and $5\frac{1}{2}$ years) have been studied in order to determine whether vision screening can be used to

***Raymond A. Sturner, Sandra G. Funk, and James A. Green*** • Department of Pediatrics, Duke University Medical Center, Durham, North Carolina 27710.

obtain clinically useful developmental data. Several studies have been performed, including initial instrument development and item selection, tests of temporal stability, interrater reliability, item sensitivity, and concurrent and predictive validity. A study of the health functioning portion of the test has been performed to assure that the vision screening portion of the test is not impaired by test alterations; time-motion estimates were also collected during that study. Finally, health practitioner acceptability has been surveyed and field testing by practitioners has been carried out to identify any obstacles to clinical utilization.

## DESCRIPTION

Standard preschool vision screening procedures have been modified to make it possible to adjust testing methods as the developmental level of the child becomes evident, and to allow for systematic recording and quantification of behavioral responses. START consists of two phases. In Phase 1, the Test Selection Phase, the child is presented with several vision testing approaches that vary in difficulty (Snellen Letter Naming, Snellen Letter Drawing, letter E card matching, letter E hand matching, and picture cards—both Allen and an experimental set). During this phase, the tester rates the child's performance and selects the most suitable vision screening approach, based on an overall judgment as to the most precise (optically correct) method to which the child is able to respond (Snellen Letter Chart before Illiterate E Chart, before Allen Picture Cards) (Brown, 1975). In Phase 2, the Test Administration Phase, the tester utilizes the approach selected to screen the child for visual acuity according to our standard protocol.

Data relating to development that were obtained from each child included the correctness of responses to each of the five vision testing approaches presented during Phase 1, as well as ratings (on a 4-point intensity scale) of specific behaviors observed during Phase 2. These included ability to follow a 3-part command, and judgment as to overall performance (e.g., persistence).

## TESTER TRAINING AND RELIABILITY

Testers have been college graduates who are not psychological or health professionals. The training procedure is not an unduly lengthy process. It involves studying a manual, watching a trained tester, and then practicing on a few children while the experienced tester observes and scores for reliability. A videotaped training procedure is currently being developed, and may be a viable alternative to hands-on tutorial.

Prior to each study, interrater reliability was obtained for each of the testers with one or two trainers, on a minimum of 15 children. In each cohort, the average agreement across items was 95% or above.

Forty-four 3- and 4-year-old children attending two private, middle-class racially mixed day care centers in the Durham, North Carolina, area were tested twice—two weeks apart—with the START protocol to assess the temporal stability or test–retest reliability of START. The second testing was performed by a tester who was not present at the time of the initial testing and who was blind to the earlier test results. The average agreement between the two ratings for each item on the test was 78%. Not surprisingly, the cognitively based items such as understanding the E match game (which had 100% agreement across the two sessions) were more stable than the more transient behavior reaction ratings, such as interest in the test (65% agreement). Many of the behavioral rating items have been omitted from later editions of the test, which should therefore be more temporally stable.

## ADEQUACY FOR VISION ACUITY SCREENING

A study was conducted to compare the START vision screening procedure with standard preschool vision screening to ensure that the modified vision testing procedure did not detract from its intended purpose as a screen for poor visual acuity.

Because the Society for the Prevention of Blindness is considered the authority for vision screening in this country, its testing protocol was chosen for comparison: The Society has recommended use of the E test (often called the "illiterate" E because the child does not have to be able to read, but merely indicates the direction of the "legs" of the E) for this age group. The subjects were 216 Head Start children aged 3 to 6 years with a median age of 4.2 years. Each child was screened by the START screen and the illiterate E test using the Society protocol, counterbalancing both order of administration and testers. As outlined earlier, the START test utilizes the most optically precise test that the child proves capable of responding to during the initial phase of the procedure. The criterion for passing the Society test was 20/40 vision in each eye. The cutoff for START testing was optically identical when chart methods were used (Snellen Letter or E), but the test distance was 20 ft for the Society test and 15 ft for START. The shorter distance was used in an attempt to avoid the need for a testing assistant to stand with the child, as seemed necessary when the child was so far away from the tester and chart. In addition, the shorter distance was used to standardize our procedure, as the guidelines for the Allen picture card test utilized by START require 15 ft on some occasions (Allen, 1957). Sev-

**Table 1.** Clinical Indexes for the Prediction of Ophthalmologist's Retest Results by START and Society Tests*

| | START | Society |
|---|---|---|
| Co-positivity | .61 | .69 |
| Co-negativity | .61 | .47 |
| Predictive value | .26 | .22 |
| Overreferral rate | .32 | .43 |
| Underreferral rate | .07 | .06 |
| Untestable rate | .07 | .13 |

*Note.* The indexes are presented to facilitate comparison of the START and Society tests; they should not be taken as representing estimates based on the whole population because of the nonrandom sampling of children.
*Untestables are included as screening failures for both tests.

enty-two children, including most test failures and some who passed the tests, were rescreened by a pediatric ophthalmologist using Allen cards, as was his practice.

The results showed that, excluding untestables, the acuity data from the two screening tests were quite similar (88% agreement), and both tests agreed well with the additional screening by a pediatric ophthalmologist (Table 1). Because the START test allowed for individualized acuity test procedures based on the child's capability, it resulted in one-half the number of untestables (7% vs. 13%). With START, individualized screening protocols reduce untestability for children who do not understand either type of E game, since they can be tested with picture cards. Additionally, individualized screening permits the use of a more precise acuity measure for those children who can respond to the letter chart by naming or drawing the letters in the air (10% in this sample). An additional study found that START fails some children who, although passed by the ophthalmologists' Allen card screen, do have mild acuity problems requiring treatment (as determined by complete ophthalmologic examination). The START took an average of 8 minutes for a 4-year-old, including scoring. Whereas this was slightly longer than the time needed to administer the Society's illiterate E protocol (2 minutes longer on the average), the lower untestable rate would decrease the number of rescreens required. In addition, START seems likely to be more cost effective, because it requires only one tester, as opposed to the four utilized by the test recommended by the Society (e.g., trainer, recorder, tester, and a person to stay with the child at the test line).

Therefore, the START screen can be recommended as a cost-effective and valid approach to preschool vision screening, apart from any consideration of the developmental data obtained (Sturner, Green, Funk, Jones, & Chandler, 1981).

## CONCURRENT VALIDITY

After preliminary item development, studies of validity were conducted over 3 successive years in a rural county of North Carolina. This county has somewhat higher education and income levels than the state as a whole, and thus more closely approximates national norms. Each year in February or March, children in this county who are to begin kindergarten the following fall are urged to attend a combined health screening and registration program. In the 3 cohorts studied, there were 1,154 $4\frac{1}{2}$ to $5\frac{1}{2}$-year-olds with approximately equal numbers of males and females and slightly more whites than nonwhites.

Each year, approximately one-third of the children–oversampling those at risk for developmental delay—were recalled after the initial START screening for concurrent developmental assessment. Stratified sampling techniques were based on an estimate of risk for developmental delay from independent screening tests—the short form of the Denver Developmental Screening Test (Sturner, Horton, Funk, Barton, Frothingham, & Cress, 1982) or a shortened form of the Minnesota Child Development Inventory (Sturner, Funk, Thomas, & Green, 1982), both developed for use in this study. The stratified sample received criterion testing using the McCarthy Scales of Children's Abilities (MSCA), except in 1 year, when the Stanford-Binet was utilized for further validation.

In order to help decide whether to alter the START items or omit some of them, item ranges and distributional properties were evaluated. Items were then correlated with the General Cognitive Index (GCI) of the MSCA to determine whether they were sensitive to the child's developmental level. Significant positive correlations were obtained in both cohorts for all items that remain in the test, except sentence reading. The correlation for this item may have been artificially low as the item had little variability, being successfully completed by very few children. Information obtained during the test selection phase of the procedure (picture naming, Snellen letter naming, drawing letters in the air) consistently showed the strongest relationships to McCarthy GCI scores ($r$'s ranged from .50 to .70, $p < .001$ in each case). Correlations for the second cohort were remarkably similar to those of the first, with those items showing the strongest correlations in the first cohort also showing the strongest relation to the criterion in the second. Altogether, differences in size and rank order of correlations appeared minor.

A collective look at the items reveals that a simple sum of vision items was found to be highly correlated with McCarthy GCI in both years ($r = .71$ and $r = .68$, respectively), and a stepwise multiple regression yielded a multiple *R* of .82 in the first cohort and .78 in the second. Discriminant analysis was performed to determine the degree to which START items could accurately distinguish those scoring more than 2 standard deviations below the mean on the McCarthy GCIs from the rest of the children (Sturner, Funk, Barton, Sparrow, & Frothingham, 1980). The cross-classification of actual McCarthy group membership with predicted McCarthy group membership showed that the START items were able to accurately identify 16 of the 19 children who actually received low scores on the McCarthy (co-positivity = .84) and 189 of the 201 who received scores of average or above (co-negativity = .94); it correctly classified 93.3% of the children (canonical *r* = .636). The discriminant analyses indicated that the excellent prediction of McCarthy group membership was possible utilizing a summative combination with approximate equal weighted component scores.

In Cohort 2, the discriminant analysis yielded similar results. Because more detailed item information was available for this cohort, it was used to devise a potential scoring system that consisted of the sum of the number of components passed, with a range of 0 to 7. Cross-tabulation of the score with GCI groupings indicated that the best prediction was obtained if the cutoff points were established at 0 to 1 points for a fail; 2 to 3 points for a questionable; and 4 or more points for a pass. Table 2 presents the resulting preliminary score classifications, cross-tabulated with the group McCarthy GCI scores, with less than 68 considered a positive case. As the table and clinical indices show, the scoring system was quite effective for predicting McCarthy grouping

**Table 2.** Concurrent Validation Scoring System for START Predicting McCarthy Group Membership

| | | McCarthy GCI score | | | |
|---|---|---|---|---|---|
| | | <68 | 68–83 | ≥84 | Total |
| START scores | Fail (0,1) | 13 | 3 | 0 | 16 |
| | Questionable (2,3) | 4 | 37 | 26 | 67 |
| | Pass (≥4) | 0 | 16 | 213 | 229 |
| | Total | 17 | 56 | 239 | 312 |

Indexes for prediction of low scorers (<68) on the McCarthy from failures on the START:

| | |
|---|---|
| Co-positivity | .76 |
| Co-negativity | .99 |
| Predictive value | .81 |
| Overreferral rate | 1.0% |
| Underreferral rate | 1.3% |
| % Agreement | 97.8% |

(predictive value = .81). Only 4 of the 17 at-risk children were not identified as failues (co-positivity = .76), and all 4 of those were classified as questionable. In addition, all 3 who failed the START but did not score in the below-68 group on the McCarthy were in the borderline (68–84) category. Overall, 97.8% were classified correctly.

An attempt was made to replicate and cross-validate this scoring method using another cohort, which received the Stanford-Binet instead of the McCarthy. The results show substantially weaker indexes. However, with one exception, overreferrals were again found in the borderline category. The weaker indexes may be a function of the fact that in the replication study some items were not scored in the same way as in earlier studies (to conserve time, picture cards were not scored singly). When the scoring was adjusted to reflect this difference, the sensitivity rose from .59 to .94.

Final selection of a scoring system is being postponed until analyses combining subjects across the years of testing can be performed, in order to have more stable estimates for the infrequent developmentally delayed children, and until predictive validation studies have been completed.

## PREDICTIVE VALIDITY

Preliminary results from school follow-up studies, although not yet complete, are encouraging. For the first cohort, follow-up reading achievement data are available for kindergarten, first, and second grades. For the two other cohorts, only first grade achievement data have been obtained. The kindergarten achievement test was the CTB-McGraw Hill Prescriptive Inventory (Level 1), which focuses on early reading-related achievement. First and second grade testing consisted of the Prescriptive Reading Inventory (Levels 2 and A). Scores on these instruments were transformed by CTB-McGraw Hill to estimate the California Achievement Test (CAT) scale and national percentile scores.

Correlational analyses showed that the START items most strongly related to achievement were basically the same cognitive items that were strongly related to concurrent criterion testing (*r*'s ranging from .46 to .53). As one would expect with an outcome measure that taps only achievement, the overall degree of relationship with the behavior items was much lower than for the cognitive items.

The pattern of relationship of the START items to first and second grade reading achievement was virtually identical to that observed in kindergarten, although diminishing somewhat from a kindergarten av-

**Table 3.** Relationship of START (Cognitive Items) and Criterion Tests to California Achievement Test Scores

| Preschool test | Kindergarten | First grade | Second grade |
|---|---|---|---|
| Cohort 1 | | | |
| START (Sum of cognitive items) | .64 | .56 | .53 |
| McCarthy GCI | .70 | .65 | .66 |
| Cohort 2 | | | |
| START (Sum of cognitive items) | | .58 | |
| McCarthy | | .63 | |
| Cohort 3 | | | |
| START (Sum of cognitive items) | | .59 | |
| Stanford-Binet IQ | | .35 | |

erage of $r$ of .49 for the best cognitive items to first and second grade average $r$'s of .42 and .39, respectively.

These item results were closely replicated across the other two cohorts, with some shift only in the lowest correlated behavioral items.

Summing across individual items, we found the cognitive portion of the START correlated well with reading achievement, with $r$'s of .64, .56, and .53 for kindergarten and Grades 1 and 2, respectively, in Cohort 1 ($N = 325$ to second grade); see Table 3. This group of items is capable of accounting for approximately one-third of the variance in reading achievement in the early schools years. The correlations between this group of START items and early school achievement compare surprisingly well with predictions from the McCarthy GCI or any of the other McCarthy Scales, and they are substantially higher than correlations obtained using the Stanford-Binet.

We are currently completing tracking in order to calculate clinical indexes (co-positivity and co-negativity) for the tests. It is possible that some of the decrement in prediction over time may be due to loss of those children doing poorly in school, because either retention or special class placement usually means that cohort equivalent achievement test scores are not available. Although the correlational data above are very encouraging, as with any screening test we are more concerned about predicting the problem cases rather than prediction across the entire range of abilities. Therefore, the clinical indexes will provide the critical test of ability of the START test to identify children with difficulties that appear later in school.

## OTHER STUDIES

START appears to be acceptable to a variety of health providers. Forty-seven health professionals at 11 different practice sites were made aware of the START procedure and surveyed by questionnaire; 88% indicated that they perceived the approach to screening to be sound. The preliminary scoring system is now being utilized at multiple clinical sites in North Carolina.

Studies of kindergarten children indicate that START is able to predict concurrent achievement in addition to developmental level (assessed by the McCarthy Scales). However, the results in this age group need replication. The possibility of extending the age range down to $3\frac{1}{2}$ years is also being explored. Additionally, a study utilizing a stereoptic testing procedure for kindergarten children indicates that excellent concurrent prediction of developmental functioning and achievement may be attained using such an adaptation (Stockton, 1981). In this study, some new items were quite predictive of developmental functioning. These included performance on a color vision test and on an acuity method requiring sustained attention to details of a visual target—the Landau Rings.

Studies describing an application of the simultaneous screening approach to preschool hearing testing have recently been published (Sturner, Green, & Funk, 1983). Screening for overall development was possible, but the sensitivity of this approach was less than that obtained by START screening. It is not yet known whether information that can be gleaned from the hearing test would provide useful complementary information to that obtained with the START.

## CONCLUSIONS

In conclusion, results of the current studies indicate that simultaneous screening for a child's health and development in pediatric practice is feasible. START is a reliable instrument for developmental screening, takes an average of 8 minutes to administer, and has both concurrent and predictive validity that is as good or better than can be attained by tests that have been designed exclusively for developmental information and are therefore less efficient. START screening also provides valid visual acuity information and has advantages of both cost effectiveness and accuracy as an acuity screen apart from any consideration of the developmental information obtained. More work is required to determine optimal scoring and training procedures.

Our major goal in exploring simultaneous screening for child health and development has been to stimulate health practitioners to utilize the so-called well-child check-up visit as a time to focus on the child's developmental functioning. As clinicians learn to catalogue meaningfully the observations of parents and children that are possible during everyday professional contacts, we believe that they will have taken a major step toward becoming adequate child development clinicians. Developmental evaluation and treatment of infants and children will interface better with primary child health care when syndromes of parent/child development that can be reliably and practically identified by health clinicians have been defined. Child development researchers might find that modified health encounters lend themselves to investigations of some developmental processes, such as those regarding stress reaction. Research conducted in these settings may be more readily translated into application than studies done in typical laboratory/experimental settings.

## REFERENCES


Allen, H. F. (1957). A new picture series for preschool vision testing. *American Journal of Ophthalmology, 44,* 38.

Bierman, J. J., Connor, A., Vaage, M., & Honzik, M. P. (1964). Pediatricians' assessment of the intellegence of two-year-olds and their mental test scores. *Pediatrics, 34,* 680.

Brown, M. S. (1975). Vision screening of preschool children. *Clinical Pediatrics, 14*(10), 968.

Korsch, B., Cobb, K., & Ashe, B. (1961). Pediatricians' appraisals of patients' intelligence. *Pediatrics, 27,* 990.

Smith, R. D. (1978). The use of developmental screening test by primary-care pediatricians. *Pediatrics, 93,* 524.

Stockton, J. S. (1981). *Simultaneous screening of school related behaviors and vision of kindergarten children.* Unpublished doctoral dissertation, Duke University.

Sturner, R. A., Funk, S. G., Barton, J., Sparrow, S., & Frothingham, T. E. (1980). Simultaneous screening for child health and development: A study of visual/developmental screening of preschool children. *Pediatrics, 65,* 1.

Sturner, R. A., Funk, S. G., Thomas, P. D., & Green, J. A. (1982). An adaptation of the Minnesota Child Development Inventory for preschool developmental screening. *Journal of Pediatric Psychology, 7,* 3.

Sturner, R. A., Green, J. A., & Funk, S. G. (1983). The relationship between developmental functioning and responses to hearing testing in preschool children. *Journal of Behavioral and Developmental Pediatrics,* 4(2), 94.

Sturner, R. A., Green, J. A., Funk, S. G., Jones, C. K., & Chandler, A. C. (1981). A developmental approach to preschool vision screening. *Journal of Pediatric Ophthalmology and Strabismus, 18,* 2.

Sturner, R. A., Horton, M., Funk, S. G., Barton, J., Frothingham, T. E., & Cress, J. N. (1982). Adaptations of the Denver Developmental Screening Test: A study of preschool screening. *Pediatrics, 69,* 3.

CHAPTER 11

# The Jansky Screening Index

## A SEVEN-YEAR PREDICTIVE EVALUATION AND COMPARATIVE STUDY

*Keith E. Barnes*

---

The Jansky Screening Index (JSI) (Jansky & de Hirsch, 1972) is a screening measure containing five subtests designed to identify those kindergarten-age children who are at risk for reading disabilities by the end of the second grade. The JSI takes approximately 20 minutes to administer and may be given by paraprofessionals or trained volunteers.

The five subtests of the JSI (letter naming, picture naming, word matching, Bender motor gestalt, and Binet sentence memory) were selected as the best predictors of later reading performance (as determined at the end of Grade 2 with the Gates Primary B Test, Gates and MacGinitie, 1965) from a pool of 19 kindergarten tests, many of which had been clinically evaluated in an earlier study by de Hirsch, Jansky, and Langford (1966). Then, in 1972, the battery was administered to a standardization sample of 402 kindergarten children. All these preschoolers spoke and understood conversational English and attended six public and two parochial (Roman Catholic) schools in two New York City school districts; however, the selection procedure was such that the children were neither randomly selected nor occupationally stratified.

Although the rationale behind the JSI was based on years of developmental research on reading disability by the test developers and their colleagues, the index itself still requires substantial additional research before it may be used as an adequately standardized screening measure. For example, there are no reliability data on the total index scores of the JSI, nor have there been any cross-validation studies on independent

*Keith E. Barnes* • Kelowna Mental Health Center, Kelowna, British Columbia, Canada V1Y 657.

samples reported in the research literature (Barnes, 1982). Furthermore, with the exception of the picture naming and letter naming subtests, the reliability coefficients for the other subtests are unacceptably low (Jansky & de Hirsch, 1972). In fact, it is possible that reducing the JSI to only the picture naming and letter naming subtests would be just as predictive of reading disability as the use of all five subtests. Another problem that is related to the use of the JSI for mass screening purposes is the necessity for collecting local norms in order to accurately determine appropriate cutoff scores. This is a crucial procedure because the selection of the cutoff scores specifically affects not only the index's sensitivity (percent of reading disorders identified) and specificity (percent of nonreading disabled identified) rates, but also its overall utility in predicting reading disability.

The present study had two major phases. The first involved cross-validation of the original Jansky and de Hirsch (1972) study on a stratified random sample of Western Canadian children. The second phase involved examination of the JSI's ability to predict later school performance. This second phase had three parts: comparison of the JSI total index with later student reading performance at the end of Grades 2 and 6; comparison of three JSI subscales administered at the end of kindergarten with end of Grade 2 and Grade 6 reading skills; and comparison of teacher ratings of reading in Grade 1 with student reading performance at the end of Grades 2 and 6.

## PHASE I: CROSS-VALIDATION OF THE JSI

### Subjects and Methods

A total of 290 children, stratified by gender, occupational status of their families' major wage earner, and geographic region, were randomly selected by a computer program. This normative sample was 31% of the total kindergarten population of the Central Okanagan School District in British Columbia. Of the 290 children selected, 143 were males and 142 were females; 209 were 5 years of age, and 81 were 6 years old. (These gender and age ratios were essentially the same as the breakdown of subjects for the 1972 JSI sample.)

The JSI was administered to this sample of students from a semirural community in Western Canada in their kindergarten year. Later, at the end of Grades 1, 2, and 6, the same children's levels of reading ability were assessed by standardized tests of reading ability and by teacher ratings. The data were then evaluated using regression, correlational, and predictive hit-rate analysis.

**TABLE 1.** Predictive Classification of White Children into Criterion Reading Groups for Barnes and Jansky and de Hirsch Studies*

Jansky & De Hirsch Study
Gates Primary B Reading Test

| Screening measure JSI total index | Problem** | No Problem** | Total |
|---|---|---|---|
| Suspect | 64 | 39 | 103 |
| Nonsuspect | 11 | 101 | 112 |
| Total | 75 | 140 | 215 |

Prevalence rate = 35%
Sensitivity 64/74 × 100 = 85%
Specificity 101/140 × 100 = 72%
Predictive value of a positive 64/103 × 100 = 62%
Predictive value of a negative 101/112 × 100 = 90%

JSI total index
Suspect = below $\bar{X}$ Nonsuspect = above $\bar{X}$

Barnes Study
Gates Primary B Reading Test

| Screening measure JSI total index | Problem** | No Problem** | Total |
|---|---|---|---|
| Suspect | 7 | 22 | 29 |
| Nonsuspect | 7 | 189 | 196 |
| Total | 14 | 211 | 225 |

Prevalence rate = 6%
Sensitivity 7/14 × 100 = 50%
Specificity 189/211 × 100 = 90%
Predictive value of a positive 7/29 × 100 = 24%
Predictive value of a negative 189/196 × 100 = 96%

JSI total index
Suspect = <27 Nonsuspect = 27 +

*Gates-MacGinitie Primary B Reading Test. **Problem = grade level < 2.3; no problem = 2.3+.

## Results

Barnes (1978) has reported a detailed comparative analysis of data from the present sample with data obtained by Jansky and de Hirsch (1972). He shows that the findings were essentially similar in terms of inter-test correlations and correlations between JSI total index scores and scores on standardized measures of reading ability at the end of Grade 1 and at the end of Grade 2. Comparative analysis for the two samples of students for the end of Grade 2 are shown in Table 1.

# PHASE II: PREDICTIVE STUDIES OF THE JSI

## Subjects and Methods

In Phase II of the study, the same Canadian subjects used in Phase I were followed up at the end of Grades 2 and 6.

The first comparison involved comparing kindergarten children's JSI total index results with their reading performance on the Gates-MacGinitie Primary B Reading Test (Gates & MacGinitie, 1965) at the end of Grade 2 and on the vocabulary and reading comprehension tests of the Canadian Tests of Basic Skills (CTBS) at the end of Grade 6 (King,

1974). The second comparison was between three subscales of the JSI (picture naming, letter naming, and word matching) and the same standardized reading tests administered at the end of Grades 2 and 6.

In a further comparison, teacher ratings at the end of Grade 1 were compared to student reading performance at the end of Grades 2 and 6, using the Gates and the CTBS as outcome measures.

**Table 2.** Comparative Analysis of Predictive Outcome for the JSI in Kindergarten with Teacher's Ratings in Grade 1 and Standardized Tests of Rading at the End of Grades 2 and 6

| | | Percentage | | | | |
|---|---|---|---|---|---|---|
| Initial screen | Measures | Prevalence | Sensitivity | Specificity | Value of + | Value of − |
| Kindergarten | End of Grade 2 | | | | | |
| JSI Picture Naming Test | Gates Primary B Reading Test | 6 | 71 | 83 | 22 | 98 |
| JSI Word Matching Test | Gates Primary B Reading Test | 6 | 57 | 85 | 20 | 97 |
| JSI Letter Naming Test | Gates Primary B Reading Test | 6 | 71 | 86 | 25 | 98 |
| JSI Total Index | Gates Primary B Reading Test | 14 | 50 | 90 | 24 | 96 |
| Kindergarten | End of Grade 6 | | | | | |
| JSI Picture Naming Test | Canadian Tests of Basic Skills | 14 | 46 | 84 | 33 | 90 |
| JSI Word Matching Test | Canadian Tests of Basic Skills | 14 | 43 | 84 | 31 | 90 |
| JSI Letter Naming Test | Canadian Tests of Basic Skills | 14 | 64 | 88 | 47 | 94 |
| JSI Total Index | Canadian Tests of Basic Skills | 14 | 50 | 92 | 52 | 92 |
| Grade 1 | End of Grade 2 | | | | | |
| Teacher ratings of overall reading | Gates Primary B Reading Test | 6 | 93 | 82 | 26 | 99 |
| Grade 1 | End of Grade 6 | | | | | |
| Teacher ratings of overall reading | Canadian Tests of Basic Skills | 14 | 61 | 86 | 43 | 93 |

### Results

Table 2 presents the longitudinal results comparing the kindergarten measures of the JSI with outcomes at the end of Grades 2 and 6. For comparison purposes the table also depicts teacher ratings at the end of first grade compared with child outcomes at the end of Grades 2 and 6. Prevalence data are based on the prevalence of problems identified by the outcome criterion measures. The remainder of the table depicts sensitivity, specificity, predictive value of a positive, and predictive value of a negative results (see Chapter 1 for calculation of predictive values).

## DISCUSSION AND CONCLUSIONS

### Phase I: The Cross-Validation Study

It is noteworthy that the prevalence of reading disorders was 35% in the New York sample and 6% at the end of Grade 2 and 14% at the end of Grade 6 in the Canadian sample. Most studies of reading disorders in the general population approximate the prevalence in the Canadian sample. These differences in prevalence rates may explain the differences in the predictive values of positives and negatives, for Galen and Gambino (1975) have demonstrated that prevalence rates are directly related to predictive values of positives (and therefore negatives). Thus, the differences in the prevalence of reading disorders may explain the differences in sensitivity, specificity, and predictive values of positives and negatives between the two samples.

### Phase II: The Predictive Studies

The comparison of the JSI total index performance at the end of kindergarten with reading performance at the end of Grade 2 yielded sensitivity and specificity rates of 50% and 90%, respectively. The sensitivity level is disappointing when compared to the original findings of Jansky & de Hirsch (1972), but may be related to a prevalence rate for reading disability that was a very low 6%. The predictive value of a positive was extremely low (24%) and suggests a potentially large number of overreferrals. A similar finding was found for end of Grade 6 reading performance, except that the predictive value of a positive was much higher (52%) and the prevalence rate had risen to the more expected level of 14%. The sensitivity level of 50% at both the end of Grades 2 and 6 is of particular concern if one wishes to use the JSI total index as a predictive screening measure of later reading disability.

In general, the performances of the three JSI subscales were more sensitive than the total index, at least for the end of Grade 2, with levels ranging from 57% to 71%; however, the predictive value of a positive remained extremely low (i.e., there were potentially large numbers of overreferrals). Unfortunately, the JSI subtest data comparing the subscales with end of sixth-grade performance had reduced sensitivity levels, with the exception of the letter naming test, which had a sensitivity level of 64%, a very impressive performance for a screening measure over a 7-year period. Although the predictive values of a positive did increase somewhat from the end of Grade 2 to the end of Grade 6, the only consistent predictive screening measure for later reading disability was the letter naming subtest.

The final comparison was teacher ratings at the end of Grade 1, with reading abilities measured with the Gates and the vocabulary and reading comprehension subscales of the CTBS at the end of Grades 2 and 6. In this regard, it is noteworthy to mention again that the prevalence of reading disorders was more than twice as high when measured with the CTBS for sixth graders than with the Gates (14% vs. 6%). Whereas the sensitivity was substantially higher with the Gates, the predictive value of a positive was low (26%), so that the predictive value of a positive with the CTBS was still higher (43%) and therefore probably more practical in that the number of overreferrals would be reduced considerably.

The foregoing investigation is presented as a naturalistic study with results that present hypotheses that warrant further investigation under more controlled conditions. One relevant investigation would be to employ a standardized reading measure at the end of Grade 2 that did not have the kind of ceiling effect the Gates Primary B obviously had. Another investigation would be a combination of independent teacher ratings with the JSI in predicting later reading ability. In combining the two, it should be possible to increase sensitivity to be higher than for either scale alone, but the degree to which the predictive values of a positive would decrease cannot be ascertained without actually conducting the study (Frankenburg & Camp, 1975). The final and perhaps most important question to answer is whether or not it makes a difference if one moves up the time of diagnosis to an earlier stage in the process of developing a reading disorder.

As a final note, although the focus of this paper has been on the predictive value of the JSI Total Index and three of its subscales, one cannot ignore the findings on the predictive efficiency of teacher ratings of readings in Grade 1. With sensitivity levels of 93% at the end of Grade 2 and 61% at the end of Grade 6, teacher ratings outperformed the JSI Total Index and its three subscales virtually at all levels.

## REFERENCES

Barnes, K. E. (1978). The Jansky Predictive Index: A cross-validational study. In W. K. Frankenburg (Ed.), *Proceedings of the Second International Conference on Developmental Screening*. Denver, Colorado: Univ. of Colorado.

Barnes, K. E. (1982). *Preschool screening: The measurement and prediction of children at risk*. Springfield, IL: Charles C Thomas.

de Hirsch, K., Jansky, J. J., & Langford, W. S. (1966). *Predicting reading failure*. New York: Harper & Row.

Frankenburg, W. K., & Camp, B. W. (1975). *Pediatric screening tests*. Springfield, IL: Charles C Thomas.

Galen, S., & Gambino, S. R. (1975). *Beyond normality: The predictive value and efficiency of medical diagnosis*. New York: Wiley.

Gates, A., & MacGinitie, W. (1965). *The Gates–MacGinitie Reading Tests*. New York: Teachers College Press.

Jansky, J., & de Hirsch, K. (1972). *Preventing reading failure: Prediction, diagnosis, intervention*. New York: Harper & Row.

King, E. (1974). *The Canadian tests of basic skills*. Don Mills, Ontario: Thomas Nelson & Sons.

CHAPTER 12

# Behavioral Risk

## AN ECOLOGICAL PERSPECTIVE ON CLASSIFYING CHILDREN AS BEHAVIORALLY MALADJUSTED IN KINDERGARTEN

*David H. Cooper and Dale C. Farran*

At school entry, generally in kindergarten, children join a milieu that holds behavioral expectations to which they must adjust. Failure in this regard may result in referral to special education classes, retention, or simply a stressful year for the maladjusted child and the teacher. In the case of referral or retention, the teacher's professional judgment is given considerable weight in classifying the child for purposes of educational placement.

### ASSESSING CHILDREN'S ADJUSTMENT TO SCHOOL

A common approach to diagnosis and classification follows from a personality-trait perspective on child psychopathology. This perspective has as its theoretical base a psychiatric tradition that views deviance as an enduring characteristic of some children. In an effort to objectify and quantify the assessment of children's social and emotional adjustment, various rating scales and checklists have been developed, which consist of behaviors to be considered in the diagnostic process. Maladjustment is typically operationalized as a range of scores derived by summing

***David H. Cooper*** • Department of Special Education, University of Maryland, College Park, Maryland 20742. ***Dale C. Farran*** • Center for the Development of Early Education, Kamehameha Schools/Bishop Estate, Honolulu, Hawaii. The work was supported by U.S. Department of Education Grant G-008201139 and NICHHD Grant HD07178-04.

across individual behavior item scores. Validation of the process typically involves determining the ability of the diagnostic instrument to reliably discriminate between groups constituted on the basis of some other diagnostic procedure. Behaviors that most reliably discriminate between groups are retained and often grouped together into components or subscales of the total instrument. Subscales are given names that convey the presumed underlying relationships of the behaviors. Examples of common subscales are conduct problems, externalizing factor, and anxiety. (For a comprehensive review of the development and validation of these procedures, see Achenbach & Edelbrock, 1978).

Efforts to demonstrate the stability of such assessments over several years have not been impressive (e.g., Cass & Thomas, 1979; Cowen, Pederson, Babigian, Izzo, & Trost, 1973). The lack of stability may be due in part to the fact that children's development and changing environmental influences move them in and out of risk (Bell, in press). Another source of errors in prediction may be the failure of the deficit model of social development, with its focus on deviance and disorder, to identify protective factors that ameliorate risk (Ramey, Yeates, & MacPhee, 1984). A third source of instability may be the lack of ecological validity of the assessment procedures. This type of validity refers to the appropriateness of the variables measured for the particular ecosystem of the subjects, and to the differential weighting of variables such that environment-specific standards are used to assess adjustment to a particular environment.

One aspect of ecologically valid classification that has received only slight attention is the contribution that children's repertoire of negative and positive behavioral skills in the classroom makes to teachers' professional judgment that a child should be referred for special services. In any given school district, school, or classroom, certain behaviors may be more critical than others. These critical behaviors may vary from setting to setting. Therefore, valid assessment of a child's adjustment should take into account the extent to which his or her behavior constitutes a risk in that environment. An ongoing effort to develop an ecologically valid assessment method is described below.

## METHOD

### Subjects

The subject pool included all kindergarten children in two public school districts. Principals in 17 of 19 schools in the two districts chose to allow teacher participation in the study; 31 of 36 eligible teachers elected to participate, resulting in a sample of 659 kindergarten students.

### *School Districts*

The demographic characteristics of the two districts differed. District A was primarily rural and agricultural, with one urban center having manufacturing and retail businesses (primarily clothing factory outlets). District B was a small, urban community with a large state university and no other major industry. Inclusion of subjects from both districts resulted in a study population featuring the rural, industrial, and agricultural aspects of District A combined with the urban, professional, technical, and service aspects of District B. This heterogeneity may permit findings to be generalized more readily than would have been possible from either district taken alone.

## Procedures

Six weeks into the school year, behavioral data were collected on all children. Teachers completed a behavioral rating scale developed specifically for this study; at midyear, they classified children according to their degree of adjustment to the kindergarten environment. The behavioral rating scale classification scheme is described below. Analyses evaluated the degree of risk for receiving a deviant midyear classification that was associated with various behaviors exhibited earlier in the year.

## Measures

### *Item Selection for the Behavioral Rating Scale*

Building on a longitudinal study of the school adjustment of poor, high-risk children, Haskins (1981) interviewed 20 kindergarten teachers. They were asked two questions: "What social skills are important for kindergarteners?" and "Name the behavior that bothers you the most in kindergarten children." Replication of the Haskins interview with a new sample of teachers revealed almost identical responses to the questions (Reinhardt, 1983).

From their responses, the Cooper-Farran Behavioral Rating Scale was developed. Each behavior to be rated was worded in a neutral manner and followed by a 7-point, bipolar scale representing the continuum of normality and abnormality for that behavior. Behavioral descriptors were provided as anchors for points 1, 3, 5, and 7 for each item in order to enhance interrater reliability (Jay & Ferran, 1981) and to help provide interpretable differences among the 7 points. (Copies of the rating instrument are available from the authors on request.) The *interpersonal skills* are reflected in behaviors primarily social in nature. Some examples are sharing materials, taking turns, aggression, and responding positively to constructive criticism. The *work-related skills* are those that tend to result in individual academic achievement, such as staying on task, listening to instructions, and completing activities in synchrony with the class. Content validity of the 39-item scale was established through pilot tests involving 80 professional educators. Intrarater reliability (consistency) over a 1-month interval was adequate; the median intraclass correlation across items was .77.

### *Subscale Structure*

Fall rating data were factor analyzed using a principal axis method and Varimax rotation. Two factors, accounting for 57% of the total variance, were retained and labeled as Interpersonal Skills (IPS) and Work-Related Skills (WRS).

### *Midyear Classification Scheme*

In February of the school year, the same 30 kindergarten teachers (one withdrew for maternity leave) who had rated the behaviors of all their students the previous fall classified each student according to social adjustment. In addition, teacher aides in each classroom completed the same questionnaire. The categories were

1. Regular kindergarten program is not appropriate. Child needs special program or help due to social behavior problems.
2. Socially very immature. Another year in kindergarten may be necessary for child to acquire appropriate social skills.
3. Slightly behind peers in most areas of social maturity. Will probably catch up this year or next.
4. Inconsistent social behavior. Sometimes shows appropriate social skills, but just as often behaves inappropriately. Or social behavior problems only in certain specific situations. Otherwise okay.
5. Infrequent behavior problems. Moderate or strong academic skills outweigh occasional lapses in behavior.
6. No noticeable behavior problem.
7. Clearly outstanding social skills.

Interrater reliability for teachers and teachers' aides on the midyear

Table 1. Means and Standard Deviations for Subscale Scores

| | Interpersonal skills | Work-related skills |
|---|---|---|
| Overall ($N$ = 659) | 5.40 (1.23) | 4.70 (1.45) |
| District | | |
| A ($N$ = 458) | 5.43 (1.21) | 4.67 (1.51) |
| B ($N$ = 201) | 5.32 (1.26) | 4.79 (1.26) |
| Sex | | |
| Females ($N$ = 310) | 5.73 (1.12) | 5.10 (1.34) |
| Males ($N$ = 349) | 5.10 (1.24) | 4.35 (1.44) |

classification was estimated by intraclass correlation. A coefficient of .70 indicated adequate reliability for this measure.

## Results

### *Behavior in the Fall*

Subscale scores were derived by summing across all items in each of two subscales and dividing by the number of items in the subscale. In this way, scores retained the original 1- to 7-point scaling. Sample means and standard deviations are given in Table 1. Differences were not found between the two school districts sampled. District A children from a mostly rural area are entirely comparable on both subscales to District B children from an urban, university community. Comparison of males and females is also shown in Table 1. Average ratings on the subscales reveal a sex difference in favor of females on both interpersonal (IPS) and work-related skills (WRS).

### *Outcome at Midyear*

Figure 1 depicts the distribution of children's midyear classifications. Again, sex differences are apparent in favor of females. It is also interesting to note that more than half of the sample had some degree of problems in the social domain, as evidenced by a classification in one of the first five categories. Sixty children, about 10%, had adjustment problems severe enough to require special education or retention. This group of 60 are referred to as *cases* of maladjustment in subsequent analyses. The other 90% of the sample are referred to as *controls*.

Comparison of the percentage of cases needing special education or retention revealed nearly identical proportions of cases and controls in the two districts. The 10% prevalence of cases in these two districts is in agreement with conservative estimates of prevalence found in the literature.

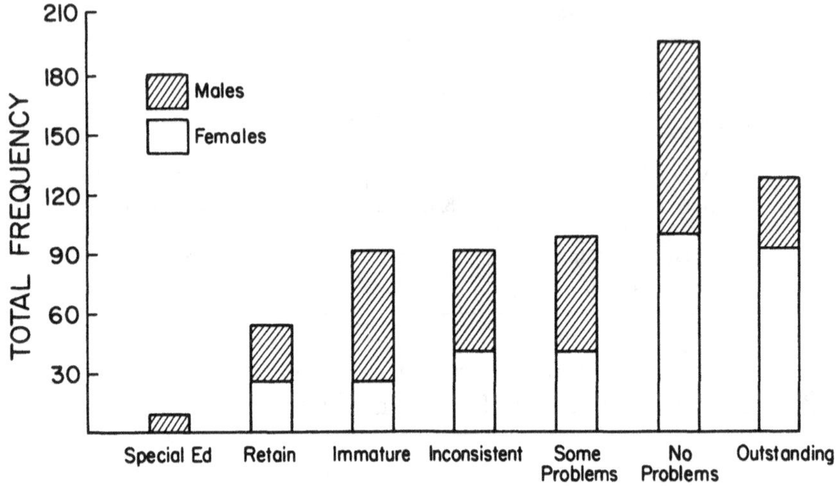


**Figure 1.** Frequency distribution of midyear classification.

## *Behavioral Risk*

A relative risk analysis was carried out (Kleinbaum, Kupper, & Morgenstern, 1982) to determine the strength of the association between behaviors and classification. For this analysis, the behavioral ratings on the two subscales were first standardized within each classroom, and then the overall sample was dichotomized at approximately the 15th percentile score, which reflected a rating of about 3 on the 7-point scale. For children low in the IPS area, the risk of classification as *maladjusted* was about 3 times as great as for children high in IPS. For low WRS, the risk was substantially higher, about 14 times as great as for children rated high on this category.

Relative risk by sex and school district were also computed. In each instance, the work-related scale was a stronger risk factor than the interpersonal scale, except perhaps in District B where the risk associated with WRS was roughly equivalent to that of IPS. This finding demonstrates the need to take an ecological perspective on risk and thus to analyze risk *within* discernible environments such as school districts.

The last analysis to be presented looks at the joint effect of IPS and WRS. This analysis is conceptually similar to interaction of effects in an analysis of variance approach. Joint effects analysis is useful in determining how much the risk of classification changes in going from an optimal rating (high ratings on both scales) to the worst rating (low on both). It affords an opportunity to examine the extent to which an intermediate rating (i.e., high rating on only *one* of the scales) may serve to protect individuals from being classified as maladjusted.

The two-by-two table shown in Figure 2 depicts data comparing a risk group to a common reference group—children with the optimal rating (i.e., high on IPS and high on WRS). The right side of the table contains the 509 children in the common reference group, representing 77% of the total sample. As shown, the reference group was compared to 55 children with low IPS but high WRS. The odds ratio .84 is not significantly different from 1, indicative of no risk. From the earlier analysis, it was shown that there was some risk associated with IPS, but the risk disappears when WRS are high.

Two explanations are possible. First, IPS and WRS may be confounded such that all the effect of IPS is accounted for by WRS variance. Though not independent, the two variables do not correlate to such a degree as to support this interpretation (phi correlation for dichotomized subscales = .38). Second, the results may suggest a protective influence of good WRS. A small but significant risk was found to be associated with low IPS; however, as shown in Figure 2, when low IPS are coupled with high WRS, the risk of being classified as maladjusted becomes nonsignificant.

Next we compared the reference group—509 children high on both IPS and WRS—to 49 children high on IPS but low on WRS. The odds ratio estimates the relative risk at 12.9. In other words, there is about 13 times greater risk when compared to the reference group in spite of *high* IPS.

Finally, the reference group was compared to the 46 worst-rated children (low on both scales). The odds ratio estimates the risk at 14.2, suggesting that adding low IPS to already low WRS only slightly increased the risk of classification. Skills assessed by the IPS subscale did not appear to make a large difference in children's classifications,

| | | Low IPS High WRS | High IPS High WRS |
|---|---|---|---|
| Maladjusted | Yes | 2 | 22 |
| | No | 53 | 487 |
| | | 55 | 509 |

Odds Ratio = .84

**Figure 2.** Joint effect of two behavioral ratings on classification as behaviorally maladjusted.

whereas the WRS subscale appeared to make a significant contribution regardless of IPS.

## DISCUSSION

Several conclusions may be drawn from these findings. The first and clearest is that kindergarten teachers' decisions about classification at midyear are almost entirely based on children's WRS. These include working independently, listening and complying, and making organized, relevant contributions to learning activities such as discussions. This is, after all, what school is all about, so it should come as no great surprise that these skills are critical for success. These findings confirm and extend earlier work by Achenbach & Edelbrock (1981), whose data suggest that poor school work in the 4- to 7-year age group may have been instrumental in determining which children were referred to mental health agencies for treatment of behavioral disorders.

The second conclusion is related to the first. We believe that the assessment of an environment and its critical behaviors is an important first step in setting behavioral objectives and goals for children about to be placed in that environment (Vincent, Salisbury, Walter, Brown, Gruenewald, & Powers, 1980). This has particular relevance to mainstreaming the handicapped and to preparing all preschool children, handicapped or not, for the demands they face on school entry. From these data, we would then be inclined to recommend an emphasis on independent, task-oriented participation as the best strategies for children to adopt in coping with the demands of kindergarten.

The type of analysis presented above follows from the adoption of an ecological perspective on deviance. It would have been possible to identify slightly different relationships between risk factors for two environments (school Districts A and B). Much of the literature on behavioral disorders is devoted to lamenting the lack of a good universally accepted definition. Clearly, trying to impose a standard definition on environments having different expectations for behavior and processes for classification would be counterproductive. It has been suggested that for useful ecologically based definition and identification of maladjustment, one must take into account the standards to which adjustment is to be compared (Hobbs, 1982; Rhodes & Paul, 1978).

These data also suggest that attention to protective factors is helpful in understanding how risk factors may operate. The fact that high WRS may have protected the children rated low on IPS was surprising and could not have been revealed if the analysis had ended at the estimation of crude odds ratios. Other possible protective factors yet to be examined are academic achievement and demographic variables such as age, race, and socioeconomic status.

Finally, these data address the meaning of risk that refers to the probability of a specified adverse outcome given the presence of an earlier detectable risk factor. In our reading of studies self-identified as "risk research," we find too little attention given to precise and replicable identification of meaningful adverse outcomes (Farran & Cooper, in press). More attention is given to finding statistically significant relationships between multiple predictors and single outcomes. Although the predictors are often measured with some depth, the outcome is often measured at only one point in time or consists only of a score on a single psychometric test.

This chapter has presented data from our study's first outcome rating. Future analysis planned for the kindergarten data include behavioral ratings, classifications, and achievement data collected at the end of the school year and first grade follow-up. At that point, the behavioral risks may shed light on the need to conduct multiple assessments of outcome due to developmental changes in the children and in teachers' altered standards for classification.

The goal of this work will continue to be understanding the outcome of behavioral maladjustment by determining what factors are taken into consideration when that outcome is assessed. In that regard, we have been focusing on an area we call behavioral risk to connote the contribution that a child's behavior makes to a subsequent classification as adjusted or not.

ACKNOWLEDGMENTS

The authors wish to thank H. A. Tyroler, University of North Carolina Department of Epidemiology, for advice on strategies for the analysis of risk data; Hardy Tew and George Gleetwood, Assistant Superintendents, for permission to conduct the research in their school districts; and Gina Walker and Pam Mann for word processing.

## REFERENCES

Achenbach, T., & Edelbrock, C. (1978). The classification of child psychopathology: A review and analysis of empirical efforts. *Psychological Bulletin, 85*(6), 1275–1301.

Achenbach, T., & Edelbrock, C. (1981). Behavioral problems and competencies reported by parents of normal and disturbed children aged four through sixteen. *Monographs of the Society for Research in Child Development, 46*(1, Serial No. 188).

Bell, R. Q. (in press). Age specific manifestations in changing psychosocial risk. In D. C. Farran & J. D. McKinney (Eds.), *Risk in intellectual and psychosocial development*. New York: Academic Press.

Cass, L., & Thomas, C. (1979). *Childhood pathology and later adjustment*. New York: Wiley.

Cowen, E., Pederson, A., Babigian, H., Izzo, L., & Trost, M. (1973). Long-term follow-up of early detected vulnerable children. *Journal of Consulting and Clinical Psychology, 41*(3), 438–446.

Farran, D. C., & Cooper, D. H. (in press). Psychosocial risk: Which early experiences are important for whom? In D. C. Farran & J. D. McKinney (Eds.), *Risk in intellectual and psychosocial development*. New York: Academic Press.

Haskins, R. (1981). *Final interview with teachers*. Unpublished manuscript, University of North Carolina at Chapel Hill.

Hobbs, N. (1982). *The troubled and troubling child*. San Francisco: Jossey-Bass.

Jay, S., & Farran, D. C. (1981). The relative efficacy of predicting IQ from mother–child interactions using ratings versus behavioral count measures. *Journal of Applied Developmental Psychology, 2*, 165–177.

Kleinbaum, D., Kupper, L., & Morgenstern, H. (1982). *Epidemiologic research: Principles and quantitative methods*. Belmont, CA: Wadsworth.

Ramey, C. T., Yeates, K. O., & MacPhee, D. (1984). Risk for retarded development among disadvantaged families: A systems theory approach to preventive intervention. In B. Keogh (Ed.), *Advances in special education: Documenting program impact* (Vol. 4). Greenwich, CT: JAI Press.

Reinhardt, B. (1983). *Important kindergarten social skills, problem behaviors, and intervention tactics*. Unpublished manuscript, University of North Carolina at Chapel Hill.

Rhodes, W., & Paul, J. (Eds.), (1978). *Emotionally disturbed and deviant children: New views and approaches*. Englewood Cliffs, NJ: Prentice-Hall.

Vincent, F., Salisbury, C., Walter, G., Brown, P., Gruenewald, L., & Powers, M. (1980). Program evaluation and curriculum development in early childhood/special education. In W. Sailer, B. Wilcox, & L. Brown (Eds.), *Methods of instruction of severely handicapped students*. Baltimore: Brooks.

CHAPTER 13

# Identification of At-Risk Infants and Preschool Children

## PUBLIC HEALTH NURSES USING A WEIGHTED MULTIFACTOR RISK ASSESSMENT FORM

*J. Helen Parkyn*

The need for Community Health Services, specifically Public health nurses (PHNs), to become involved in a program of planned identification and follow-up of infants and preschool children at risk for developmental delays, failure to thrive, neglect or abuse, or physical or emotional problems secondary to other handicaps has a mandate from many sources. The World Health Organization, in its position paper "Risk Approach for Maternal and Child Health Care" (1978), outlines a managerial strategy to improve the coverage and quality of maternal and child health services based on the measurement of individual and community risk. This strategy attempts to "ensure a minimum of care for all while providing guidelines for the diversion of limited resources to those who most need them" (p. 18).

The 1980 report of the Canadian Standing Senate Committee on Health, Welfare, and Science (1980) on the child at risk recommended

> that Provincial and Territorial governments establish or expand in-home support services for parents, and in particular that they establish or expand health visitor programs to offer in-home assistance to parents and/or children identified as being at risk. (p.55)

The recently published Provincial Study of Severely Handicapped Chil-

*J. Helen Parkyn* • South Central Health Unit, Kamloops, British Columbia, Canada V2C 2T8. This project is being carried out with the cooperation of the British Columbia Ministry of Health and the British Columbia Health Care Research Foundation.

dren (Talbot, 1981) outlined the major responsibility as belonging to Community Health Services, with PHNs identified as being involved in developmental assessment.

The current project is significant for two main reasons, one of which relates to human suffering and the other to cost factors. In a time when it is becoming increasingly obvious that it will not be possible to provide all services to everyone, there is a particular need to ensure that available resources are allocated to those most in need. Ensuring that extra services are received by those at highest risk in an organized manner is essential. In addition, it must be remembered that not identifying, preventing, and/or intervening early has a very considerable cost, apart from the suffering involved, in the form of rehabilitation and remediation in later years.

## CURRENT STATE OF EXISTING PROGRAMS

The desirability of early identification has led to a wide variety of attempts to detect and follow families at risk, but most of these methods have proven unsatisfactory. Some examples of identification strategies tried to date by Canada's PHNs follow.

1. Use of a single factor assessment form. Unfortunately, single factors alone have not proven useful. The main problem with this type of assessment form is that if all risk factors are considered in an unweighted fashion, up to half of the infant population may be categorized as at risk, and follow-up becomes impractical.

Some assessment forms consider only a limited number of risk factors, but these are usually physical risk factors (Clemmens, 1982), whereas social factors, which are omitted, compound all other factors. Furthermore, social factors are often the main indications of children at risk for abuse, neglect, failure-to-thrive, and psychosocial retardation.

2. Use of voluntary open preschool screening clinics. There are a number of problems with this approach. First, only a small percent of all preschool children are seen in these programs. Second, families in the target population (i.e., those at risk) are probably less likely than the average family to attend a voluntary clinic. Third, if this approach did in fact cover a significant percent of the population, it would prove extremely costly to screen the numbers in question.

3. Assessment of risk by individual health workers based on their own judgment. This has the drawback that the assessment may be extremely variable and very subjective.

## DEVELOPMENT OF THE WEIGHTED MULTIFACTOR RISK ASSESSMENT FORM

The current project began in 1980 in the South Central Health Unit of the Province of British Columbia. The model for the assessment form was the work of Aubry and Pennington (1973) and Aubry and Nesbitt (1969) on the identification of high-risk pregnancies using a weighted multifactor semi-objective tool. This model addresses many of the problems of identifying children at risk. With a priority ranking established from the scoring, the percentage of children to be followed can vary depending on an agency's staff resources, but the highest risk children are always served first. The form was designed for completion by staff public health nurses from information received from hospital liaison and home visits.

The first draft of the instrument was prepared by a development committee following an extensive literature review. Only factors supported by other studies or considerable written expert opinion were included. (Item 18 on the form, "Other and Specify," does allow an element of individual judgment by PHNs, who can note additional factors that may create stress in a particular family.) The initial weighting of factors was based on the literature and on the committee's judgment regarding each factor's degree of association with the severity and frequency of expected adverse outcomes. For example, all individual factors given a score of 9 were those known to be predictive of serious outcomes with or without any other contributary factor. The instrument's first draft was field tested by the 15 PHNs of one school district, and a second draft was taken to various experts from the fields of pediatrics, genetics, and psychology for critique, with a view to establishing a level of consensus about choice of factors. Expert consultations resulted in minimal changes in the factors listed, and some reorganization and increased precision of definitions (e.g., the definition of a low Apgar score). A third draft was then prepared and field tested. (The 15 PHNs who had used the first draft also carried out this testing in the same school district.)

During both field tests, reliability checks were conducted by the development committee, which compared a limited number of factors on both the completed assessment forms and the birth notices. There was more than 90% accuracy in the assessment form completion according to the factors available on the birth notices.

Our current draft of the instrument reflects subsequent minor revisions that have clarified the ordering of factors and that take into account a recent literature review (see Figure 1). Throughout the process

Child's Name: ______________________ Birthdate: ______________________

Please Circle Score as Determined by Assessment

I CHILDREN WITH KNOWN HANDICAP

1. Congenital Anomaly
   - (a) Major, e.g., Down's syndrome, spina bifada, etc. .......... 9
   - (b) Moderate, e.g., cong. ab. hips, cleft palate, hypospadias .......... 6
2. (a) Major illness or handicap acquired during first 2 years of life e.g., cerebral palsy, severe head injury .......... 9
   - (b) Moderate illness or handicap acquired during first 2 years of life e.g., meningitis .......... 6

II DEVELOPMENTAL RISK FACTORS

3. Low Birth Weight
   - (a) Under 1,500 g any reason .......... 9
   - (b) 1,500–2,000 g less than 38 weeks .......... 5
   - (c) 2,000–2,500 g less than 38 weeks .......... 2
   - (d) 1,500–2,500 g 38 weeks plus .......... 7
4. Bilirubin level over 20 m .......... 9
5. Complications of Pregnancy
   - (a) Infections that can be transmitted in utero to fetus (e.g., rubella, toxoplasmosis) in first 4 months .......... 9
   - (b) Drugs – e.g., alcohol – diagnosed in mother .......... 9
6. Complications of Labor and Delivery
   - (a) Labor requiring mid and high forceps including breech delivery with forceps .......... 3
   - (b) Infant trauma or illness (e.g., convulsions, respiratory distress syndrome) .......... 6
   - (c) Apgar at 5 minutes only if less than 7 Deduct Apgar score at 5 minutes from 10 points .......... —
7. Family history of a relevant handicap (e.g., deafness, mental retardation) 6
8. Delayed on developmental assessment in first 2 years of life .......... 9

III FAMILY INTERACTION RISK FACTORS

9. Age of Mother
   - (a) 15 and under .......... 9
   - (b) 17 and under .......... 6
   - (c) 19 and under .......... 3
10. Social Situation
    - (a) Father of infant not resident but other support available .......... 1
    - (b) Father not resident and no support .......... 5
    - (c) Father resident, no other social support, or isolation by language or geography .......... 3
11. On Social Assistance .......... 3
12. No Prenatal Care before 6th Month .......... 4
13. Mental Illness or Retardation in Mother and/or Father
    - (a) Schizophrenia or manic depression .......... 9
    - (b) Post-partum depression .......... 6
    - (c) Mental retardation of parent .......... 6

**Figure 1.** PHN at-risk assessment form.

14. Prolonged Maternal Separation (5 days or more)
    (a) with frequent infant contacts ........ 2
    (b) little or not infant contact ........ 4
15. Assessed Lack of Bonding
    (a) Eye contact, touching, etc. absent ........ 9
    (b) Eye contact, touching, etc. minimal ........ 6
16. Failure to Thrive falling below the 5th percentile, when born with birth weight above 2500 g. Assess weight individually if birth weight below 2500 g ........ 7
17. Repeated hospitalization (3 plus in a year) in first 2 years of life ........ 3
18. Other: e.g., marital distress, financial difficulty, low education status, difficulty raising an older child, et.
    Specify: Score 0–9 _

9 and over High Risk; 6–8 Moderate Risk; 3–5 Low Risk TOTAL _

**Figure 1.** (*continued*).

of the development of the instrument, there have only been two changes in the actual choice of factors. An item regarding bilirubin levels for premature infants was deleted due to studies published in 1982, and an item regarding illness or handicap acquired in the first 2 years was divided into major and moderate subsections.

Reliability and validity testing have begun in a study involving one school district (#24). This district covers more than 70% of the populations of the South Central Health Unit, where newborns may be considered representative of the province as a whole based on 1980 vital statistics (Vital Statistics, 1980). As was noted earlier, there are 15 staff PHNs servicing this school district. Six have a nursing degree and nine a public health nursing diploma, which is a typical cross-section of educational preparation of PHNs. In addition, the caseloads are representative of most Health Units in the province. Thus, the district provides a cross-section of both living circumstances and service availability.

In our current study, the weighted multifactor At-Risk Assessment Form is designed for completion by general staff PHNs and is based on the following information:

1. Birth notice. A copy of each birth notice is received at the health unit within an average of 5 days after the birth of a child. This notice is sent to the PHN prior to the postnatal home assessment visit.

2. Postnatal notes. A British Columbia Provincial Postnatal Notes form is completed on approximately the second day postnatally in the hospital by a Health Unit staff member. The form is brought directly to the Health Unit and sent to the PHN before the home visit.

3. Home visit. A minimum of one home visit is made by the PHN to assess the newborn infant and family. This visit is usually made within 2 weeks of hospital discharge of the infant except where unusual

circumstances prevail (e.g., extreme geographic isolation). This postnatal home visit is a routine part of public health nursing practice in the British Columbia Provincial Health services, and results in more than 95% of all newborns being visited.

Consent of selected families to participate in the testing is being obtained. There is little difficulty in obtaining such consent, as newborn-visits by PHNs are extremely well accepted by the public.

Interrater reliability is being tested by comparing assessment scores between the following:

1. Experienced staff PHN and experienced staff PHN
2. Expert PHN and experienced staff PHN
3. Expert PHN and beginning staff PHN

Each nurse involved has received a similar orientation to the use of the assessment form. In each situation, one of the staff nurses is carrying out the postnatal home assessment with the second nurse as a nonparticipant observer.

The observer who visits the homes with the staff PHNs also reviews the same birth notices and liaison slips. Whereas ideally the second nurse would complete a home postnatal assessment at a different time from the first nurse, this would be seen as very unusual by the public as compared with the not uncommon event of two nurses visiting together. The nurses separately score the At-Risk Assessment Form following the home visit and before any discussion between them takes place.

In conclusion, a weighted multifactor assessment form has been developed for PHNs to use in identifying children at risk. There appears to be a consensus among experts on the choice of factors, as these have remained almost unaltered throughout the process of development. A study is currently in progress to assess the reliability of the form.

## REFERENCES

Aubry, R., & Pennington, J. (1973). Identification and evaluation of high-risk pregnancy: The perinatal concept. *Clinical Obstetrics and Gynecology, 16*(1), 3.

Aubry, R., & Nesbitt, R. E. (1969). High risk obstetrics II: Value of semi-objective grading system in identifying the vulnerable group. *American Journal of Obstetrics and Gynecology, 103*, 972–985.

Clemmens, D. (1982). High risk follow-up program of the infant and family in the community. *Canadian Journal of Public Health,* May/June *73*, 163–166.

Standing Senate Committee on Health, Welfare, and Science. (1980). *Child at risk*. Hull, Quebec, Canada: Canadian Government Publishing Centre.

Talbot, T., Brock-Dunbar, P., Sheps, S., & Stull, S. (1981). *Provincial study of severely handicapped children*. Unpublished report for the Ministry of Health, Victoria, British Columbia, Canada.

*Vital statistics of the province of british columbia*. (1980). Victoria, British Columbia, Canada: Queen's Printer for British Columbia.

World Health Organization, Task Force on Risk Approach for Improved Maternal and Child Health and Family Planning. (1978). Geneva.

CHAPTER 14

# Developmental Review

## A NEW APPROACH TO EARLY INTERVENTION EMPHASIZING PARENTAL INVOLVEMENT

*Harry Ireton*

---

The importance of involving parents in the assessment of their young children's development has long been recognized as an integral part of developmental screening (Frankenburg & Dodds, 1967) and diagnosis (Gesell & Amatruda, 1954). This paper describes a method for reviewing young children's developmental progress that stresses parent involvement and the utilization of parental information about the child's development. The purpose of the Development Review is to review the child's progress with the parent (usually the mother) in a way that is beneficial for the parents of both normally functioning and developmentally disabled children. In addition, it includes a mechanism for identifying children who are developmentally delayed.

Although parent involvement has been mandated in the United States through legislation for Early Periodic Screening, Diagnosis, and Treatment (EPSDT), and the Education of All Handicapped Children's Act (P.L. 94-142), professionals have been slow to respond to the challenge of including parents in screening. Instead, most professionals have preferred to rely mainly on developmental testing of the child. Failure to make more use of parental information appears to be related to professionals' distrust of parents' "subjective" reports, pediatricians' time constraints, and psychologists' emphasis on tests as measures of childrens characteristics.

Although for the most part, professionals have not sought out or created systematic methods for obtaining and utilizing parental infor-

---

*Harry Ireton* • Department of Family Practice and Community Health, University of Minnesota, Minneapolis, Minnesota 55455.

mation about their children's development, some systematic methods for utilizing parental information do exist. The Denver Developmental Screening Test (DDST) includes items that may be passed either by parent report or professional observation (Frankenburg & Dodds, 1967); the Prescreening Developmental Questionnaire (Frankenburg, van Doorninck, Liddell, & Dick, 1976) is based exclusively on parent observation and report; the Developmental Profile II (Alpern, Boll, & Shearer, 1980) provides a structured interview format for obtaining current developmental information from the parent; the Minnesota Child Development Inventories (Ireton & Thwing, 1974, 1979, 1980a) obtain the mother's report of the child's current development, readiness skills, adjustment, and symptoms. All of the above were developed in a systematic fashion and validated against independent measures.

A comprehensive review of preschool screening (Lichtenstein & Ireton, 1984) suggests that, in the aggregate, various "methods of observation" (including parents' reports of daily behavior and concerns about the child, professional observation of the child and parent–child interaction, plus brief, formal tests) provide the soundest basis for reviewing each child's development and for identifying children with significant developmental problems. Parent reports can be obtained by means of questionnaires, interviews, and/or developmental inventories, depending on the ability and willingness of the parent to respond to the various modalities.

The utility of parental information, of course, depends on the accuracy of the information that is provided. The reliability and validity of parental reports is a complex function of the type of information requested, certain characteristics of the parent, and the method used to obtain the information. A review of research (McShane, 1973) suggests that parents are most likely to provide trustworthy information when the information requested pertains to the child's *current, observable* behavior, and when the method employed is *structured* and includes clear instructions and specific items. Parent comprehension of the request for information is a major factor. Less obvious but of importance is the parent's opportunity to observe the child's functioning and the parent's sophistication about child development (Gottfried, Guerin, Spencer, & Meyer, 1983).

## THE DEVELOPMENTAL REVIEW CONCEPT

The concept of the Developmental Review emerged from a series of conferences on developmental screening sponsored by the American Association of Psychiatric Services for Children, the outcome of which is described in a report titled "Developmental Review in the EPSDT

Program" (Huntington, 1977). The Developmental Review is conceived as an enabling process for both parents and children. It is based on the recognition that a child is as likely to be advanced in some areas of development as it is that a child may be delayed in some areas. It is designed to provide a means by which all parents can be helped to understand how their children are doing, and to obtain information and support that can enable them to be more effective and comfortable as parents. At the same time, it includes a mechanism by which children with significant developmental delays and potential school problems can be at least tentatively identified.

The Developmental Review is based on a philosophical and conceptual shift from the screening model as follows: A major limitation of developmental screening is that development is not like a disease entity, to be judged as present or absent. Development describes the evolution of certain abilities and the complex processes that underlie this evolution. The rate of development of a particular ability is not necessarily consistent over time, nor does the rate of development in one area necessarily parallel the rate of development in another area. For young children, the "range of normal" is difficult to define, and predicting future functioning is hazardous. Parents wonder, "How is may child doing?" and sometimes worry, "Is my child normal?" Information addressing these questions and concerns may be hard to come by, and parents may be left to deal with their anxiety as best they can. At any given time, a child will be demonstrating a particular array of abilities and will be more or less adjusted to his or her environment. At the same time, the parent will be more or less satisfied with the child's progress, will possibly be concerned or worried about the child's development or well-being, or will at least have questions regarding the child.

What is needed is a procedure for reviewing each child's developmental progress with parents, and for responding to their questions and concerns in a way that enables them to become better parents. This developmental review needs to assume a positive orientation that goes beyond the concept of "screening for defects." What parents need most is affirmation of their children's developmental achievements, and emotional support of their roles as parents. They also need information about child care and child development, and an opportunity to raise questions and express their concerns about their child. In addition, if the child is developmentally handicapped or has other problems, the child and parents will need special assistance.

The Developmental Review process stresses parent involvement by keying on the mother's description of her child's current behavior, and her questions and concerns, if any. It also includes direct observation of the child. Developmental Review has a clearly defined clinical structure. The parent interview, child observation, and interpretation of results are conducted according to a specified format with reference to a Developmental Map of milestones for the first 5 years.

From the initial contact with parents, Developmental Review emphasizes the importance of parent involvement and the value of parents' observations of the child's functioning. Parents are informed, in words and by attitude, that "you know a lot about your child, and we need to know what you know about your child in order to understand him or her." Parents' involvement in the process of describing and understanding the child then serves as the bridge to the development of a working relationship or partnership between the parents and the professional.

Developmental Review focuses on describing the child's current developmental achievements in five areas of development: gross motor, fine motor, language, self-help, and social-emotional. Language development is broken down into expressive language, language comprehension, and speech articulation. Parental information about the child is obtained first by means of a brief questionnaire and then through a structured interview. The child's positive attributes as well as parental concerns regarding the child are solicited. The interview with the parent and the observation of the child are accomplished with specific attention paid to the questions and/or concerns initially raised by the parent.

In conducting the parent interview and the observation of the child, the evaluator refers to what is called a *Developmental Map* (Figure 1). The items of the Developmental Map are observable behaviors that were selected to provide milestones in the five areas across the first 5 years. For the most part, these items (for example, items that also appear in the Minnesota Child Development Inventory or DDST) have established age norms. In the interview, the parent is first given a brief opportunity to describe the child's current development, in the parent's own words. Next, depending on the parent's spontaneous description, the interviewer asks for additonal description in each of the five areas. Finally the interviewer asks about specific behaviors in each area from the Developmental Map around the child's age level. At the same time, the child is observed in a free play situation where blocks, paper and pencil, and so on are available. Then the child's achievements in each area are compared with expected development for the child's age and are interpreted as *advanced, within age expectations, questionable,* or *delayed* (Figure 2).

## METHOD

A pilot project (Stone, Ireton, & Runquist, 1979) evaluated the efficiency of Developmental Review (time, ease of administration), its impact on parents, and, to some degree, its validity for identifying delayed children. The project was conducted at a number of EPSDT sites in Minnesota, Ohio, and Texas in order to include both urban and rural sites and public and private providers. In some sites, it was possible to compare Developmental Review results with the results obtained by screening with the DDST. A questionnaire for those conducting Developmental Reviews was completed by 28 professionals, of whom 74% were nurses, and 17% physicians. The time to complete the procedure, including information gathering, interpretation, and follow-up discussion, averaged 38 minutes. Developmental Review procedures were rated as both more time-consuming and more comprehensive than the DDST. Practical utility for generating data for referral decisions are rated by the professionals as about the same, whereas parent acceptance as perceived by the professionals tended to be higher for the Developmental Review.

Comments by participating professionals included the following. "The parents really like it.... They enjoy having their opinions asked.... This encouraged parents to talk.... Some parents seem so eager to talk to a professional about their children.... They appreciated receiving a copy of the Developmental Map." Overall effectiveness was rated as "useful or very useful" by 73% of professionals. Parents themselves (about 95%) felt comfortable with the procedure, believed that their questions and concerns had been heard, and said they would recommend the procedure to other parents.

Validity data for the procedure are based on 599 children, of which 71% were English-speaking, 8% were Spanish-speaking, and 21% were bilingual. Age range of the sample was fairly evenly distributed from birth through 5 years of age, and both sexes were equally represented. Incidence of apparently delayed development was 6% for the group as a whole, and ranged from 0 to 22% across sites. Of the 28 children viewed as possibly delayed, 21 were boys and 7 were girls. For those children referred for follow-up evaluation, 70% were considered developmentally delayed. The 6% incidence rate and the 70% delayed rate paralleled the rates in a comparison group of 928 children screened by the DDST at the same sites prior to the use of the Developmental Review.

## DISCUSSION

This study of the efficacy and validity of the Developmental Review procedure was carried out under serious constraints and with limited training of the professionals who utilized the procedure (which consisted mainly of their being provided with instructions and the materials). The validity data are limited to follow-up of a small number of

| AGE | GROSS MOTOR | FINE MOTOR | LANGUAGE | SELF-HELP | SOCIAL-EMOTIONAL |
|---|---|---|---|---|---|
| 0–6 | Lifts head & chest high<br>Supports head (no lag)<br>Rolls over back to front | Clasps hands together<br>Reaches toward objects<br>Picks up toy with one hand | Vocalizes, coos, chuckles<br>Vocalizes spontaneously, social | Comforts self with thumb or pacifier | Social smile<br>Distinguishes mother from others<br>Initiates social contact |
| 6–9 | Sits alone--erect, steady without support | Transfers toy from one hand to other<br>Picks up objects with thumb and finger grasp | Wide range of vocalizations (vowel sounds, consonant-vowel combinations)<br>Says mama, dada | Feeds self cracker | Pushes things away he/she doesn't want |
| 9–12 | Crawls on hands & knees<br>Stands alone well<br>Walks with support | Picks up small objects-precise thumb & finger grasp | Says mama, dada as names for parents<br>Understands "no," "stop," etc. | Holds own bottle **or** drinks from a cup | Plays social games - peek-a-boo, pat-a-cake, bye-bye<br>Expresses several emotions clearly<br>Objects to separation |
| 12–18 | Walks alone<br>"Dances" to music | Stacks two or more blocks<br>Scribbles | Uses one or two words as names of things or actions<br>Points to familiar things<br>Points to parts of the body | Cooperates in dressing<br>Feeds self with spoon | Plays simple ball games<br>Hugs parent |
| 18– | Runs well, rarely falls<br>Kicks ball forward | Builds tower of four or more blocks<br>Makes imitative strokes (vertical, circular) | Uses words to express wants<br>Uses 2-3 word phrases or sentences<br>Names pictures of familiar objects<br>Follows simple directions | Eats with spoon, spilling little | Kisses with pucker<br>Imitates adult activities<br>"Helps" with simple household tasks |

| Age | | | | | |
|---|---|---|---|---|---|
| 2-0 to 3-0 | Rides tricycle, using pedals<br>Walks up and down stairs--one foot per step | Holds crayon with fingers<br>Handles small toys skillfully<br>Draws complete circle | Uses pronouns for self and others<br>Talks in simple sentences<br>Speech understandable ½ of time<br>Tells use of familiar objects | Puts on simple garment<br>Washes and dries hands<br>Toilet trained | Refers to self as I or me<br>Tells first & last name<br>Plays with children<br>Shows sympathy |
| 3-0 to 4-0 | Hops on one foot, without support | Draws a person that has at least **three** parts<br>Draws a cross (+) | Tells stories about daily experiences<br>Knows three colors<br>Understands concepts--big & little, etc.<br>Understands 2-3 prepositions<br>Counts 4 objects, answers "how many" | Washes & dries hands & face<br>Combs or brushes hair | Knows sex (own and opposite)<br>Plays cooperatively with others |
| 4-0 to 5-0 | Hops--one foot, repeatedly<br>Skips<br>Dances--skillfully<br>Good balance & coordination | Draws a person that has at least **six** parts<br>Draws a square with good corners<br>Prints a few letters | Talks in sentences<br>Completely understandable<br>Defines familiar words | Dresses & undresses without help, except for tying shoes | Plays role in "make-believe" play<br>Follows simple game rules |

**Figure 1.** Developmental Map of the first 5 years.

1. Calculate the child's age by subtracting his birthdate from the date the Developmental Review was completed. See example below: The child has passed the age of 3 years, 1 month, but is not yet 3 years, 2 months. His age is recorded as 3-1. Drop the days after calculating the age, not before. For children under age 2, the age is recorded in months. For example, a child whose age is calculated as 1 year 7 months is recorded as 19 months.

| | | | | | | | |
|---|---|---|---|---|---|---|---|
| Date Completed | 1978 | ~~7~~ 6 | ~~8~~ 38 | Date Completed | ____ | ____ | ____ |
| Birthdate | 1975 | 5 | 14 | Birthdate | ____ | ____ | ____ |
| Age | 3 | 1 | 24 | Age | ____ | ____ | ____ |

2. Draw a horizontal line across the Developmental Map at the child's age level.

3. For each area of development, mark the individual items reported by the mother or observed in the clinic. It may be necessary to mark only the more mature items in each area rather than all items.

4. For each area of development, compare the child's behavioral age level to his actual age level. In this way, it is possible to appreciate whether the child's behavior is above, within, or below age expectations.

5. Use the following developmental status categories to determine whether the child, in each area, is

   A = Advanced—displays behavior characteristic of children significantly older than himself (behavior above age interval).

   WA = Within age expectations—displays behavior at age interval or within age range (one interval below).

   (?) = Questionable development—displays behavior at a level which is less mature than children significantly younger than himself. Fails to demonstrate behaviors within his age interval *and* fails to demonstrate behaviors at the next younger age interval. For example, a 13-month-old who is not walking (12–18 months) and not crawling (9–12 months).

   DD = Definitely delayed—over 50% delayed, for example, a 2-year-old who is not displaying the behavior of a 1-year-old; example, a 2-year-old who is not walking, a 4-year-old who is not using word combinations, etc.

6. Record the classification in the space at the bottom of the Developmental Map. *When in doubt*, record two categories, for example: A/WA; Wa/(?); (?)/DD. Underline ratings for those areas of development where the rating is either (?) or DD.

**Figure 2.** Developmental Map interpretative guidelines.

children, and do not include any follow-up evaluation of the incidence of children who "passed" the Developmental Review. Nevertheless, the results are promising in that they found incidences of positives and true positives comparable to the DDST. The Developmental Review procedures show considerable promise for involving parents in the process and encouraging parents to be more aware of and more enabling of their child's development. The most meaningful conclusions at this point are that the concept and methodology are deserving of serious consideration, but need refinement, and subsequently formal research, to test their validity and utility.

The authors wish to stress that, at this point, the Developmental Review process is a prototype for a systematic means of reviewing a child's development. Neither the items of the Developmental Map nor the guidelines for interpretation of results should be taken literally until further research is done with this method. The logic and process of Developmental Review could probably be used by professionals in its present form if the professional is knowledgeable about early childhood development (i.e., milestones, and the range of normal) and experienced in working with young children.

Developmental review, by virtue of its intent and format, is more time-consuming than developmental screening. It is probably best viewed as a parent education or anticipatory guidance tool. It would appear to stand at an intermediate level between brief screening and in-depth developmental assessment.

Given the present narrowly defined goals of most screening programs, it is unrealistic to expect that the Developmental Review method would be used *in toto*. However, it is our hope that the concept of Developmental Review will at least affect the way that screening is viewed, especially in terms of the way that parent information is regarded and utilized, and the way a child's development is viewed and characterized. Furthermore, if future trends are in the direction of placing higher priorities on preventative services, on family involvement in promoting child development, and on regarding all children as "special," the shift toward Developmental Review will be a logical one.

## REFERENCES

Alpern, G. D., Boll, T. J., & Shearer, M. (1980). *Developmental Profile II.* Aspen, CO: Psychological Development Publications.

Frankenburg, W. K., & Dodds, J. B. The Denver Developmental Screening Test. *Journal of Pediatrics, 71,* 181–191.

Frankenburg, W. K., van Doorninck, W. J., Liddell, T. N., & Dick, N. P. (1976). The Denver Prescreening Developmental Questionnaire. *Prediatrics, 57,* 744–753.

Gesell, A. L., & Amatruda, C. S. (1954). *Developmental diagnosis.* New York: Hoeber.

Gottfried, A. W. Guerin, D., Spencer, J. E., & Meyer, C. (1983). Concurrent validity of the Minnesota Child Development Inventory in a nonclinical sample. *Journal of Consulting and Clinical Psychology, 51,* 643–644

Huntington, D. (1977). *Developmental review in the EPSDT program* (HCFA 77-24537). Washington, DC: U.S. Development of Health, Education, and Welfare, The Medicaid Bureau.

Ireton, H., & Thwing, E. (1974). *The Minnesota Child Development Inventory.* Minneapolis, MN: Behavior Science Systems.

Ireton, H., & Thwing, E. (1979). *The Minnesota Preschool Inventory.* Minneapolis, MN: Behavior Science Systems.

Ireton, H., & Thwing, E. (1980a). *The Minnesota Infant Development Inventory.* Minneapolis, MN: Behavior Science Systems.

Ireton, H., & Thwing, E. (1980b). *The Minnesota Preschool Inventory Form* 3, 4. Minneapolis, MN: Behavior Science Systems.

Lichenstein, R., & Ireton, H. (1984). *Preschool screening: Identifying young children with developmental and educational problems.* New York: Grune & Stratton.

McShane, M. (1973). *The utility of parent reports in clinical practice and research with children.* Unpublished manuscript. (Available from H. Ireton, Mayo Box 381, University of Minnesota Health Sciences, Minneapolis, MN 55455).

Stone, N. W., Ireton, H., & Runquist, R. (1979). *Procedures for the assessment and review of development: A field study* (HCFA 77-500-0031). Washington, DC: The American Association of Psyhiatric Services for Children. No. 77-500-0032.

CHAPTER 15

# The Texas Preschool Screening Inventory

## A SIMPLE SCREENING DEVICE FOR LANGUAGE AND LEARNING DISORDERS

*Julian S. Haber and Marylee Norris*

Of the more than 4 million children in the United States classified as educationally handicapped (Martin, 1980), more than half are classified as having hearing, speech, or learning disabilities. Many of these youngsters have subtle deficits not readily identified by routine pediatric examination. Furthermore, most of the available screening examinations are somewhat laborious and not well suited for routine office use (Smith, 1978).

In 1980 it came to the attention of the Committee on Handicapped Children of the Texas Pediatric Society and the Texas Chapter of the American Academy of Pediatrics that many youngsters were failing one, two, or even more grades of school before they were referred for proper psychometric testing. Because many children have a checkup by a health professional before they enter elementary school, the Committee sought to develop an instrument that would identify youngsters with potential school problems.

The Texas Preschool Screening Inventory (TPSI) which resulted (Haber, 1981) is a simple preschool screening device for identifying children who need further assessment for language and learning disabilities. It is designed to be given in an office setting by paramedical personnel in less than 10 minutes.

*Julian S. Haber and Marylee Norris* • Miller Speech and Hearing Clinic, Division of Communication Pathology, Texas Christian University, Fort Worth, Texas 76129.

## METHOD

### Subjects in the Validation Study

Eighty-one subjects were used for initial validation studies. These children were students at Starpoint School, the Miller Speech and Hearing Clinic, Texas Christian University, and/or the Fort Worth Independent School District. All were currently enrolled in programs for language and learning disabled students.

### Field Tests

In addition, field tests were performed in physician's offices. This group contained 282 subjects (who are an ongoing sample). All tests were administered by licensed practical nurses, registered nurses, and occasionally by the physicians. Family income levels were variable; parents of 104 of the subjects earned between 0 and $19,000; 142 earned between $20,000 and $39,000; and 36 earned more than $40,000.

### Special Populations

Two subgroups were also examined. One consisted of 53 Head Start subjects (an ongoing sample) from urban areas who were tested at Miller Speech and Hearing Clinic. Assessment was performed by junior and senior undergraduate students and graduate students enrolled in the Communication Pathology Department at Texas Christian University. All subjects were also tested with the Hannah–Gardner Test of Verbal and Nonverbal Language Functioning (Hannah & Gardner, 1978).

Table 1 provides details of the sex, ages, and races of children in the groups.

### Measures

The TPSI is composed of eight subtests in areas that are important for successful school performance. They are auditory memory, visual memory, auditory sequencing, articulation, sound discrimination, rotations and reversals, following instructions, and prepositions. The eight subtests are described below.

***Auditory Memory.*** This subtest is based on the writings of Zimmerman, Steiner, and Pond (1979), McCarthy (1972), and Gesell (1956). The examiner states, "Listen to what I say and repeat the numbers when I stop talking." The numbers are given in sequences of 3 (i.e., 3-4-2),

**Table 1.** Characteristics of Study Subjects

| | Validation study ($N$ = 81) | Physicians' offices field test ($N$ = 282) | Head Start urban subgroup ($N$ = 53) |
|---|---|---|---|
| Male | 54 | 168 | 30 |
| Female | 27 | 114 | 23 |
| 4 yrs. | 23 | 84 | 40 |
| 5 yrs. | 21 | 114 | 13 |
| 6 yrs. | 37 | 84 | — |
| White | 55 | 248 | 6 |
| Black | 19 | 18 | 44 |
| Mexican-American | 7 | 10 | 3 |
| Asian | — | 6 | — |

sequences of 4 (i.e., 7-2-8-1), sequences of 5 (i.e., 2-1-5-7-6). This task is scored in the following manner: For a sequence of 3, a 4-year-old should be able to repeat 2 out of 3 attempts; for a sequence of 4, a 5- or 6-year-old should be able to repeat 2 out of 3 attempts; and for a sequence of 5 numbers, a 6-year-old should be able to repeat at least 2 out of 3 occasions.

***Visual Memory.*** A 4-year-old is presented with four objects in sequence, a 5-year-old with five objects in sequence, and a 6-year-old with six objects in sequence. The child is permitted to watch the sequential order for 15 seconds, after which the objects are scrambled. The child is asked to replicate them in order.

***Auditory Sequencing (Syntax).*** This subtest results from the work of Wiig and Semel (1980). The child is given sentences of increasing length and complexity to repeat for each age level. The child is instructed, "Repeat these sentences exactly as I say them." Then the examiner says for a 4-year-old: "I like to eat red apples." For the 5-year-old the following phrase is added: "Tommy went to the store to get food for his cat." The phrase added for the 6-year-old is "Mrs. Jones asked John to bring home some bread and butter."

The task is scored as follows: A 4-year-old should repeat the first sentence correctly. A 5-year-old should be able to reproduce the second sentence correctly with only one or two word displacements. A 6-year-old is required to produce all three sentences correctly. In addition, if a child articulates the sentences poorly, the articulation subtest is performed (that subtest may be omitted if the child articulates the sentences well).

***Articulation.*** Helmick and Mason (1977) have discussed this subtest. The child is told to repeat the following words: K-Kite, G-Goat, R-Rabbit, L-Leaf, J-Jar, Th-Thumb, S-Socks, Z-Zoo, Ch-Church, Sh-Shoes. If the child scores below age level on the articulation subtest, further evaluation with an articulation screening instrument is recommended.

***Sound Discrimination.*** Hammill and Newcomer (1977) and Wigg and Semel (1976) influenced the development of this subtest in which the child is presented with a series of similar-sounding words and asked to differentiate which pairs sound the same and which do not sound the same. The examiner instructs the subject as follows: "If I say girl-girl these are the same words and sound the same. If I say share-chair, these are not the same words and do not sound the same. We share toys but a chair is something we sit in. Even though the words rhyme, they are not the same word and do not sound the same."

The task is scored as follows: One or two misses is normal at age 4; at ages 5 and 6, the child is permitted one miss.

***Rotations and Reversals.*** The work of Kinsbourne and Caplan (1979) was influential in this subtest. Children who have not completed kindergarten are asked to copy the following symbols: ○, +, ▭,
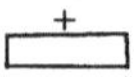.

A 4-year-old should be able to copy one of the four symbols, a 5-year-old should be able to copy two, and a 6-year-old should be able to copy three of the four.

Children who have completed kindergarten are instructed, "Please print the following words in lower case ('little,' not capital letters) when I say the words . . . boy, girl, moon, no, good, saw, bad, pop . . . . And now please write the following numbers: 16, 85, 92, 37, 45." If a child cannot spell, he or she is asked to print the letters b, g, m, n, o, d, p. If a child does not understand the dual number system, the numbers 1 through 10 may be presented separately.

A child still in kindergarten normally rotates and reverses these letters. By the end of kindergarten, two reversals in the entire series are acceptable. By the middle of the first grade, there should be no rotations or reversals in the words and numbers presented in this subtest.

***Following Instructions.*** This is divided into the ability to follow a two-part and three-part instruction. The child is told by the examiner: "Give the block to me and then sit down." Next, the youngster is instructed, "Walk to the door, touch your nose, and then sit down,"

A 4-year-old should be able to follow the two-part instruction. A 5-year-old and 6-year-old should be able to follow the three-part instruction.

*Prepositions.* The child is handed a block and instructed to put it under the table and then on top of the table. All age groups should be able to do this task.

*Scoring.* The entire screening test (task, examiner's instructions, and scoring procedure) is listed on both sides of a single sheet of paper. The scoring is by age and task. The highest age of achievement in each category is checked by the examiner. However, any subtest should be stopped when a child reaches his or her chronological age level.

Individual examiners may wish to exercise their own judgment when a child scores below age level on a single subtest. However, a child is only considered to be at high risk for language and learning disabilities when scoring below age level on two or more subtests.

## PROCEDURE

Children in the validation group were diagnosed as language or learning disabled utilizing criteria established by the Texas Education Agency according to rules set forth in P.L. 91–142. Their scores on standard achievement tests were greater than 1 *SD* below expectancy based on their cognitive ability. The WISC-R was administered to the 5- and 6-year-olds and the WIPPSI to the 4-year-olds. Achievement tests utilized were the WRAT, Woodcock Johnson, or Piat. In the prekindergarten children, the Zimmerman Preschool Language Scale was used to determine expressive, receptive, and mean language ages. A child was considered to be language disabled if any of the above was greater than 1 *SD* below cognitive ability.

Examiners were senior students and graduate students from the Division of Communication Pathology at Texas Christian University. The results of the subjects' initial psychometric testing was unknown to the examiners.

Subjects tested in physician's offices were randomly selected during the course of routine physical examinations at ages 4, 5, and 6. These were recorded and then reported to our group at TCU. Each subject was followed up within 1 year after the initial testing.

## RESULTS

### Validation Study

Of the 81 subjects in the validation group with educationally diagnosed, known language and learning disabilities, 78 (96.2%) failed to perform at age level in two or more subtests and were, therefore, regarded as in the high-risk category. Three children performed below age level on one subtest, and no subjects passed all subtests at age level.

### Field Tests

Following the validation study, the TPSI was administered to 282 subjects in the offices of private physicians engaged in general pediatrics. These were located in Fort Worth and Bedford, Texas. Fifty-five subjects (20%) scored below age level on two or more subtests. There was no follow-up on 6 of these subjects, but 37, after psychometric testing by their respective schools, were placed in various special education classes. Four were felt to have severe behavior problems without any significant educational deficit. There were 8 children falsely identified.

During the field test, 13 high-risk students were identified at ages 4 and 5 (in each group, 2 were falsely identified). There were 29 high-risk youngsters at age 6 (4 of them falsely identified). Thirty high-risk youngsters were identified in the 0 to $19,000 income group, 18 in the $20,000 to $39,000 income group, and 7 in the over $40,000 income group. Racially, 53 whites and 2 blacks were at risk. The mean time to administer the instrument during field testing was 7.4 minutes.

### Special Population

The urban Head Start sample from day care centers consisted of 53 subjects. Thirteen (24.5%) failed two or more subtests. Twelve subjects were commonly identified by the TPSI and the Hannah–Gardner (1978). One subject was identified by the Hannah–Gardner and not the TPSI, and one by the TPSI and not the Hannah–Gardner.

## DISCUSSION

The eight subtests of the TPSI were chosen because they include some of the key components of language necessary for adequate school performance. In designing the TPSI, we intended to create a simple instrument capable of identifying children at risk for learning and language disabilities. The test was constructed to be administered by various paraprofessional personnel (such as aides, teachers, nurses, and so on) with a minimum of instruction in less than 10 minutes. As the results indicate, the test identifies children at risk both when validated with a group of educationally identified language and learning disabled children as well as with various samples of unknowns in the field. The average time of administration was 7.4 minutes, which certainly is acceptable for most office uses. Indeed, due to its simplicity, the authors hope that the TPSI can be used much as one would use an eye chart, audiogram, or urinalysis or blood pressure instrument.

The study attempted to include all socioeconomic and certain ethnic subgroups so as to avoid the mistakes and pitfalls of some other instruments (Dunn, 1980; Kirk, McCarthy, & Kirk, 1968). The authors do not recommend use of this test where the predominant language in the home is Spanish, as this group was not adequately studied. A bilingual version of the TPSI is currently being prepared; it will be extensively field-tested among bilingual children in the not-too-distant future.

It is important that professionals utilizing the TPSI realize that this is merely a screening device and not a definitive measure. Prognostications should not be made to parents on the basis of the TPSI; rather, children at risk should be referred to their appropriate local school agency for further delineation of the potential problem.

> Indeed, the concept of a screening and evaluation are separate issues. Screening is a process whereby the child's performance is judged against a set standard or expectation for chronologic age or other factor. Failure of a screening exam only indicates a need for evaluation. It does not identify the child as being handicapped. However, the child who fails a screening exam should be identified to the Educational Agency as a child in need of a full evaluation. (Powers, 1981, p. 1)

Although the TPSI was designed specifically for use in physicians' offices, the authors feel that it has multiple purposes. Among these are in preschool screening programs, transitional testing between kindergarten and first grade, screening when the teacher is unsure whether to refer a child, and to help indicate to a reluctant parent that a child might need further psychometric evaluation. It is our feeling that it is important to identify these problems before a child actually begins formal school instruction, as failure to do so may impact negatively on a child's health and well-being for a lifetime.

## SUMMARY

1. The TPSI is a simple screening test designed to be given in a minimal amount of time by examiners with varying degrees of professional training.

2. In field testing to date on various ethnic and socioeconomic groups, the TPSI has efficiently identified children at high risk for learning and language disabilities.

3. Children identified as being at risk by the TPSI should be referred to their local education agency for further testing.

4. A bilingual (Spanish-English) version is under preparation and should be available within a year.

## REFERENCES

Dunn, L. (1980). *Peabody Picture Vocabulary Test*. Circle Pines, MN: American Guidance Service.

Gesell, A. (1956). Developmental schedules. New York: Psychological Corp.

Haber, J. S. (1981). *Texas Preschool Screening Inventory*. Austin, TX: Texas Pediatric Society.

Hamhill, D. D., & Newcomer, P. L. (1977). *Test of Language Development*. Austin, Texas: Univ. of Texas Press.

Hannah, E., & Gardner, J. (1978). *Hannah–Gardner Test of Verbal and Nonverbal Language Functioning*. Northridge, CA: Lingua Press.

Helmick, J., & Mason, R. (1977). Speech screening of children in the dental office. *Journal of American Dental Association, 94*, 709–771.

Kinsbourne, M., & Caplan, P. (1979). *Children's learning and attention problems*. Boston, MA: Little Brown.

Kirk, S., McCarthy, J., & Kirk, W. (1968). *Illinois Test of Psycholinguistics*. Urbana, IL: Univ. of Illinois Press.

Martin, E. (1980). *2nd Annual Report to Congress: Public Law 94–142, The Education for All Handicapped Children's Act*. State Program of Implementation Studies, Branch of the Office of Special Education, Washington, DC.

McCarthy, D. A. (1972). *Manual for the McCarthy Scale of Children's Abilities*. New York: Psychology Corp.

Powers, J. (1981). *Task force on Public Law 94–142*. Evanston, IL: American Academy of Pediatrics.

Smith, R. D. (1978). The use of developmental screening test by primary care physicians. *Journal of Pediatrics, 93*, 524–527.

Wiig, E., & Semel, E. (1976). *Language disabilities in children and adolescents*. Columbus, OH: Charles E. Merrill.

Wiig, E., & Semel, E. (1980). *Language assessment and intervention for the learning disabled*. Columbus, OH: Charles E. Merrill.

Zimmerman, I. L., Steiner, V. G., & Pond, R. E. (1979). *Preschool Language Scale*. Columbus, OH: Charles E. Merrill.

Miller Speech and Hearing Clinic, Division of Communication Pathology, Texas Christian University, Fort Worth, Texas 761290.

# PART III

## SELECTIVE FOLLOW-UP OF AT-RISK POPULATIONS

CHAPTER 16

# A Risk Index to Predict Learning Problems in Preterm and Full-Term Children

*Linda S. Siegel*

---

Learning problems, that is, significant difficulties in one or more school subjects in spite of normal intelligence, are estimated to exist in 10% to 16% of the population (Gaddes, 1976), and as such are an important problem for those concerned with the physical and mental health of children. Early prediction of learning difficulties would be useful, for remediation could be provided at a time when it is likely to be most effective and less costly. Existing systems of prediction of problems have been very complex, have failed to provide information about an individual child, or have been used only with infants and not children of school age (Broman, Nichols, & Kennedy, 1975; Caputo, Taub, Goldstein, Smith, Dalack, Pursner, & Siberstein, 1974; Field, Hallock, Ting, Dempsey, Dabiri, & Shuman, 1978; Littman & Parmelee, 1978; Ramey, Stedman, Borders-Patterson, & Mengel, 1978; Smith, Flick, Ferriss, & Sellman, 1972).

A risk index has been developed in an attempt to identify young children likely to be at risk for learning problems. The index involves a relatively small set of reproductive, perinatal, and demographic variables, and predicts aspects of cognitive and language development in children at 2 years (Siegel, Saigal, Rosenbaum, Morton, Young, Berenbaum, & Stoskopf, 1982), 3 years (Siegel, 1982a), and 5 years (Siegel, 1982b). This chapter examines the ability of the risk index to predict achievement test scores at 6 years and to detect children whose scores

---

*Linda S. Siegel* • Department of Special Education, Ontario Institute for Studies in Education, Toronto, Ontario, Canada M5S 1V6.

are in the below-average range. The ability of the infant tests to predict achievement test scores at 6 years is also examined.

Previous studies have found that the Bayley Scales (Bayley, 1969) and Uzgiris-Hunt Scale (Uzgiris & Hunt, 1975) predict subsequent scores and discriminate children who will show developmental delay (Siegel, 1979, 1981, 1982c, 1983a). With heterogeneous samples, others have also found moderate correlations with tests of intellectual functioning in middle childhood (e.g., Ramey, Cambell, & Nicholson, 1973; Wilson, 1978a,b). It was expected that the accuracy of the risk index's prediction of developmental functioning and delay could be improved with the use of infant tests. In addition, a measure of the environment—Bradley and Caldwell's (1976) Home Observation for the Measurement of the Environment (HOME)—was used to assess environmental influence on development. It was expected that developmental outcome would not be determined by a single factor, but that measurement of a variety of biological and environmental factors would be necessary for the successful prediction of later learning disorders.

## METHODS

### Subjects

All the infants whose birth weights were ≤1,500 g and who were born and/or treated at the McMaster University Health Sciences Centre Neonatal Intensive Care Unit in the period of July 1, 1975 to June 1976 were enrolled for a longitudinal prospective study. The comparison group of full-term infants consisted of demographically similar infants (Siegel *et al.*, 1982) who were born after uncomplicated singleton deliveries, and who have experienced a normal perinatal course. The preterm and full-term infants were matched for socioeconomic factors, parity, sex, and age of the mother at the birth of the infant.

There were 44 full-term and 42 preterm children available for testing at 6 years. Most of the children who were not available from the original sample had moved outside the area. However, 10 preterm children and 1 full-term child from the total sample had sequelae (blindness, severe retardation, and/or cerebral palsy) such that it was not meaningful to administer developmental tests. Four of the preterm infants died in the first 12 months following their discharge from the Neonatal Intensive Care Unit.

The demographic characteristics of the children who were available for study at 6 years were as follows: Hollingshead (1957) SES, percentage class 3 to 5; 81% were preterm and 63.2% were full-term; 50% of the preterm children were male, whereas 60.5% of the full-term children were male; and 37.5% of the preterm were firstborns, whereas 40.5% of the full-term children were firstborn. The groups were not significantly different on these variables ($\chi^2$). The mean maternal age for both groups was 26.1 years. The preterm children had a mean birth weight of 1.20 kg and a mean gestational age of 30.5 weeks.

### Developmental Testing

The children were seen at 4, 8, 12, 18, 24, 36, 48, 60, and 72 months. Chronological age was used as the basis for developmental testing, although scores corrected for the degree of prematurity were also considered when possible. The Bayley Scales of Infant Development (Bayley, 1969) was administered at 4, 8, 12, 18, and 24 months; a modified version of the Uzgiris–Hunt Scale (Uzgiris & Hunt, 1975) was used at 4, 8, 12, and 18 months; the Reynell Developmental Language Scales (Reynell, 1969) was given at 24, 36, and 48 months; and a battery designed to predict learning disabilities (Satz, Taylor, Friel, & Fletcher, 1978) was administered at 48 and 60 months. In addition, the Wechsler Intelligence Scale for Children—Revised (WISC-R) (Weschler, 1974), the Wide Range Achievement Test (WRAT) (Jastak & Jastak, 1978), the Grammatic Closure subtest of the Illinois Test of Psycholinguistic Abilities (ITPA) (Kirk, McCarthy, & Kirk, 1968), and the Connors Parent questionnaire (Goyette, Connors, & Uhrich, 1978) were administered at 5 and 6 years.

The Grammatic Closure subtest of the Illinois Test of Psycholinguistic Abilities measures the child's understanding of some regular and irregular aspects of English syntax. A scaled score based on age is used for this test. The WRAT provides measures of reading, spelling, and arithmetic.

The Satz battery (Satz *et al.*, 1978), designed to predict learning disabilities, was administered at 4 and 5 years and consists of five tests, as follows:

1. The Peabody Picture Vocabulary Test (PPVT) (Dunn, 1959). This is a vocabulary test in which the child must identify which of four pictures depicts a given word. Results are typically reported in terms of IQ scores.

2. The Beery Developmental Test of Visual-Motor Integration (VMI) (Beery, 1967). For this test, the child has to copy an increasingly difficult series of geometric forms. Performance is compared with age norms and an IQ equivalent can be calculated based on the child's chronological age.

Three other tests included recognition discrimination, alphabet recitation, and finger localization.

## Risk Index Variables

Reproductive, perinatal, and demographic variables were used for each child. The reproductive variables were birth order (gravidity), amount of maternal smoking during pregnancy (none, less than 10, 10 to 20, and over 20 cigarettes per day), and number of previous spontaneous abortions. The perinatal variables included birth weight; 1-minute and 5-minute Apgar scores; and, for the preterm infants, gestational age, severity of respiratory distress (RDS), birth asphyxia, and apnea. These terms were defined as follows: Severe RDS involved assisted ventilation, X-ray evidence of RDS, and/or oxygen levels higher than 80%; moderate RDS included assisted ventilation, continuous positive airway pressure (CPAP), and/or oxygen levels between 40% and 80%; and mild RDS consisted of oxygen levels less than 40%. A 1-minute Apgar score of less than 5 was defined as asphyxia. For apnea, a measure of the number of days in which apneic spells occurred was used, with periods of apnea greater than 20 seconds. Hollingshead (1957) socioeconomic status, sex, and maternal and paternal educational levels were also included in the analyses.

# RESULTS

When the scores of the preterm and full-term children on the WRAT, PPVT, ITPA Grammatic Closure, Beery VMI, and the Conners Parent Questionnaire Learning Problem Scale were compared, the preterm children had significantly lower scores on the WRAT Spelling and Arithmetic subtests, the Beery VMI, the ITPA Grammatic Closure, and the Conners Learning Problem Index. The WRAT Spelling subtest and the Beery VMI involve copying shapes and are measures of eye–hand coordination. A number of investigators have reported difficulties with eye–hand coordination in very low birth weight children (Hunt, Tooley, & Harvin, 1982; Siegel *et al.*, 1982; Siegel, 1983b; Wallace, Escalona, McCarton-Daum, & Vaughan, 1982). These preterm children also had greater difficulties with some aspects of language at earlier points in their development (Siegel *et al.*, 1982). The Conners score indicates that parents of preterm children rated their children as having more learning problems than did parents of full-term children.

## Specific Learning Disabilities

A *learning disability* is defined as having difficulties in some area of of academic achievement in spite of normal intellectual functioning or IQ. A learning disability was defined as a low achievement test score

**Table 1.** Percentage of Children with Specific Learning Disabilities

| | If WISC-R IQ ≥ 90 | | If WISC-R IQ ≥ 80 | |
|---|---|---|---|---|
| | Full-term (*N* = 40) | Preterm (*N* = 32) | Full-term (*N* = 43) | Preterm (*N* = 38) |
| WRAT | | | | |
| Reading | 10.0 | 9.4 | 14.0 | 10.5 |
| Spelling | 2.5 | 28.1** | 4.7 | 28.9** |
| Arithmetic | 5.0 | 15.6 | 7.0 | 18.4 |
| Beery VMI | 30.8 | 59.4* | 33.3 | 57.9* |
| PPVT | 0.0 | 0.0 | 0.0 | 5.7 |
| ITPA | 8.3 | 16.0* | 15.4 | 19.4 |

*$p < .05$ for significance of difference between full-term and preterm infants. **$p < .01$ for significance of difference between full-term and preterm infants.

(≤25th percentile) in spite of IQ test scores in the normal range. The percentage of children who were delayed in these areas using a cutoff score of a WISC-R Scale IQ ≥90 or ≥80 (the choice is arbitrary) are shown in Table 1. The pattern of results was the same for both cases; more of the preterms were delayed in WRAT Spelling, and the Beery VMI indicating specific problems with perceptual motor functioning.

## Prediction of Subsequent Development

Stepwise linear multiple regression analyses were conducted using the risk index variables as predictors and the WRAT subtests as outcome variables. This statistical technique allows us to examine the relative contributions of variables to a particular outcome and enables us to assess the combined correlatives of several variables with the outcome. The results (Table 2) show that the correlation between these variables and the outcome measures was significant. Although environmental factors were significant components of the regression analyses, the indicators of the severity of perinatal insult (e.g., RDS, asphyxia, apnea) were also important.

## Predicting Delays in Academic Achievement

In order to predict a learning disability, I used linear stepwise discriminant function analyses. This statistical technique allows the determination of a set of cutoff scores that separate the children likely to be at risk from the larger population. A score of 25th percentile on one of the subtests of the WRAT was considered an indication of a possible learning disability. The ability of the risk index variables to predict per-

**Table 2.** Results of the Multiple Regression Analysis of Risk Index Prediction

| Full-term | | Preterm | |
|---|---|---|---|
| | Reading | | |
| Birth order<br>Maternal education<br>Maternal smoking<br>Apgar—1 minute<br>Sex | .57 | SES<br>Apgar—1 minute<br>IVH<br>Sex<br>RDS | .71 |
| | Spelling | | |
| Maternal education<br>Apgar—1 minute<br>Birth order<br>Apgar—5 minutes<br>SES | .54 | Apnea<br>Asphyxia<br>SES<br>RDS<br>Sex | .71 |
| | Arithmetic | | |
| Previous spontaneous abortions<br>SES<br>Sex<br>Apgar—5 minutes<br>Maternal smoking | .43 | Asphyxia<br>SES<br>Gestational age<br>Apgar—5 minutes<br>Sex | .62 |

formance is shown in Table 3. As can be seen, rate of children falsely identified as not being at risk when they in fact were was low. Most of the children who would show a problem could have been detected. However, the rate of children falsely identified as being at risk who were not was slightly higher.

## Prediction of Achievement Scores with Learning Infant Tests

The correlations of the Bayley Scales with the WRAT, Beery VMI, PPVT, and the ITPA Grammatic Closure as shown in Tables 4 and 5. As can be seen from these tables, the Psychomotor Development Scale (PDI) had higher correlations with the outcome variables earlier in development (4, 8, and sometimes 12 months), whereas the Mental Development Scale (MDI) had higher correlations at 18 and 24 months. In infancy, the Bayley Scales may be providing an indication of the level of maturation of the nervous system, and the Beery may be providing similar information at an older age.

**Table 3.** Prediction of Delay on the WRAT at 6 Years

| | True negative | True positive | False negative | False positive | Percentage correct prediction |
|---|---|---|---|---|---|
| | | | Reading | | |
| Full-term | 35 | 4 | 1 | 3 | 90.7 |
| Preterm | 35 | 3 | 0 | 4 | 90.5 |
| | | | Spelling | | |
| Full-term | 35 | 2 | 0 | 6 | 86.1 |
| Preterm | 19 | 12 | 2 | 6 | 79.5 |
| | | | Arithmetic | | |
| Full-term | 35 | 2 | 1 | 5 | 86.1 |
| preterm | 23 | 9 | 1 | 9 | 76.2 |

## Correlations of Preschool Tests with Outcome Variables

The correlations of the Reynell Language Scales and the Stanford Binet with the WRAT and other outcome variables revealed that scores on these preschool tests were significantly correlated with the 6-year scores. Typically, the correlations were statistically significant, but in the

**Table 4.** Correlations of the Bayley Scales in Infancy with the WRAT at 6 Years ($N$ = 67–82)

| | Time of administration of the Bayley (months) | | | | |
|---|---|---|---|---|---|
| Bayley scale | 4 | 8 | 12 | 18 | 24 |
| | | | WRAT reading | | |
| MDI | ns | ns | ns | .33 | .27* |
| PDI | .21* | .22* | .19* | ns | ns |
| | | | WRAT spelling | | |
| MDI | .29** | .28** | .35*** | .41*** | .31** |
| PDI | .51.*** | .41*** | .36*** | ns | .25* |
| | | | WRAT arithmetic | | |
| MDI | .22* | ns | .26* | .28** | .28** |
| PDI | .37*** | .28** | .39*** | ns | .30* |

*$p$ < .05. **$p$ < .01. ***$p$ < .001.

**Table 5.** Correlations of the Bayley with the PPVT, ITPA, and Beery VMI at 6 Years ($N$ = 67–82)

| | Time of administration of the Bayley (months) | | | | |
|---|---|---|---|---|---|
| Bayley scale | 4 | 8 | 12 | 18 | 24 |
| | | | PPVT | | |
| MDI | ns | ns | .24* | .38*** | .44*** |
| PDI | .28** | .24* | .23* | ns | .26* |
| | | | ITPA | | |
| MDI | ns | ns | ns | .38*** | .52*** |
| PDI | .21* | .24* | ns | ns | ns |
| | | | Beery | | |
| MDI | .37*** | .40*** | .43*** | .35*** | .35*** |
| PDI | .41*** | .29*** | .49*** | ns | .36*** |

*$p < .05$. **$p < .01$. ***$p < .001$.

moderate range. However, the Reynell language measures (Expression and Comprehension) were quite highly correlated with the ITPA and PPVT, both of which are measures of various aspects of language development.

The correlations of the components of the Satz battery administered at 4 years with the 6-year measures were significant. The Beery and the Recognition Discrimination were most consistently correlated with the outcome measures, although the PPVT at 4 years was correlated with the language measures (ITPA and PPVT) at 6 years.

The multiple correlations of the Satz battery administered at 4 years with WRAT percentile scores were as follows: reading, .58; spelling, .57; and arithmetic, .51. In the case of reading, alphabet recitation was the most important variable, whereas for spelling and arithmetic, the Beery Visual Motor and the Recognition Discrimination task were the most important. The reading score was more closely related to language measures, whereas the spelling and arithmetic scores were related to perceptual and eye–hand coordination measures. If a cutoff score of less than the 25th percentile on a WRAT subtest was used, the five tests of the Satz battery correctly classified 76.1% for the reading scores, 70.7% for the spelling scores, and 66.2% for arithmetic scores.

The multiple correlations of the five variables in the Satz battery administered at 5 years with the WRAT percentile scores was .68 for reading, .67 for spelling, and .64 for arithmetic. The Beery Visual Motor Integration had the highest individual correlation in all cases. If a cutoff score of less than the 25th percentile on the WRAT was used, the Satz battery was reasonably accurate at predicting the children with significantly low scores. The overall classification rates were 88.4% for reading, 81% for spelling, and 85.1% for arithmetic. Obviously, the Satz battery was more accurate at 5 years than 4 years.

### Environmental Influences

When correlations of the HOME scale administered at 12, 36, and 60 months were compared with outcome variables, there were few indications of environmental effects early in development, although these effects became more pronounced later on. The Beery VMI scores were not correlated with any environmental measures, whereas the language measures (PPVT, WRAT Reading, and ITPA) were. The Beery may be sensitive to the level of maturation of the nervous system as noted earlier, and thus is not the type of measure that would be sensitive to environmental influence. The language measures, on the other hand, may reflect environmental influences. (See Table 6.)

## DISCUSSION

The findings of this study indicate that it is possible to predict with some degree of success which infants will show subsequent learning problems. The system that was successful in this study used biological and environmental variables that were combined in a risk index.

The system utilized is a multifactor one. No single isolated factor,

**Table 6.** Correlations of HOME Total Score with the 6-Year Tests

| | Time of administration of the HOME (months) | | |
|---|---|---|---|
| | $12^a$ | $36^b$ | $60^c$ |
| WRAT | | | |
| Reading | ns | .26* | .40*** |
| Spelling | .21* | .26* | .40*** |
| Arithmetic | ns | .24* | .26* |
| PPVT IQ | .28* | .28* | .37*** |
| ITPA Grammatic Closure | ns | .39** | .44*** |
| Beery VMI | ns | ns | ns |

$^a n = 56$. $^b n = 44$–$46$. $^c n = 69$–$71$.
$^*p < .05$. $^{**}p < .01$. $^{***}p < .001$.

even prematurity, can account for very much of the variable in the outcome. Similar results were reported by Bee *et al.* (1982). Although Bee *et al.* did not find that perinatal variables were high correlated with outcome measures, it should be noted that they had primarily healthy children, little variation, and consequently these measures had virtually no chance of predicting outcome. There was, of course, more variation in the preterm group in the present study. A system of considering a variety of factors simultaneously has proved useful in understanding high-risk parenting also (Riccuiti & Dorman, 1983). Although the risk index was reasonably successful, there was a higher proportion of children falsely identified as at risk than was desirable. Some sort of intervention would have been recommended for these children; such intervention might be beneficial, so that if errors in prediction are to occur, it is probably better that they are in the direction of overidentification. There were few children with later learning problems missed; most of the children with low scores were detected.

The difficulties noted in the preterm children in this study may be an indicator of a potential learning disability, specifically a problem with writing, spelling, arithmetic, and/or spatial concepts, such as that described in Siegel and Feldman (1983).

Perceptual motor problems have been noted as being associated with prematurity (e.g., Caputo, Goldstein, & Taub, 1981; Hunt, 1981; Hunt *et al.*, 1982; Siegel, 1983b; Taub, Goldstein, & Caputo, 1977). This pattern is similar to that noted by Mednick (1977), who found that full-term children who had certain transient symptoms in the neonatal period (e.g., respiratory distress, convulsions) had lower scores than controls on perceptual motor tasks, though there were no differences between the groups on intelligence test scores.

The relationship of environmental influences to subsequent language development was stronger than the relationship of environmental influences to visual-motor and perceptual development. This is a pattern the author has found in a previous study (Siegel, 1984), and suggests the need to consider specific rather than global outcomes when examining relationships. Language of the type measured by the PPVT, which is a vocabulary test, and the ITPA Grammatic Closure, which measures the correct use of inflections, are the type of functions for which the environment may provide specific models. On the other hand, motor and visual-perceptual development can be expected to be less susceptible to specific environmental influences.

## SUMMARY

The purpose of this study was to develop a risk index that would predict learning problems in school-age children. It was intended that the risk index, composed of demographic, environmental, and perinatal variables, be effective and relatively simple and practical to use. The contribution of infant tests and a systematic measure of the environment, the HOME scale, to the prediction of developmental problems was investigated. The subjects in this study were 47 children who had been born prematurely and of very low birth weight (less than 1,500 g) and 44 children who had been full-term infants and who weighed greater than 2,500 g at birth. The groups were matched on socioeconomic status, sex, birth order, and maternal age at the time of the birth.

The children were administered the WISC-R and a variety of achievement tests at 6 years. They had been administered the Bayley Scales at 4, 8, 12, 18 and 24 months, the Reynell Language Scales at 2, 3, and 4 years, the Stanford-Binet at 3 years, the Satz battery (to predict possible learning disabilities) at 4 and 5 years, and the HOME scale at 1, 3, and 5 years.

A risk index composed of a variety of demographic, reproductive, and perinatal variables was developed. Demographic variables included sex, socioeconomic status (Hollingshead, 1957), maternal and paternal educational levels, and maternal smoking history during pregnancy; the reproductive variables included number of previous spontaneous abortions, number of previous preterm births, and birth order of the child; and the perinatal variables included 1-minute and 5-minute Apgar scores and (for the preterm group) apnea, severity of respiratory distress, gestational age, and birth weight.

Stepwise linear multiple regression analyses were conducted using the variables in the risk index as predictors and WRAT reading, spelling, and arithmetic percentile scores as outcome variables. The risk index was significantly correlated with the outcome measures and was successful at detecting developmental problems with relatively low rates of false identification. The infant tests, while significantly correlated with the outcome variables, did not contribute very much to the predictive accuracy of the risk index. The HOME scale was more highly correlated with language than visual or perceptual motor measures.

## Acknowledgments

The author wishes to thank Lorraine Hoult, Denise Marshall, and Wendy McHugh for their help with data collection and analyses; their research was supported by grants from the Ontario Mental Health Foundation and the March of Dimes Birth Defects Foundation, and the Natural Sciences and Engineering Research Council of Canada. The author also wishes to thank the Special Enquiries and Grievance Committee of the McMaster University Faculty Association for their invaluable assistance with this project.

## REFERENCES


Bayley, N. (1969). *Bayley Scales of Infant Development*. New York: Psychological Corp.

Bee, H. L., Barnard, K. E., Eyres, S. J., Gray, D. A., Hammond, M. A., Spietz, A. L., Snyder, D., & Clark, B. (1982). Prediction of IQ and language skill from perinatal status, child performance, family characteristics, and mother–infant interaction. *Child Development, 53*, 1134–1156.

Beery, K. E. (1967). *Developmental Test of Visual Motor Integration*. Chicago: Follett.

Bradley, R. H., & Caldwell, B. M. (1976). The relation of infant's home environment to mental test performance at 54 months: A follow-up study. *Child Development, 47*, 1172–1174.

Broman, S. H., Nichols, P. L., & Kennedy, W. A. (1975). *Preschool IQ: Perinatal and early developmental correlates*. Hillsdale, NJ: Erlbaum.

Caputo, D. V., Goldstein, K. M., & Taub, H. B. (1981). Neonatal compromise and later psychological development: A ten year longitudinal study. In S. L. Friedman & M. Sigman (Eds.), *Preterm birth and psychological development*. New York: Academic Press.

Caputo, D. V., Taub, H. B., Goldstein, K. M., Smith, N., Dalack, J. D., Pursner, J. P., & Silberstein, R. M. (1974). An evaluation of the parameters of maturity at birth as predictors of development at one year of life. *Perceptual and Motor Skills, 39*, 631–652.

Dunn, L. (1959). *Peabody Picture Vocabulary Test*. Circle Pines, MN: American Guidance Service.

Field, T. M., Hallock, N., Ting, G., Dempsey, J., Dabiri, C., & Shuman, H. H. (1978). A first year follow-up of high-risk infants: Formulating a cumulative risk index. *Child Development, 49*, 119–131.

Gaddes, W. H. (1976). Prevalence estimates and the need for definition of learning disabilities. In R. M. Knights & D. J. Bakker (Eds.), *The neuropsychology of learning disorders: Theoretical approaches*. Baltimore: University Park Press.

Goyette, G. H., Conners, C. K., & Ulrich, R. F. (1978). Normative data on the revised Connors Parent and Teacher Rating Scales. *Journal of Abnormal Child Psychology, 6*, 221–236.

Hollingshead, A. B. (1957). Two factor index of social position. Unpublished manuscript, Yale University, New Haven, CT.

Hunt, J. V. (1981). Predicting intellectual disorders in childhood for preterm infants with birth weights below 1501 grams. In S. L. Friedman & M. Signman (Eds.), *Preterm birth and psychological development*. New York: Academic Press.

Hunt, J. V., Tooley, W. H., & Harvin, D. (1982). Learning disabilities in children with birth weights less than 1500 grams. *Seminars in Perinatology, 6*, 280–287.

Jastak, J. F., & Jastak, S. R. (1978). *Wide Range Achievement Test*. Wilminton, DE: Guidance Associates.

Kirk, S. A., McCarthy, J. J., & Kirk, W. D. (1968). *Illinois Test of Psycholinguistic Ability*. Urbana, IL: Univ. of Illinios Press.

Littman, B., & Parmelee, A. H. (1978). Medical correlates of infant development. *Pediatrics, 61*, 470–474.

Mednick, B. R. Intellectual and behavioral functioning of 10- to 12-year-old children who showed certain transient symptoms in the neonatal period. *Child Development, 48*, 844–853.

Ramey, C. T., Campbell, F. A., & Nicholson, J. E. (1973). The predictive power of the Bayley Scales of Infant Development and the Stanford-Binet Intelligence Test in a relatively constant environment. *Child Development, 44*, 790–795.

Ramey, C. T., Stedman, D. J., Borders-Patterson, A., & Mengel, W. (1978). Predicting school achievement from information available at birth. *American Journal of Mental Deficiency, 82*, 525–534.

Reynell, J. (1969). *Reynell Developmental Language Scales*. Windsor, Berkshire, England: NRER.

Riccuiti, H. N., & Dorman, R. (1983). Interaction of multiple factors contributing to high-risk parenting. In R. A. Hoekelman (Ed.), *Minimizing high-risk parenting* (Pediatric Round Table No. 7). Media, PA: Hart Publishing.

Satz, P., Taylor, G. G., Friel, J., & Fletcher, J. (1978). Some developmental and predictive precursors of reading disabilities: A six year follow-up. In A. L. Benton & D. Pearl (Eds.), *Dyslexia: An appraisal of current knowledge*. New York: Oxford Univ. Press.

Siegel, L. S. (1979). Infant perceptual, cognitive, and motor behaviors as predictors of subsequent cognitive and language development. *Canadian Journal of Psychology, 33,* 382–395.

Siegel, L. S. (1981). Infant tests as predictors of cognitive and language development at two years. *Child Development, 52,* 545–557.

Siegel, L. S. (1982a). Reproductive, perinatal, and environmental factors as predictors of the cognitive and language development of preterm infants. *Child Development, 53,* 963–973.

Siegel, L. S. (1982b). Reproductive, perinatal, and environmental variables as predictors of development of preterm (< 1501 grams) and fullterm children at 5 years. *Seminars in Perinatology, 6,* 274–279.

Siegel, L. S. (1982c). Early cognitive and environmental correlates of language development at 4 years. *International Journal of Behavioral Development, 5,* 433–444.

Siegel, L. S. (1983a). Correction for prematurity and its consequences for the assessment of the very low birth weight infant. *Child Development, 54,* 1176–1188.

Siegel, L. S. Predicting possible learning disabilities in preterm and full-term infants. In T. Field & A. Sostek (Eds.), *Infants born at risk: Physiological and perceptual processes*. New York: Grune & Stratton.

Siegel, L. S. (1984). Home environmental influences on cognitive development in preterm and full-term children. In A. W. Gottfried (Ed.), *Home environment and early cognitive development*. San Diego: Academic Press.

Siegel, L. S., & Feldman, W. (1983). Nondyslexic children with combined writing and arithmetic learning disabilities. *Clinical Pediatrics, 22,* 241–244.

Siegel, L. S., Saigal, S., Rosenbaum, P., Morton, R. A., Young, A., Berenbaum, S., & Stoskopf, B. (1982). Predictors of development in preterm and full-term infants: A model for detecting the "at risk" child. *Journal of Pediatric Psychology, 7,* 135–148.

Smith, A. C., Flick, G. L., Ferriss, G. S., & Sellman, A. H. (1972). Prediction of developmental outcome at seven years from prenatal, perinatal, and postnatal events. *Child Development, 43,* 495–507.

Taub, H. B., Goldstein, K. M., & Caputo, D. V. (1977). Indices of neonatal prematurity as discriminators of development in middle childhood. *Child Development, 48,* 797–805.

Uzgiris, I., & Hunt, M. V. (1975). *Assessment in infancy: Ordinal scales of psychologial development*. Urbana: Univ. of Illinois Press.

Wallace, I. F., Escalona, S. K., McCarton-Daum, D., & Vaughan, H. G. Jr. (1982). Neonatal precursors of cognitive development in low birth weight children. *Seminars in Perinatology, 6,* 327–333.

Wechsler, D. (1974). *Weschler Intelligence Scale for Children—Revised*. New York: The Psychological Corp.

Wilson, R. S. (1978a). Sensorimotor and cognitive development. In F. D. Minifie & L. L. Lloyd (Eds.), *Communicative and cognitive abilities: Early behavioral assessment*. Baltimore: University Park Press.

Wilson, R. S. (1978b). Synchronies in mental development: An epigenetic perspective. *Science, 202,* 939–948.

CHAPTER 17

# Neonatal Brazelton and Bayley Performance at 12 and 18 Months of Infants with Intraventricular Hemorrhage

*Juarlyn L. Gaiter, Helga Binder, Cheryl Naulty, and Sharon Murray*

Intraventricular hemorrhage (IVH) is the most common brain lesion documented at autopsy in 40% to 50% of preterm infants with birth weights less than 1,500 g (Papile, Burstein, Burstein, & Kofler, 1978). The incidence of IVH remains high in the very low birth weight preterm population because of improved survival rates of infants with increasingly shorter gestations in whom IVH insult can be expected (Shinnar, Molteni, Gammon, D'Souva, Altman, & Freeman, 1982). Ultrasonographic studies conducted within 2 to 10 days of preterm birth can detect IVH in approximately one-third of infants of very low birth weight (less than 1,500 g) (Ahmann, Lazzara, Dykes, Brann, & Schwartz, 1978; Papile *et al.*, 1978).

Results of follow-up studies of premature infants with IVH indicate that IVH is highly associated with subsequent motor dysfunction and cerebral palsy (Ment, Scott, Ehrenkranz, Rothman, Duncan, & Warshaw, 1982; Schechner, Ross, & Auld, 1980; Williamson, Desmond, Wilson, Andrew, & Garcia-Prats, 1982); higher incidence of neurodevelopmental dysfunction (Palmer, & Dubowitz, Leven, & Dubowitz,

*Juarlyn L. Gaiter, Helga Binder, Cheryl Naulty, and Sharon Murray* • Children's Hospital National Medical Center, Washington, DC 20016. Preparation of this manuscript was funded in part by a grant No. 12-24 from the March of Dimes-Birth Defects Foundation to the first author.

1982); and abnormal developmental functioning at 12 months of age or older (Gaiter, 1982; Papile, Munsick-Bruno, & Schaefer, 1983; Shinnar *et al.*, 1982).

Currently, there are two major hypotheses concerning the ways in which IVH influences subsequent development.

1. *Severity hypothesis* advocates that it is only the more severe grades of IVH that have long-term adverse effects (e.g., Grades III and IV—ventricular dilation and sequelae of progressive hydrocaphalus requiring shunts—Horbar, Pasnick, Leahy, & Lucey, 1982; Palmer *et al.*, 1982; Papile *et al.*, 1978, 1983).

2. *Marker for risk hypothesis* proposes that regardless of the degree of IVH there is a persistent pattern of identifiable delays in the performance of IVH infants as compared with infants who did not evidence IVH (Bozynski *et al.*, 1982; Fitzhardinge, Pape, & Arstikaitis, 1976; Krishnamoorthy, Shannon, & DeLong, 1979; Papile, Munsick, Weaver, & Techa, 1979).

A corallary hypothesis is that the trauma *per se* bears little association with later outcome if recovery rate is not taken into account. The infants most at risk for compromised developmental functioning are those for whom the trauma and attendant medical complications resulted in a protracted hospital stay with numerous setbacks (Dubowitz & Dubowitz, 1981; Markestaad & Fitzhardinge, 1981).

The purpose of this investigation was to empirically test the validity of these hypotheses to determine which appears to best explain the affects of IVH on subsequent developmental outcome. Assessments were made during the newborn period using Brazelton's (1973) Neonatal Behavioral Assessment Scale, thereby providing heretofore unavailable data concerning effects of IVH during the newborn period. Assessments were also conducted at 12 and 18 months of age using the Bayley Scales of Mental and Motor Development (Bayley, 1969).

## STUDY SAMPLE

The 30 preterm infants studied were transported to the Children's Hospital National Medical Center tertiary care nursery with the primary diagnosis of hyaline membrane disease (lung disease commonly associated with preterm birth and very low birth weight). All infants were appropriate for gestational age and required assisted ventilation for management of their respiratory disease. Within their first week in the nursery, infants received CT scans for the identification and grading of IVH. Sixteen of the 30 infants had intraventricular hemorrhage and 14 controls matched on neonatal variables (i.e., birth weight, gestational age, Apgar scores, etc.) did not have this diagnosis. All infants were also participants in a longitudinal, multidisciplinary investigation of the relationship between multiple early medical, sociobehavioral and cognitive factors, and later learning disabilities. The sample of 30 newborns was selected for study because of the availability of early Brazelton data at 40 weeks (corrected age). As a group they were representative of the larger group under study.

A summary of the neonatal characteristics of the sample is shown in Table 1. There were no significant differences between the IVH and control infants on neonatal variables. The preterm infants studied came mostly from low- to middle-class home environments. There were 6 black and 8 white families in the control group and 6 black and 10 white families in the hemorrhage sample.

Of the 16 IVH infants, CT scan studies revealed that 2 infants had a Grade I hemorrhage. Six infants had a Grade II hemorrhage and 8 infants had a Grade III hemorrhage. Three of these 6 severe cases (Grade III IVH) were treated with ventriculoperitoneal shunts for the management of progressive hydrocephalus. A summary of the neontal complications sustained by the entire sample of infants is shown in Table 2. Both the IVH and control group babies had major medical complications that included hyperbilirubinemia, episodes of recurrent apnea, bradycardia, and sepsis.

## NEWBORN AND INFANT ASSESSMENTS

### The Brazelton Neonatal Assessment

Testers administered Brazelton's (1973) Neonatal Behavioral Assessment Scale (BNBAS) to all infants to assess neurobehavioral organization capabilities at 40 weeks (corrected gestational age). Infant performance was scored in six behavioral clusters: Habituation, Orientation, Motor Performance, Range of State, Regulation of State, and Autonomic Regulation (Lester, Als, & Brazelton, 1978). For each cluster a mean score with values ranging from 1 to 9 was derived. Low scores indicated inferior performance on a given cluster and a score of 5 (midpoint) represented low average functioning. An additional score reflected the total number of abnormal reflexes.

### The Bayley Scales of Infant Development

All infants were administered the Bayley Scales of Mental (MDI) and Motor Development (PDI) (Bayley, 1969) by a trained examiner who was unaware of the composition of the IVH and control groups at the time of the assessments. Bayley data at 12 months corrected age were available for 15 IVH and 13 control infants, respectively. Two infants (1

**Table 1.** Summary of Neonatal Characteristics

| Characteristic | Group: IVH infants ($n$ = 16) | Group: Control infants ($n$ = 14) |
|---|---|---|
| Mean birth weight (g) | 1,201.81 (212) | 1,225.20 (308) |
| Mean gestational age (wk) | 30 (1.5) | 30 (2.1) |
| Median 5 minute Apgar | 6 | 6 |
| Mean head circumference (cm) | 26.37 (1.8) | 27.16 (2.6) |
| Mean days in hospital | 65 (41) range = 30–171 | 54 (21) range = 35–112 |
| Mean age of mother | 26 | 27 |

*Standard deviations shown in parentheses.

**Table 2.** Summary of Neonatal Complications (Number and Percentages of Cases)

| Complications | Group: IVH infants ($n$ = 16) | Group: Control infants ($n$ = 14) |
|---|---|---|
| Sleep apnea | 10 (62%) | 9 (64%) |
| Apnea monitor ( home) | 4 (25%) | 5 (36%) |
| Bradycardia | 10 (62%) | 9 (64%) |
| Bronchopulmonary dysplasia | 6 (37%) | 4 (28%) |
| Hyaline membrane disease | 16 (100%) | 14 (100%) |
| Patent ductus arteriosus | 6 (37%) | 1 (7%) |
| Meningitis | 1 (6%) | 2 (14%) |
| Seizures | 5 (31%) | 0 (—) |
| Sepsis | 8 (50%) | 9 (64%) |
| Necrotising entercolitis | 4 (25%) | 4 (28%) |
| Placenta previa | 3 (19%) | 1 (7%) |
| Emergency C-section | 2 (12%) | 3 (21%) |
| Placenta abruptio | 2 (12%) | 1 (7%) |
| 5 min. Apgar 6 (birth asphyxia) | 7 (44%) | 4 (28%) |
| Retrolental fibroplasia | 5 (31%) | 1 (7%) |
| Pneumonia | 2 (12%) | 0 (—) |
| Pneumothorax | 4 (25%) | 2 (14%) |
| Cor pulmonale | 4 (25%) | 0 (—) |
| Anemia | 3 (19%) | 5 (36%) |
| Hyperbilirubinemia | 11 (69%) | 11 (78%) |
| Microcephaly | 3 (19%) | 0 (—) |
| Hydrocephalus | 9 (56%) | 0 (—) |
| Failure to thrive | 4 (25%) | 2 (14%) |

IVH and 1 control) missed their 12-month appointments. AT 18 months, 13 and 14 Bayley tests were available for the control and IVH samples (3 infants missed appointments).

The Kohen-Raz (1976) subscale analysis of the Bayley compared the performance of the control and IVH infants on differentiated measures of functioning. The Kohen-Raz, an empirically derived scoring system of items from the Bayley Mental Scale, has five subscales: Eye–Hand Coordination, Manipulation, Object Relations, Imitation–Comprehension, and Vocal-Social. A developmental age (in months) is derived for each of the subscales. Additionally, a neurological examination was administered to all infants at 18 months corrected age.

## RESULTS

### Brazelton Cluster Performance

No significant differences were found between the performance of the IVH and control infants on the Brazelton cluster. Scores for both groups at 40 weeks (corrected age) revealed depressed neurobehavioral organization. Poorest scores were Range of State, State Regulation, Motor, Autonomic, and Orientation. Best scores (low average for both groups) were for Habituation. The lowest mean score earned by the IVH infants was Range of State followed by the Motor, Regulation of State, Orientation, and Autonomic clusters. For the controls, Range of State was also the lowest mean cluster score followed by the Regulation of State, Motor, and Autonomic clusters.

### Bayley Mental and Motor Performance (12 Months)

There were no significant differences between the mean Bayley mental scores (MDI) for the IVH and control groups (see Table 3). Of the 13 control infants, only 1 infant scored less than 85 on the mental scale. In contrast, 4 IVH infants earned scores of less than 85 at 12 months. There was a significant difference between the 2 groups on the mean Bayley Motor Scale (PDI) that favored the control infants ($t = 3.08$, $df = 27$, $p < .01$). No control infant earned a motor score less than 85 compared to 7 infants in the IVH group.

### Kohen-Raz Subscale Data (12 Months)

No significant differences were evident in mean age levels of the Kohen-Raz comparing the control and hemorrhage samples. Slight differences in each of the five subscales favored the controls who performed one month above their corrected age (12 months) for the Vocal-Social subscale. The controls were age-appropriate in performance on the Eye–Hand, Object Relations, and Imitation–Comprehension subscales. However, they showed an approximate 2-month delay on the Manipulation subscale. IVH infants were age-appropriate in Imitation–Comprehension and were less than a month below their corrected age on the Eye–Hand, Object Relations, and Vocal-Social subscales. Like the controls, the IVH infants were approximately two months below age level in performance on the Manipulation subscale.

## Bayley Mental and Motor Scale Performance (18 Months)

At 18 months there were no significant differences between the IVH and control infants on the Bayley Mental Scale (MDI) (see Table 3 for Bayley data). Of the 14 IVH infants tested at 18 months, 5 had Bayley mental scores which were less than 85, compared to 3 of the 13 control infants. There was a significant difference between the performance of the control and the IVH infants on the Bayley Motor Scale (PDI) ($t = 2.47$, $df = 25$, $p < .05$). No control infant earned a motor score of less than 85. Four IVH infants scored less than 85 on the Bayley Motor Scale.

**Table 3.** Mean Bayley Mental and Motor Scores at 12 and 18 Months

| Mean Bayley scores | Group | |
|---|---|---|
| | IVH infants ($n = 14$) | Control infants ($n = 13$) |
| | 12 months | |
| MDI | 98.28<br>(21.04)<br>range = 50–126 | 109.15<br>(15.31)<br>range = 66–130 |
| PDI | 87.64<br>(19.90)<br>range = 50–125 | 108.92**<br>(13.80)<br>range = 86–133 |
| | 18 months | |
| MDI | 95.57<br>(23.59)<br>range = 50–138 | 103.54<br>(20.31)<br>range = 70–124 |
| PDI | 87.21<br>(21.15)<br>range = 50–107 | 104.31*<br>(11.76)<br>range = 88–129 |

*Note.* Standard deviations are shown in parentheses.
*Significant group difference ($p < .05$). **Significant group difference ($p > .01$).

### Kohen-Raz Subscale Data (18 Months)

There were no significant differences between the IVH and control infants on the Kohen-Raz subscales at 18 months. There were, however, slight differences on all five subscales that again favored the controls. The mean score of the control group for the Imitation–Comprehension subscale was almost 2 months above age appropriate performance. Control infants were 6 and 7 months delayed on the Manipulation and Object Relations subscales, respectively. On the Eye–Hand coordination subscales, controls were delayed by 1 month and showed a 6-month delay on the Vocal-Social subscale. The IVH infants had a similar pattern of delayed performance on the Manipulation (8 months) and Object Relations (6 months) subscales. They were age-appropriate on the Imitation–Comprehension subscales but were delayed by 2 months on both the Eye–Hand and Vocal-Social subscales.

### Neurological Findings

At approximately 18 months, neurological examinations revealed the following: 3 IVH and 8 control infants had normal neurological exams. Six of the IVH infants had cerebral palsy (quadriplegia, $n = 1$ spastic diplegia, $n = 2$; hemiplegia, $n = 3$), whereas no control infant had this diagnosis. Four control infants and 2 IVH infants had no focal neurological deficits but evidenced clear functional asymmetries (mild hemisyndromes) by better performance or preference for one side of the body. Three IVH infants showed generalized delay in neurologic functioning characterized by clumsiness and poor balance. Attentional and behavioral deficits were noted in 2 IVH and 2 control babies.

### Severity of IVH

To evaluate the hypothesis that severe IVH (ventricular dilatation and progressive hydrocephalus) is more closely associated with poor behavioral outcome in contrast to IVH (without dilatation), the developmental performance of Grade III IVH infants was compared with those with Grades I and II. Separate *t*-test analyses of Brazelton cluster data, Beyley MDI and PDI scores at 12 and 18 months, and Kohen-Raz subscales revealed no statistically significant differences between the performance of Grade III and Grades I and II IVH infants.

Both IVH groups performed poorly on five of the six Brazelton clusters ( highest mean scores for IVH Grade III = 5.0; IVH Grade I and II = 5.53). The most severely depressed performance for both groups was on the Range of State cluster (means of 3.69 and 3.67), and best scores were for the Habituation cluster (5.0 and 5.53, low average), respectively. Grade III IVH infants, however, had twice as many abnormal reflexes as Grades I and II infants (4 vs. 2).

## DISCUSSION

Several provocative findings have emerged from this study regarding IVH and preterm infant performance on the Brazelton and Bayley scales. The failure to find significant differences in 40-week Brazelton performances between the hemorrhage and non-IVH infants was unexpected. The Brazelton data documented severe CNS depression evidenced by the inability of both groups of infants to regulate state changes or to experience a range of states. The presence of IVH did not have the effect of further depressing behavioral organization during the newborn period in this sample of critically ill, preterm babies. Alternatively, the Brazelton scale may not be sensitive enough to detect the possible differences in performance of infants with and without hemorrhage insult. However, the Brazelton data clearly identified poor state control as well as autonomic instability in this sample of infants who had sustained major medical complications and intensive care therapy.

Even at 40 weeks corrected age, control of responsiveness and autonomic and state functions typical of full-term infants were not evident in preterm infants may not result from preterm birth *per se,* but that Pasternak (1982) reported a similar pattern of depressed Brazelton performance in preterm infants compared with healthy full-term infants at 40 weeks. They found that the Brazelton performance of sick preterm, sick full-term, and full-term infants hospitalized with sick mothers were all inferior compared with that of normal term babies. From these results Holmes *et al.* concluded that incompetent behavioral functioning in preterm infants may not result from preterm birth *per se,* but that medical complications (i.e., severity of illness) may significantly influence recovery to adequate functioning. Consequently, preterm newborn behavioral organization may be adversely affected by protracted care in an intensive care nursery environment (i.e., separation from parents, routine handling, lack of adequate rest, continuous exposure to high levels of illumination, etc.). In this study, on the average, both IVH and control groups of preterm infants had been hospitalized for approximately 3 months.

The Bayley Scales of this study revealed differences between the hemorrhage and non-IVH infant at 12 and 18 months in motor development but not in mental development. These results, though tentative, support the "marker for risk hypothesis" concerning the relation between IVH and subsequent development. The link between IVH and inferior motor development has been previously reported with confirmation that the common site for IVH is near motor centers in the fetal brain (Wigglesworth & Pape, 1979). Thus, IVH is likely to result in varying degrees of cerebral palsy as was evident in this study. However, control infants who also sustained severe medical insults evidenced subtle motor deficits (fine motor delays, poor balance, eye–hand dyscoordination, attentional and behavioral difficulties), further suggesting that illness in combination with prolonged hospitalization influences dysfunction. Although this study had a relatively small sample, data indicate that the effects of IVH on infant developmental performance may be confounded with the effects of other major medical complications (such as perinatal asphyxia, seizures, bronchopulmonary dysplasia, hyperbilirubinemia, etc.). Thus, the combined effects of IVH and medical complications may significantly depress not only the rate of recovery from early trauma but subsequent follow-up measure of cognitive and motor performance (Gaiter, 1982).

Although IVH is a serious neonatal trauma, its presence in combination with other life-threatening, debilitating conditions significantly contributes to the pattern of developmental dysfunction found in later infancy. This study, therefore, suggests that follow-up research investigations should abandon simplistic explanations of infant neurobehavioral dysfunction based on the identification of a single salient early trauma.

Sameroff and Chandler (1974) have theorized that after 18 months a complex interaction of infant behavioral and constitutional characteristics combines with socioenvironmental factors to determine both the velocity and quality of infant growth. Before 18 months, however, stable and progressive physiologic organization and the ability to recover from life-threatening illness appear necessary for subsequent competent infant functioning.

## REFERENCES

Ahmann, P. A., Lazzara, A., Dykes, F., Brann, A. W., & Schwartz, J. F. (1978) IVH: Incidence and outcome. *Annals of Neurology, 4,* 186.

Bayley, N. (1969). *Bayley Scales of Mental and Motor Development.* New York: Psychological Corp.

Bozynski, M. E., Nelson, M. N., Genaze, D. R., Chilcote, W. S., Ramsey, R. G., Clasen, R. A., O'Donnell, K. J., & Meier, W. A. (1982, December). *Longitudinal follow-up by ultrasound of intracranial hemorrhage and ventriculomegaly in relation to developmental outcome in infants weighing less than 1200 grams at birth.* Paper presented at the Conference on Perinatal Intracranial Hemorrhage, Ross Laboratories, Washington, DC.

Brazelton, T. B. (1973). *Neonatal Behavioral Assessment Scale.* Philadelphia: J. B. Lippincott.

Dubowitz, L. M., & Dubowitz, V. (1981). The neurological assessment of the preterm and full-term newborn infant. *Clinics in Developmental Medicine* (No. 79). London: Heineman.

Fitzhardinge, P. M., Pape, K., & Arstikaitis, M. (1976). Mechanical ventilation of infants of less than 1501 grams birth weight: Health, growth, and neurologic sequelae. *Journal of Pediatrics, 88* 531.

Gaiter, J. L. (1982). The effects of intraventricular hemorrhage on Bayley Developmental performance in preterm infants. *Seminars in Perinatology, 6,* 305.

Holmes, D. L., Nagy, J. N., Slaymaker, S., Sosnowski, R. J., Prinz, S. M., & Pasternak, J. S. (1982). Early influences of prematurity, illness, and prolonged hospitalization on infant behavior. *Developmental Psychology, 18,* 744.

Horbar, J. D., Pasnick, M., Leahy, K., & Lucey,, J. F. (1982). Factors associated with periventricular-intraventricular hemorrhage. *Pediatric Research, 16,* 292.

Kohen-Raz, R. (1976). Scalogram analysis of some developmental sequences as measured by the Bayley Scale of Mental Development. *Genetic Psychology Monographs, 76,* 3–21.

Krishnamoorthy, K., Shannon, D., DeLong, G. (1979). Neurologic sequelae in the survivors of neonatal intraventricular hemorrhage. *Journal of Pediatrics, 64,* 233.

Lester, B. M., Als, H., & Brazelton, T. B. (1978). *Scoring criteria for seven clusters of the Brazelton scale.* Unpublished manuscript. Boston, MA: Child Development Unit, Children's Hospital Medical Center.

Markestaad, T., & Fritzhardinge, P. M. (1981). Growth and development in children recovering from bronchopulmonary dysplasia. *Journal of Pediatrics, 98,* 597.

Ment, L. R., Scott, D. T., Ehrenkranz, R. A., Rothman, S. G., Duncan, C. C., & Warshaw, J. B. (1982). Neonates of 1250 grams birth weight: Prospective neurodevelopmental evaluation during the first year post-term. *Pediatrics, 70,* 292.

Palmer, P., Dubowitz, L. M. S., Levene, M. I., & Dubowitz, V. (1982). Development and neurological progress of preterm infants with intraventricular-hemorrhage and ventricular dilitation. *Archives of Diseases in Children, 57,* 748–753.

Papile, L. A., Burstein, J., Burstein, R., & Koffler, H. (1978). Incidence and evolution of subependymal and intraventricular hemorrhage: A study of infants with birth weights less than 1500 grams. *Journal of Pediatrics, 92,* 529.

Papile, L. A., Munsick-Bruno, G., & Schaefer, A. (1983). Relationship of cerebral intraventricular hemorrhage and early childhood neurologic handicaps. *Journal of Pediatrics, 103,* 273.

Papile, L. A., Munsick, G., Weaver, N., Techa, S. (1979). Cerebral intraventricular hemorrhage in infants less than 1500 grams: Developmental follow-up at one year. *Pediatric Research, 13,* 527.

Sameroff, A., & Chandler, M. J. (1974). Reproductive risk and the continuum of caretaking casualty. In F.D. Horowitz (Ed.), *Review of child development research* (Vol. 4). Chicago: Univ. of Chicago Press.

Schechner, S., Ross, G., & Auld, P. (1980). *Developmental follow-up at one year post-term of infants with intracranial hemorrhage.* Proceedings of Perinatal Intracranial Conference. Columbus, OH: Ross Laboratories.

Shinnar, S., Molteni, R. A., Gammon, K., D'Souva, D. J., Altman, J., & Freeman, J. M. (1982). Intraventricular hemorrhage in the premature infant. *New England Journal of Medicine, 306,* 1464.

Wigglesworth, J. S., & Pape, K. (1979). *Hemorrhage, ischemia, and the perinatal brain.* Philadelphia: J. B. Lippincott.

Williamson, W. D., Desmond, M. M., Wilson, G. S., Andrew, L., & Garcia-Prats, J. A. (1982) Early neurodevelopmental outcome of low birth weight infants surviving neonatal intraventricular hemorrhage. *Journal of Perinatal Medicine, 10,* 34.

# PART III

## EXPERIMENTAL EFFORTS

CHAPTER 18

# An Experimental Selective Screening Device for the Early Detection of Intellectual Deficit in At-Risk Infants

*Joseph F. Fagan III, Lynn T. Singer, and Jeanne E. Montie*

Attempts have been made to predict intellectual functioning during childhood from various indices of infant sensorimotor development, such as the Gesell Developmental Schedules (Gesell & Amatruda, 1954), the Cattell Infant Intelligence Scale (Cattell, 1960), the Griffiths Scale of Mental Development (Griffiths, 1954), and the Bayley Scales of Mental Development (Bayley, 1969). The basic result has been that infant mental tests based on sensorimotor functioning have been found ineffective in predicting later intelligence (e.g., McCall, Hogarty, & Hurlburt, 1972). For example, correlations obtained between tests of infant sensorimotor development given during the 3- to 7-month period and standard intelligence tests at 3 years or beyond average about .18 for high-risk and clinical samples (Fagan & Singer, 1983).

Our explanation for the low correlation between early sensorimotor functioning and later intellectual performance is based on the fact that standard tests of infant intelligence measure the development of simple sensory and motor skills, which are not related to differences in intelligence later in life. We therefore assumed that to predict later intelligence, the task is to sample infant behaviors that tap processes known to be related to later intelligence. On later intelligence tests, children are

*Joseph F. Fagan III, Lynn T. Singer, and Jeanne E. Montie* • Department of Psychology, Case Western Reserve University, Cleveland, Ohio 44106.

asked to abstract or identify similarities and differences among stimuli, to retain new information, to categorize stimuli, and to retrieve useful information. Thus, to the extent that is possible to ask an infant to exhibit such processes as discrimination, abstraction, identification, retention, and categorization, it should be possible to develop a valid test of infant intelligence.

## STUDIES OF EARLY COGNITIVE FUNCTIONING

The study of early cognitive functioning has been based largely on observation of the infant's visual behavior. From birth, infants tend to look at some stimuli more than others. The procedure for determining the infant's visual fixation is to place the infant in front of a stage on which targets are secured. An observer, looking through a peephole centered between the targets, observes the corneal reflection of a target over the pupils of the infant's eyes and records the length of fixation paid to each target (Fantz, 1956). One such naturally occurring example of differential fixation is the infant's devotion of more attention to a novel than to a previously seen target (Fagan, 1970). Preference for novel over previously exposed targets shows that the two targets are discriminable, and also indicates that the infant can recognize or identify one of the targets as familiar.

Studies of infant's preferences for visual novelty have shown that the infant is able to act intelligently. *Intelligent* action on the part of the infant means that the infant displays processes that are also employed by children and adults to solve problems on intelligence tests. The ability to detect similarities among otherwise diverse stimuli, for example, would seem to be a basic intellectual process. Such abstraction is necessary if two or more objects are to be treated as equivalent, a behavior that serves as an operational definition of categorization (Mervis & Rosch, 1981).

The solution of various tasks on standard intelligence tests requires the ability to abstract common features as well, and the study of responsiveness to novelty has made it possible to demonstrate that the infant is also capable of abstraction. Specifically, the infant separates attributes, notes invariants in form over transformations in perspective, sees similarities across different representations, is capable of transferring information across modalities, and can form prototypes (Fagan, in press). If such processes of abstraction represent intelligent activity later in life, it is justifiable to assume that their exercise early in life represents intelligent activity on the part of the infant.

## VALIDITY OF VISUAL PREFERENCE TESTS

The fact that infants appear to behave in an intelligent manner raises the question of whether or not individual differences in response to novelty are predictive of later intelligence.

Variations in novelty preference during infancy have indeed been found to be related to later intelligence. Concurrent validity for the extent of an infant's visual preference for a novel target as a measure of intelligence is provided by studies where groups of infants expected to differ in intelligence later in life have been compared for their ability to recognize a previously seen stimulus. With few exceptions (Cohen, 1981; Fagan, Fantz, & Miranda, 1971), the infant groups differ in their preference for a novel visual target. This conclusion is true for offspring of highly intelligent parents as compared to offspring of women of average intelligence (Fantz & Nevis, 1967), for comparisons of normal infants to infants with Down's syndrome (Cohen, 1981; Miranda & Fantz, 1974), and when term and preterm infants are compared (Caron & Caron, 1981; Rose, 1980; Rose, Gottfried, & Bridger, 1979; Sigman & Parmalee, 1974).

In addition to studies providing concurrent validity, published reports are available in which the relationship between tests of early novelty preference and later intelligence have been explored for individuals. Specifically, studies by Yarrow, Klein, Lomonaco, and Morgan (1975), Fagan (1981), Fagan and McGrath (1981), Lewis and Brooks-Gunn (1981), Fagan and Singer (1983), and Caron, Caron, and Glass (1983) include tests of predictive validity for 12 samples of infants drawn from essentially normal populations (i.e., infants not at risk for later cognitive deficit). For each of the 12 samples, a significant association holds between early novelty preferences and later intelligence. Preferences for visual novelty during infancy yield moderate predictive validity coefficients (ranging from .33 to .66 across the 12 samples, with a median of .40).

The general finding appears to be quite robust, occurring despite many subject and procedural variations from study to study. Moreover, the median correlation of .40 obtained in these studies very likely underestimates the predictive validity of infant novelty preference tests. One source of attenuation was the restricted range of intelligence within which predictions were made. A second source of attenuation of predictive validity for each sample was the small number of visual novelty preferences (from one to five tests of preference) administered from sample to sample. For example, Fagan and McGrath (1981) and Fagan (1981), who account for 6 of the 12 coefficients, report a median estimated reliability of .42 for a novelty score composed of an average of 3.5 novelty preferences. In other words, it would be reasonable to assume that future tests based on samples with a wider range of intellectual outcome and on novelty preference scores based on more pairings of previously exposed and novel targets should yield higher preditive validity coefficients than those obtained so far. In any case, substantial concurrent and predictive validity exists for the assumption that tests of visual novelty preference administered during infancy reflect intelligent activity.

## THE SELECTIVE SCREENING DEVICE

Given that sufficient evidence exists to link early novelty preferences to later intelligence, a major goal of our research since 1977 has been to develop an infant intelligence test based on tests of visual novelty preference (Fagan & Singer, 1983). Briefly, the test is based on paired-comparison tests of the infant's differential fixation to novel over previously exposed targets.

The basic component of the test is a novelty problem. Each novelty problem consists of a pairing of two stimuli immediately following exposure to one of the two stimuli. We felt that the most advantageous approach to standard assessment was to allow each infant the same amount of study fixation, and then to test for preferences by pairing a novel and previously seen target. Following this procedure with a variety of tasks allowed each infant a composite novelty preference score derived from many items. Some 1,800 home visits to infants were made in order to discover which combination of standard study times and stimulus pairings would lead, at each of four ages (12, 16, 22, and 29 weeks of corrected age), to a set of three novelty problems that could easily be administered during a single session and that could be solved individually. The result was a standard, 12-item test of infant novelty preference called the Fagan Test of Infant Intelligence (Fagan, 1981), which may be administered between 3 and 7 months of age.

### Methods

Two studies were undertaken to test the predictive validity) of the 12-item selective screening device based on visual preference for novelty for the early detection of cognitive deficit when applied to groups of at-risk infants. Infants were considered to be at risk for cognitive deficit if they came from populations where the incidence of low IQ scores at 3 years of age (i.e., IQ less than 70) was greater than a normal population.

#### *Population*

The population included 58 at-risk infants, who were divided into two samples. The first sample was composed of 20 infants diagnosed a failure-to-thrive. The second sample included 38 infants considered to be at risk for any one of a variety of reasons, such as prematurity, intrauterine growth retardation, treated hypothyroidism, a diagnosis of failure-to-thrive, or a history of maternal diabetes.

### *Procedure*

The procedure was to expose the infant to a target until a predetermined amount of fixation time had accumulated to the target (e.g., 30 seconds). Following the study period, the previously exposed stimulus was paired with a novel stimulus. The 20 infants in the first sample received 4 such novelty tests at 5 or 7 months, and the 38 infants in the second sample received at least 7 and as many as all 12 novelty tests during visits at 3, 4, 5, and 7 months. Each infant's novelty preference score was defined as the mean percent of total fixation paid to novel targets over tests.

In addition to novelty preference tests, the 20 infants in the first sample and 6 infants in the second sample were given the Bayley Scales of Mental Development (Bayley, 1969) between 6 and 8 months of age. Intellectual outcome at 3 years for all 58 children was assessed by administering the Stanford–Binet (Terman & Merrill, 1973), the Peabody Picture Vocabulary Test (Form L) (Dunn & Dunn, 1981), or, if necessary, by giving the Bayley and estimating IQ by dividing the age attained on the test by chronological age.

### **Results**

At 3 years of age, the 20 failure-to-thrive children comprising the first sample yielded a group mean of 73.0, standard deviation (*SD*) 16.9, range ($r$) of 27 to 98. As to prediction from infancy, the novelty preference scores correctly identified 7 out of 8 (or 88%) of the children with IQs of 70 or less, as may be seen from the data listed in Table 1. Such high co-positivity was not accomplished at great cost to co-negativity, as the test also correctly identified 83% of the normal children. Correlating the infant novelty preference scores with 3-year IQ scores yielded a predictive validity coefficient of .53 ($df$ 19, $p < .01$). Early novelty preference tests also proved to be valid in predicting low IQs in the second sample of 38 at-risk children. Their average IQ at 3 years was 99.9 (*SD* 24.9, $r = 25$ to 135). As Table 1 shows, the co-positivity of the early recognition tests was 100%, predicting 5 out of 5 children with 3-year IQs of 70 or less. The test was also quite high in co-negativity, correctly identifying 94% as normal. Predictive validity was high and significant at $r = .54$ ($df$ 37, $p < .0001$). The data given here, although encouraging, should be treated as preliminary data given the small sample sizes (20

**Table 1.** Co-Positivity and Co-Negativity of Tests for Visual Novelty Preference for the Prediction of Intellectual Deficit at 3 Years

| Age of testing<br>Group tested | 5–7 months<br>Failure-to-thrive children<br>($N$ = 20) | | 3–7 months<br>At-risk children<br>($N$ = 38) | | 3–7 months<br>Children also with Bayley scales ($N$ = 26) | |
|---|---|---|---|---|---|---|
| Outcome | Retarded | Normal | Retarded | Normal | Retarded | Normal |
| Risk prediction | 7 | 2 | 5 | 2 | 10 | 3 |
| Normal prediction | 1 | 10 | 0 | 31 | 1 | 12 |
| Co-positivity | 88% | | 100% | | 91% | |
| Co-negativity | 83% | | 94% | | 80% | |

and 38) and the relatively high incidence of intellectual deficit in the sample as a whole. Moreover, cutoff scores for risk based on early novelty preferences varied from sample to sample and were selected to maximize co-positivity and co-negativity. We are in the process of validating these initial findings and developing a standard cut off score for novelty preferences in order to specify risk.

As noted earlier, 26 of the 58 children in the sample had also been assessed with the Bayley Scales during infancy, an assessment that allowed a direct comparison of the predictive power of novelty preference tests with that of a conventional test of sensorimotor development. The 26 children given both types of assessment turned out to be a particularly compromised group with a mean IQ of 71.2 (*SD* 25.1, with a range from 25–115). As may be seen from the data in Table 1, prediction from early novelty preference scores for this subsample of 26 children was highly co-positive, with 91% of the children correctly identified as retarded, and highly co-negative in identifying 80% as normal at 3 years. The predictive validity coefficient for the novelty preference test was high and statistically significant at .54 ($df$ 25, $p < .01$).

In contrast, as noted in Table 2, the Bayley Scales administered at about 8 months were low in co-positivity with MDI scores $\leqslant 75$ correctly identifying only 45% of the delayed children. The scales were low in co-negativity also, as they correctly identified only 53% of the normals. The correlation of the 8-month Bayley scores with the 3-year IQ scores was not significantly greater than chance, at $r = .26$.

In summary, tests of visual novelty preference administered between 3 and 7 months appear to constitute a valid screening device for the early detection of intellectual deficit in at-risk populations. Moreover, early tests of visual novelty preference appear to be clearly superior to conventional sensorimotor tests of infant intelligence in predicting later intellectual deficit.

**Table 2.** Co-Positivity and Co-Negativity of the Bayley Scales Given at 6 to 8 Months for the Prediction of Intellectual Deficit at 3 Years ($N$ = 26)

| | | Outcome | |
|---|---|---|---|
| | | Retarded | Normal |
| Prediction | Risk | 5 | 7 |
| | Normal | 6 | 8 |

Note. Co-positivity = 45%; co-negativity = 53%.

## PRACTICAL APPLICATIONS

The primary use for an early selective screening device based on novelty preferences would be to identify those individuals most at risk for later intellectual deficit. Presumably those individuals would be drawn from groups of infants suspected to be at risk due to various prenatal or perinatal conditions. No doubt normal development would be predicted for the majority of infants screened, and families could then be encouraged to treat their infants as intellectually normal and would be spared the uncertainty and anxiety of waiting until the child is 2 or 3 years old for an accurate intellectual assessment. Families of infants suspected of ultimate impaired cognitive development could be given emotional support and guided toward early intervention programs.

In a more general vein, early novelty preference tests could be used to rank various risk factors such as low birth weight, fetal and infant growth retardation, intraventricular hemorrhage, hypoglycemia, neonatal seizures, prenatal exposure to potential teratogens, etc., according to the likelihood that a certain risk condition or combination of conditions would result in impaired intellectual development. Treatment and prevention efforts could then be concentrated on the alleviation of risk factors most likely to lead to intellectual deficits.

Aside from identifying individuals at risk for later intellectual deficit and from identifying circumstances associated with such risk, the other major use for a valid test of infant intelligence would be to provide an assessment of the effects of intervention. Intervention designed to prevent or alleviate cognitive deficit is only possible when the victims and the causes of such deficit can be identified. At the moment the factors underlying the majority of cases of intellectual retardation are unknown. One reason for this lack of knowledge is that researchers have had to wait for years to discover if intellectual deficit is present. In other words, there has been a problem of "lost signs," such that researchers have not been able to discover which of a myriad of factors over the years might singly or in combination lead to cognitive malfunction. A valid early test of intelligence would mitigate such problems by allowing early identification of candidates for intervention, by facilitating early differentiation among the many possible contributors to intellectual deficit, and by permitting rapid assessment of intervention programs.

## SUMMARY

Conventional tests of infant intelligence based on individual differences in sensorimotor development have failed to predict later intelligence, perhaps because sensorimotor functioning is not related to intelligence *per se*. If intelligence is to be predicted from infancy, the task is to tap the same cognitive processes at early and at later points in development. Tests of the infant's preference for novel visual targets involves cognitive processes similar to those employed to solve later tests of intelligence. The assumption that variations in early visual novelty preferences are indicative of intelligence has empirical support. Normal infants are more apt to prefer visual novelty than are infants considered to be at risk for later intellectual deficit, and significant relationships have been demonstrated between the extent of infant's visual preferences for novel targets and later performance on standard tests of intelligence.

## REFERENCES

Bayley, N. (1969). *The Bayley Scales of Infant Development*. New York: Psychological Corp.

Caron, A. J., & Caron, R. F. (1981). Processing of relational information as an index of infant risk. In S. L. Friedman & M. Sigman (Eds.), *Preterm birth and psychological development*. New York: Academic Press.

Caron, A. J., Caron, R. F., & Glass, P. (1983). Responsiveness to relational information as a measure of cognitive functioning in nonsuspect infants. In T. Field & A. Sostek (Eds.), *Infants born at risk*. New York: Grune & Stratton.

Cattell, P. (1940). *The measurement of intelligence in infants and young children*. New York: Science Press. (Reprinted by the Psychological Corp., 1960.)

Cohen, L. B. (1981). Lags in the cognitive competence of prematurely born infants. In S. L. Friedman & M. Sigman (Eds.), *Preterm birth and psychological development*. New York: Academic Press.

Dunn, L. M., & Dunn, L. M. (1981). *Peabody Picture Vocabulary Test-Revised: Manual for forms L and M*. Circle Pines, MN.: American Guidance Service.

Fagan, J. F. (1970). Memory in the infant. *Journal of Experimental Child Psychology, 16*, 424–450.

Fagan, J. F., Fantz, R. L., & Miranda, S. B. (1971, April). *Infants' attention to novel stimuli as a function of postnatal and conceptional age*. Paper presented at the meeting of the Society for Research in Child Development, Minneapolis, MN.

Fagan, J. F. (1981, April). *Infant memory and the prediction of intelligence*. Paper presented at Society for Research in Child Development meeting, Boston, MA.

Fagan, J. F., & McGrath, S. K. (1981). Infant recognition memory and later intelligence. *Intelligence, 5,* 121–130.

Fagan, J. F., & Singer, L. T. (1983). Infant recognition memory as a measure of intelligence. In L. P. Lipsitt (Ed.), *Advances in infancy research* (Vol. 2). Norwood, NJ: Ablex.

Fagan, J. F. (in press). A new look at infant intelligence. In D. K. Detterman (Ed.), *Current topics in human intelligence*. Norwood, NJ: Ablex.

Fantz, R. L. (1956). A method for studying early visual development. *Perceptual and Motor Skills, 6,* 13–15.

Fantz, R. L., & Nevis, S. (1967). The predictive value of changes in visual preference in early infancy. In J. Hellmuth (Ed.), *The exceptional infant* (Vol. 1). Seattle, WA: Special Child Publications.

Gesell, A., & Amatruda, C. S. (1954). *Developmental diagnosis*. New York: Paul B. Holber.

Griffiths, R. (1954). *The abilities of babies*. New York: McGraw-Hill.

Lewis, M., & Brooks-Gunn, J. (1981). Visual attention at 3 months as a predictor of cognitive functioning at 2 years of age. *Intelligence, 5,* 131–140.

McCall, R. B., Hogarty, P. S., & Hurlburt, N. (1972). Transitions in infant sensorimotor development and the prediction of childhood IQ. *American Psychologist, 27,* 728–748.

Mervis, C. B., & Rosch, E. (1981). Categorization of natural objects. *Annual Review of Psychology, 32,* 89–115.

Miranda, S. B., & Fantz, R. L. (1974). Recognition memory in Down's syndrome and normal infants. *Child Development, 45,* 651–660.

Rose, S. A. (1980). Enhancing visual recognition memory in pre-term infants. *Developmental Psychology, 16,* 85–92.

Rose, S. A., Gottfired, A. W., & Bridger, W. H. (1979). Effects of haptic cues on visual recognition memory in full-term and pre-term infants. *Infant Behavior and Development, 2,* 55–67.

Sigman, M., & Parmalee, A. H. (1974). Visual preferences of 4-month-old premature and full-term infants. *Child Development, 45,* 959–965.

Terman, L. M., & Merrill, M. A. (1973). *Stanford–Binet Intelligence Scale: 1973 norms edition*. Boston: Houghton-Mifflin.

Yarrow, L. J., Klein, R. P., Lomonaco, S., & Morgan, G. A. (1975). Cognitive and motivational development in early childhood. In B. X. Friedlander, G. M. Sterritt, & G. E. Kirk (Eds.), *Exceptional infant* (Vol. 3). New York: Brunner/Mazel.

*CHAPTER 19*

# Sound Localization and Screening

## IS THERE A BRIDGE AND IS IT WORTH CROSSING?

*Joseph W. Sullivan*

In this volume, Fagan and Rock present findings from their measure of visual novelty preference in infants 3 to 7 months of age, indicating that their measure is more predictive of 3-year intelligence scores than standardized measures of sensorimotor performance. Fagan and Rock's findings provide support for Zelazo's (1979) proposal that the use of an information processing approach (i.e., the ways in which infants process visual and auditory information) will be a more valid measure of underlying cognitive development than the prevalently used assessments of sensorimotor development. The assumption is that the early information processing abilities are more closely related to the processes assessed by subsequent measures of intelligence. In this chapter, I describe research that is studying the efficacy of using auditory processing abilities for the identification of those infants from a high-risk population who are truly at risk for subsequent developmental problems. The chapter is divided into two sections. The first section provides some necessary background and the rationale for the approach being taken. In the second section, a study employing 4-month-old infants as subjects is presented as an example of the research that is being done as part of this project.

## BACKGROUND AND RATIONALE

The auditory process chosen for the study was sound localization. *Sound localization* refers to the judgments of the direction and distance

***Joseph W. Sullivan*** • Rocky Mountain Child Development Center, Department of Psychiatry, University of Colorado School of Medicine, Denver, Colorado 80207.

of a sound source from the organism (Moore, 1977). In this case acoustic stimulation provides information about the auditory space the organism inhabits. The organism's ability to locate the source of a sound is seen as a basic and adaptive skill that evolved to allow the organism to detect, for example, the position of preditors, prey, mates, and distressed offspring (Gibson, 1966).

Sound localization requires binaural input if it is to be accurate. That is, the acoustic information arriving at the two ears is compared in order to determine the spatial location of sound. Primarily two binaural cues provide this spatial information: (a) the time difference ($\Delta_t$) of the arrival of the sound at each ear; and (b) the intensity difference ($\Delta_i$) of the sound arriving at each ear. These cues and how they are used will be discussed in more detail in the second section. What is important to understand at this point is that the input from the two ears must be processed and compared somewhere along the auditory pathway. The most likely places that these comparisons occur are at the superior olivary complex and the inferior coliculus. As such, sound localization is a more complex and higher order auditory process than has typically been used in studies of infant auditory processing abilities. It is precisely these qualities that may make sound localization a viable candidate for identifying the truly at-risk infant.

**Sound Localization in Infants**

The traditional view of the infant's ability to localize sounds was that this ability did not develop until 5 to 6 months of age (Chun, Pawsett, & Forster, 1960). Wertheimer (1961), however, was the first to demonstrate that an infant, within minutes after birth, will move its eyes in the direction of a sound. Subsequent studies attempting to replicate Wertheimer's results using direction of eye movements as the dependent measure met with mixed success (Butterworth & Castillo, 1976; Crassini & Broerse, 1980; Hammer & Turkewitz, 1966; McGurk, Tunure, & Creighton, 1977; Mendelson & Haith, 1976; Turkewitz, Birth, & Cooper, 1972a,b; Turkewitz, Birth, Moreau, Levy, & Cornwell, 1966).

The emergence of Brazelton's (1973) Neonatal Behavioral Assessment Scale (NBAS) added a new dimension to sound localization research. The NBAS contains several items that assess the newborn infant's ability to turn its head in the direction of a sound. Data collected on a sample of 1,388 infants indicate that the average response is a head turn toward the sound (Horowitz, Sullivan, & Byrne, in preparation). These data indicate that the experimental studies using eye turns may have, in fact, underestimated the newborn's abilities. The procedures employed in the NBAS (i.e., long stimulus presentation—20–40 sec.; low intensity of stimulation; and careful manipulation of the infant state) probably contributed to the enhanced performance. Recent experimental studies incorporating these procedures have met with consistent success in demonstrating head turning to sounds in the newborn period (Alegria & Norrot, 1978; Clifton, Morrongiello, Kulig, & Dowd, 1981; Field, Muir, Pilon, Sinclair, & Dodwell, 1980; Field, DeFranco, Dodwell, & Muir, 1979; Muir, Abraham, Forbes, & Harris, 1979; Muir & Field, 1979; Sullivan & Ingram, 1983; Turner & McFarlane, 1978).

An important finding that somewhat reconciles the early data (e.g., Chun *et al.*, 1960) and the current data on infant sound localization is that sound localization appears to follow a U-shaped developmental function over the first 4 to 5 months of life. In their longitudinal study, Muir *et al.* (1981) found that the infants turned toward sounds during the first weeks of life, but at around 20 days of age there began a marked decline in head turning, reaching its lowest level at about 80 days of age. By 120 days of age, however, there was a rapid recovery of head turning on almost all trials. There was also a change in the quality of the head turns with the infants' turning briskly and accurately toward the sounds at 120 days of age. Muir *et al.* (1981) speculated that this U-shaped function may represent a shift from a reflexively based behavior at birth to a voluntary, cortically mediated behavior by 4 months of age.

## Significance of Sound Localization as a Screening Tool

Although sound localization is an interesting and important research topic in its own right, the focus of this chapter is also on its function as a method for identifying infants who are at risk for future developmental problems. At this point it would appear appropriate, therefore, to outline the relationships that may exist between early sound localization abilities and subsequent development, especially subsequent language development.

A common interpretation that pervades the infant sound localization literature is that the infant's turning of its eyes and head in the direction of a sound evidences an integration of the visual and auditory modalities. That is, the infant turns toward the sound because it expects to see something. Therefore, according to this view, the ability to localize sounds is not only evidence of complex auditory processing abilities but also of the early capacity for intermodal perception.

This latter feature of sound localization, although very intriguing, is not, as yet, fully supported by the research. It does seem safe to say, however, that orienting the eyes and head in the direction of a sound will, at the least, provide the opportunity for the infant to begin appreciating the relationship between visual and auditory components of objects and events. And, as has been pointed out by Sonksen (1979), the inability to do this, as in the case of blind infants, may have adverse effects on language development. Further ties between early abnormal localization and subsequent language problems have been documented for otherwise normal infants. Pollock (1981) found that 44% of the children who evidenced early atypical localization responses also had some degree of subsequent language delay. Swift, Swift, Camp, and Silvern (1981) also found a relationship between atypical localization at 6 to 9 months of age and delayed language at 4 years of age.

Elsewhere, based on extensive review of the research literature Sullivan and Horowitz (1983) argued that the infant's intermodal perceptual abilities in conjunction with the contiguous (and sometimes synchronous) multimodal stimulation provided by the infant's social environment are important factors in the equation for the development of early nonverbal language abilities. Certainly sound localization, at some as yet precisely specified level, is an important component of the infant's very early intermodal abilities.

The high-risk population for which sound localization may be most applicable as a screening device is that of prematurely born infants. There are several lines of evidence that lend support to this contention. First, longitudinal studies that have measured language outcomes of preterm infants have found evidence of delays in the language development of these infants (Beckwith, 1977; Cohen & Beckwith, 1976; Field, 1979; Field, Dempsey, & Shuman, 1979). A second line of research has also found deficits at 12 months of age in the preterm infant's intermodal perceptual abilities (Rose, 1981; Rose, Gottfried, & Bridger, 1978, 1979). A third, in a study using the Einstein Neonatal Neurobehavioral Assessment Scale (Kurtzeburg, Vaughn, Daum, Grellong, Albin, & Rotkin, 1979), found that the major difference between term and preterm neonates was a significant deficit in the preterm's ability to localize sounds—a deficit that could not be accounted for by differences in alertness or general motor performance.

These findings taken as a whole form what appears to be a set of potentially related deficits for the population of infants born prematurely. Although one cannot infer a causative relationship at this time (it is equally possible that the two phenomena may be parallel and unrelated), the findings certainly present an intriguing and promising picture. What is not known is what is the cause of these deficits. One possibility is that during the course of the premature birth or due to factors subsequent to birth (e.g., asphyxia, intraventricular hemorrhage, hyaline membrane disease, and ototoxic drugs) the brain may have suffered insult sufficient to cause long-lasting damage.

Another possibility is that the deficits are the result of the iatrogenic effects of the intensive care nursery (Cornell & Gottfried, 1976; Gottfried, Wallace-Landes, Sherman-Brown, King, Coen, & Allen, 1980; Korones, 1976; Lawson, Daum, & Turkewitz, 1977; Lucey, 1977). Long-term adverse effects may have resulted from the infant's prolonged exposure to an environment that does not provide the types of stimulation optimal for normal development. It is quite possible that these two factors may in fact interact. That is, infants who are compromised by factors related to premature birth are then exposed for long periods of time to an environment that may exacerbate the negative effects rather than provide stimulation that would serve to compensate for the early trauma.

An additional feature of sound localization that may be relevant to screening is the developmental changes that occur in localization abilities over a relatively short period of time (i.e., within the first 6 months of life). Kopp and Parmalee (1979) found in their comprehensive review that none of the research attempting to predict adverse outcome using measures of the preterm infant's perceptual processes had assessed the *same* process at several points in time. Rather, the process was measured only once or different processes were measured at different ages. Important information as to how the perceptual process changed over time was lost. The U-shaped developmental function found for sound localization may be ideal for assessing change over a relatively short span of time. The suggestion that the U-shaped function is the result of a subcortical to cortical shift in the control of the behavior may indicate that this is a period that is sensitive for illuminating underlying deficits. Divergence from the typical developmental function may serve to identify those infants who are truly at risk.

### An Example: Psychophysics of Sound Localization in 4-Month-Old Infants

Research with adult subjects has demonstrated that the accuracy of aurally localizing a sound varies systematically as a function of frequency (Stevens & Newman, 1936). Gulick (1971) compared, in graphic form, the results of the Stevens and Newman (date) study with the data describing the frequency-dependent changes in the effectiveness of the acoustic cues employed for sound localization (viz., $\Delta_t$ and $\Delta_i$). The results of this comparison are presented in Figure 1.

The reason there is a shift in cue effectiveness as frequency increases is due to changes in the relationship between sound wavelength and head size. In the case of low frequency sounds the sound waves are long enough that only a portion of the entire sound wave will fit between the two ears, thereby simplifying the calculations of time of ar-

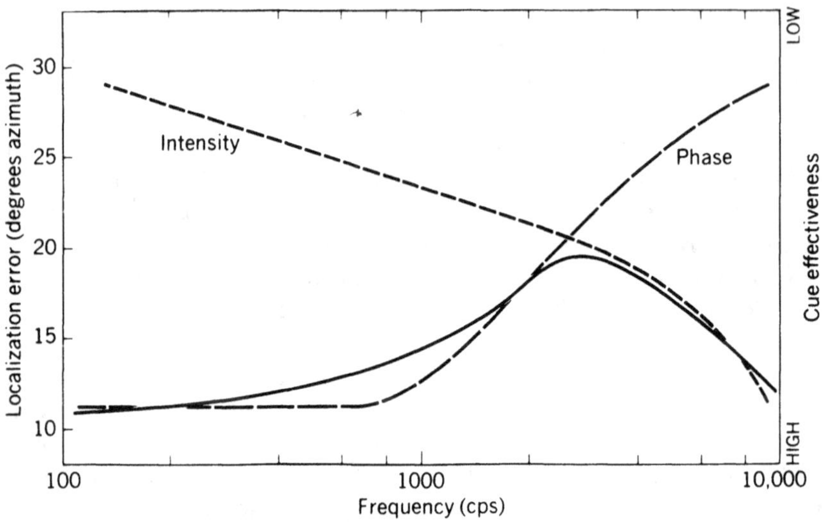


**Figure 1.** Cue effectiveness in adults as a function of frequency. Relative cue effectiveness is in arbitrary units for intensity and phase (dashed lines) as a function of frequency. *Note.* From *Hearing: Physiology and psychophysics* by W. L. Gulick, 1971, London: Oxford University Press. Copyright 1971 by Oxford University Press. Reprinted by permission.

rival differences. In addition, these long sound waves can bend around the head, thereby suffering very little loss in the intensity of the sound arriving at one ear versus the other. As frequency increases the length of the sound wave decreases as does the effectiveness of $\Delta_t$ as a cue. Conversely, as the sound wave becomes shorter it loses its ability to bend around the head, but rather is partially reflected, creating differences in the intensity of the sound arriving at each ear. For example, a 250 Hz tone eminating from a source 90° to the right of midline will result in approximately a 2 dB (SPL) difference in intensity of the sound arriving at the left versus the right ear. A 10,000 Hz tone will result in approximately a 20 dB difference.

The effect of these changes on subject performance can be seen by examining the solid line in Figure 1. The subjects are accurate in localizing the low and high frequency tones but do poorly in the middle frequencies. The frequency (3,000 Hz) localized with the least accuracy also coincides with the crossover point between the two cues (i.e., at the point where both $\Delta_t$ and $\Delta_i$ are of equal effectiveness).

The purpose of the present study was to determine whether the accuracy of 4-month-old infants' localization could be represented by a similar psychophysical function. We would expect *a priori,* however, that there should be a rightward shift in the infants' function due to differences in the diameter of the infant versus adult head. The 4-month-old, for example, should have $\Delta_t$ available at higher frequencies than the adult.

A total of 36 healthy, full-term infants were tested. Twelve infants (6 male and 6 female) were randomly assigned to one of three frequency conditions: Low Frequency (250, 500, 800, & 1,000 Hz); Mid Frequency (2,000, 3,000, 4,000, & 5,000 cps); and High Frequency (8,000, 10,000, 12,000, & 16,000 Hz). The infants within each condition were presented four trials at each of the four frequencies. The sounds emanated from speakers located 90° to the right and left of the infant's midline. One of six orders was randomly assigned for each frequency (e.g., LRLR, RLLR, LLRR) such that there were always two left and two right trials. The order of presenting the four frequencies within conditions was counterbalanced across infants with each frequency falling equally often in the first and last position. The stimuli were generated by taking a sample of "*pink*" noise (i.e., a noise whose intensity is inversely proportional to frequency over a specified range to give constant energy per octave) and filtering it using a Bruel & Kjaer $\frac{1}{3}$ Octave Graphic Spectrum Equalizer (Model 125) to produce narrow bands of noise at the above-mentioned frequencies. All stimuli were presented at 70 to 75 dB as measured at the infant's ear. Infant head turns were coded from video tapes as either (a) no turn—0° to 29° from midline; (b) 30° head turn—30° to 49°; (c) 50° head turn—50° to 79°; and (d) 80° head turn—80° to 90°. Interrater reliabilities were all above 85%.

The results are presented in Figure 2. Necessary adjustments have been made in the adult curve to account for the differences in head sizes between infants and adults.

The infant data plotted in Figure 2 represent the most accurate category of correct head turns (i.e., turns greater than 80° from midline). There were very few incorrect head turns of this magnitude. It was felt

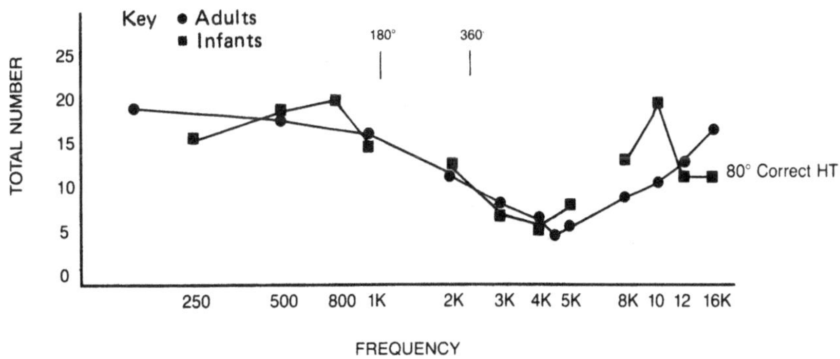


**Figure 2.** Cue effectiveness in infants as compared with adults.

that this category of head turns might be the most sensitive to change in the frequency of the sounds. Indeed, as can be seen in Figure 2, the function obtained from the 4-month-olds closely approximates the smoothed adult function. It does appear, however, that the infant function rises more sharply at the higher frequencies than does the adult function. The discrepant data points at 12,000 and 16,000 Hz may not be valid due to difficulty encountered in accurately reproducing and presenting acoustic stimuli in this frequency range. Further analysis using all correct head turns produced similar results.

It appears, therefore, that by 4 months of age the infant's use of the binaural acoustic cues for localization approximates that of the adult. This is true when corrections are made for the differences in head size between the infant and adult. We are currently replicating this study using a within-subjects design in which each infant will receive stimuli at 250, 1K, 2K, 3K, 4K, 5K, 8K, and 10K Hz.

## CONCLUSIONS

In this chapter an experimental approach that may prove effective for the early identification of infants who are at risk has been outlined. The approach taken was based on the assessment of auditory processing abilities of infants from birth to 4 to 5 months of age. We suggest that ultimately we will need to go beyond the strategies outlined in this and the Fagan and Rock chapters. The most impressive results are likely to be obtained from the assessment of information processing in multiple modalities as measured at critical transition periods during early development. The infancy period may be ideally suited for this strategy given the rapid development that occurs during a short period of time.

The emphasis on testing more than one modality stems from the hypothesis that risk factors may not have global effects that are equally harmful to all systems (see Garmezy, Chapter 3). Exposure to ototoxic medication, for example, may be more detrimental to the auditory system; whereas prolonged exposure to pure oxygen has its primary effect on the visual system. The occurrence of intraventricular hemorrhage, on the other hand, may effect the different systems in different infants. An assessment strategy that focuses on only one modality may, therefore, identify some infants but not others. Additionally, the integration of information gathered by the various modalities is also important to assess. The findings reported by Rose (1981) and Rose, Gottfried, and Bridger (1978, 1979) have already demonstrated deficits in 12-month-old premature infants' ability to perform intermodal perceptual tasks.

We are currently conducting studies that compare the sound localization of full-term and preterm samples of infants. These studies are employing both cross-sectional and longitudinal designs. Once the differences and similarities between these populations have been mapped-out, we need to embark on a long-term, longitudinal study to determine the relationship between the early differences and subsequent developmental problems.

## REFERENCES


Alegria, J., & Noirot, E. (1978). Neonate orientation behavior towards human voice. *International Journal of Behavior Development, 1,* 291–312.

Beckwith, L. (1977, March) *Development of conversation competency related to caregiver-infant interaction.* Paper presented to the American Psychological Association, San Francisco.

Brazelton, T. B. (1973). Neonatal Behavioral Assessment Scale. *National Spastics Society Monograph.* Philadelphia: Lippincott.

Butterworth, G., & Castillo, M. (1976). Coordination of auditory and visual space in newborn human infants. *Perception, 5,* 155–160.

Chun, R. W. M., Pawsat, R., & Forster, F. M. (1960). Sound localization in infancy. *Journal of Nervous and Mental Disease, 130,* 472–476.

Clifton, R., Morrongiello, B., Kulig, J., & Dowd, J. (1981). Developmental changes in auditory localization in infancy. In R. Aslin, J. Alberts, & M. Petersen (Eds.), *Sensory and perceptural development: Influences of genetic and experimental factors.* New York: Academic Press.

Cohen, S. E., & Beckwith, L. (1976). Maternal language in infancy. *Developmental Psychology, 12,* 371–372.

Cornell, E. H., & Gottfried, A. W. (1976). Intervention with premature infants. *Child Development, 47,* 32–39.

Crassini, B., & Broerse, J. (1980). Auditory-visual integration in neonates: A signal detection analysis. *Journal of Experimental Child Psychology, 29,* 144–155.

Field, J., DeFranco, D., Dodwell, P., & Muir, D. (1979). Auditory-visual coordination in $2\frac{1}{2}$-month-old infants. *Infant Behavior and Development, 2,* 113–122.

Field, J., Muir, D., Pilon, R., Sinclair, M., & Dodwell, P. (1980). Infants' orientation to lateral sounds from birth to three months. *Child Development, 51,* 295–298.

Field, T. M. (1979). Interaction patterns of preterm and term infants. In T. M. Field, A. M. Sostek, S. Goldberg, & H. H. Shuman (Eds.), *Infants born at risk.* New York: Spectrum.

Field, T. M., Dempsey, J. R., & Shuman, H. H. (1979). Developmental assessment of infants surviving the respiratory distress syndrome. In T. M. Field, A. M. Sostek, S. Goldberg, & H. H. Shuman (Eds.), *Infants born at risk.* New York: Spectrum.

Gibson, J. J. (1966). *The senses considered as perceptual systems.* Boston: Mifflin.

Gottfried, A. W., Wallace-Lande, P., Sherman-Brown, J. K., Coen, C., & Allen, K. (1980, April). *Physical and social ecology of newborn special care units.* Paper presented at the International Conference on Infant Studies, New Haven, CT.

Gulick, W. L. (1971). *Hearing: Physiology and psychophysics.* London: Oxford Univ. Press.

Hammer, M., & Turkewitz, G. (1975). Relationship between effective intensity of auditory stimulation and directional eye turns in the human infant. *Animal Behavior, 23,* 287–290.

Horowitz, F. D., Sullivan, J. W., & Byrne, J. M. (Manuscript in preparation). *The behavioral atlas of the newborn.* University of Kansas, Lawrence, Kansas.

Kopp, C. B., & Parmelee, A. H. (1979). Prenatal and perinatal influences on behavior. In J. Osofsky (Ed.), *Handbook of infant development.* New York: Wiley.

Korones, S. B. (1976). Disturbances and infant rest. In J. D. Moore (Ed.), *69th Ross Congress on Pediatric Research: Iatrogenic problems in intensive care.* Oltro.

Kurtzberg, D., Vaughan, H. G., Daum, C., Grellong, B. A., Albin, S., & Rotkin, L. (1979). Neurobehavioral performance of low-birthweight infants at 40 weeks conceptual age: Comparison with normal full-term infants. *Developmental Medicine and Child Neurology, 21,* 590–607.

Lawson, K., Daum, C., & Turkewitz, G. (1978). Environmental characteristics of a neonatal intensive care unit. *Child Development, 48,* 1633–1639.

Lucey, J. F. (1977). Is intensive care becoming too intensive? *Pediatrics Neonatalogy Supplements, 59,* 1064.

McGurk, H., Turnure, C., & Creighton, S. J. (1977). Auditory-visual coordination in neonates. *Child Development, 48,* 138–143.

Mendelson, M. J., & Haith, M. M. (1976). The relation between audition and vision in the human newborn. *Monographs of the Society for Research in Child Development, 41*(4).

Moore, B. C. (1977). *Introduction to the psychology of hearing.* Baltimore, MD: University Park Press.

Muir, D., Abraham, W., Forbes, B., & Harris, L. (1979). The ontogenesis of an auditory localization response from birth to four months of age. *Canadian Journal of Psychology, 33,* 320–333.

Muir, D., & Field, J. (1979). Newborn infants orient to sounds. *Child Development, 50,* 431–436.

Pollock, D. Cited in Swift, E. W., Swift, W. J., Camp, B. A., & Silvern, L. W. (1981). Predictive value of early testing of auditory localization for language development. *Developmental Medicine and Child Neurology, 23,* 306–312.

Rose, S. A. (1981). Lags in cognitive competence of prematurely born infants. In S. L. Friedman & M. Sigman (Eds.), *Preterm birth and psychological development.* New York: Academic Press.

Rose, S. A., Gottfried, A. W., & Bridger, W. H. (1978). Cross-modal transfer in infants: Relationship of prematurity and socio-economic background. *Developmental Psychology, 14,* 643–652.

Rose, S. A., Gottfried, A. W., & Bridger, W. H. (1979). Effects of haptic cues on visual recognition memory in full-term and preterm infants. *Infant behavior and Development, 2,* 55–67.

Sonksen, P. M. (1979). Sound and the visually handicapped baby. *Child: Care, health, and development, 5,* 413–420.

Stevens, S. S., & Newman, E. B. (1936). The localization of actual sources of sound. *American Journal of Psychology, 48,* 297–306.

Sullivan, J. W., & Horowitz, F. D. (1983). Infant intermodal perception and maternal multimodal stimulation: Implications for language development. In L. P. Lipsitt & C. K. Rovee-Collier (Eds.), *Advances in infancy research* (Vol. 2). New Jersey: Ablex.

Sullivan, J. W., & Ingram, E. (1983, April). *Factors contributing to newborn sound localization.* Paper presented to the Society for Research in Child Development, Detroit, MI.

Swift, E. W., Swift, W. J., Camp, B. W., & Silvern, L. W. (1981). Predictive value of early testing of auditory localization for language development. *Developmental Medicine and Child Neurology, 23,* 306–312.

Turkewitz, G., Birth, H. G., & Cooper, K. K. (1972a). Patterns of response to different auditory stimuli in the human newborn. *Developmental Medicine and Child Neurology, 14,* 487–491.

Turkewitz, G., Birth, H. G., & Cooper, K. K. (1972b). Responsiveness to simple and complex auditory stimuli in the human newborn. *Developmental Psychobiology, 5,* 7–19.

Turkewitz, G., Birth, H. G., Moreau, T., Levy, L., & Cornwall, A. C. (1966). Effect of intensity of auditory stimulation on directional eye-movements in the human neonate. *Animal Behavior, 14,* 93–101.

Turner, S., & Macfarlane, A. (1978). Localization of human speech by the newborn baby and the effects of pethidine ("meperidine"). *Developmental Medicine and Child Neurology, 20,* 727–734.

Wertheimer, M. (1961). Psychomotor coordination of auditory and visual space at birth. *Science, 134,* 1692.

Zelazo, P. R. (1979). Reactivity to perceptual-cognitive events: Application for infant assessment. In R. B. Kearsley & I. E. Sigel, (Eds.), *Infants at risk: Assessment of cognitive functioning.* New Jersey: Lawrence Erlbaum.

CHAPTER 20

# The Development of Temperament in Very Low Birth Weight Children

*Jo Hermanns, Bernard Cats, and Lya den Ouden*

The survival rate of very low birth weight (VLBW) children—generally defined as 1,500 g or less at birth—has improved considerably in the last few decades. In the Netherlands, for example, 60% to 70% of these children now survive the hazardous neonatal period (van Doornik, Cats, Versluys, de Saint Aulaire, & van de Woerd, 1980). However, they continue to be at risk for later developmental problems. Three interdependent groups of variables are held responsible for the less-than-favorable prognosis for many VLBW children. They are as follows:

1. The prematurity or dysmaturity as such. The untimely born child is not prepared for the life outside the uterus, and especially has problems with respiration and the regulation of body temperature.
2. The suboptimal physical condition that results from the low birth weight and leads to such problems as an increased susceptibility for infection.
3. The effect that the several weeks or months spent in the incubator separated from the parents has on the psychological development of the child.

As a result of such factors, a number of VLBW children later demonstrate moderate to severe handicaps, such as motoric disturbances and mental retardation. The majority do not show readily observable deviations from the normal pattern of physical and psychological development; however, even in this normal group there is increased risk for

*Jo Hermanns* • Department of Developmental Psychology, University of Utrecht, Utrecht, Netherlands. *Bernard Cats and Lya den Ouden* • Department of Neonatology, University of Utrecht, Utrecht, Netherlands.

disturbances in the parent–child relationship, a factor that results in a relatively high percentage of child abuse in VLBW children (Hunter, Kilstrom, Kraybill, & Loda, 1978; Jeffcoate, Humphrey, & Loyd, 1979; Klein & Stern, 1971).

It is our hypothesis that at least part of the parent–child interactional problems have to do with the VLBW child's characteristic behavioral style. For example, in a number of studies it has been found that the behavioral interaction between a mother and her preterm infant is less smooth and synchroneous than with a full-term child (Di Vitto & Golberg, 1980; Field, 1977b). Preterm babies seem to be less active and more fussy, and are harder to make eye contact with. Their parents seem to invest more than the normal amount of energy in interactions without affecting the child's behavior.

To explore our hypothesis that the behavioral style of the child influences the behavior of the parents, we are engaged in the longitudinal study of mother–child interactions. This chapter briefly examines the results of a study that followed VLBW children until the age of 2 to 4 years; it focuses on the behavioral style (temperament) of nonhandicapped children.

## THE POPULATION OF VLBW CHILDREN

The follow-up population involved a group of VLBW children who were admitted to the neonatal intensive care unit of the Wilhelmina Kinderziekenhuis in Utrecht from 1976 to 1979. From 118 survivors (out of 170 live births), parents of 92 of the children responded to a request to participate in the study. The age of the children at the time they were studied ranged from 14 to 46 months, with a mean age of 30 months. The birth weights varied from 700 g to 1,500 g (mean = 1,190 g). On the average, the children were 10 weeks premature. Twelve children were small for gestational age. The socioeconomic background of their families was comparable to that of the overall Dutch population.

The instruments used in this follow-up study were a Dutch standardization of the Denver Developmental Screening Test (DDST) (Cools & Hermanns, 1979); the Toddler Temperament Scale (TTS) (Fullard & McDevitt, 1978) for measuring behavioral style; an interview with the parents; and a pediatric examination.

Nineteen (21%) of the 92 children had abnormal or questionable DDST results (corrected for prematurity). Nine of the children were found to have severe handicaps that probably will result in the requirement of life-long institutional care. The other 10 children had moderate to mild handicaps such as mild spastic diplegia or developmental delay for which the prognosis is still unclear.

## EVALUATION OF TEMPERAMENT IN VLBW CHILDREN

The results of the temperament questionnaire are discussed here only for those children who had normal DDST results. When we also excluded those instances where foreign parents had language problems, the number of behavioral style questionnaires included in the study was reduced from a possible 79 to 60.

In the current study, we chose to describe the behavior of the child in terms of the concept of "temperament" as first formulated by Thomas and Chess (1977). This concept refers to individual style; it refers to the *how* of the behavior of the child, rather than to the *what* or the *why*. The Toddler Temperament Scale (TTS) has nine dimensions that include approximately 90 questions for the parents concerning everyday life experiences with their child (Fullard & McDevitt, 1978).

These include the following:

1. *Activity level* is the motor component present in a given child's functioning and the diurnal proportion of active and inactive periods. Questionnaire items are motility during bathing, eating, playing, dressing, and handling.

2. *Rhythmicity (regularity)* includes the predictability and/or unpredictability in time of any function. It can be analyzed in relation to the sleep–wake cycle, hunger, feeding patterns, and elimination schedule.

3. *Approach or withdrawal* is the nature of the initial response to a new stimulus, be it a new food, new toy, or new person. Approach responses are positive, whether displayed by mood expression (smiling, verbalizations, etc.) or motor activity (swallowing a new food, reaching for a new toy, active play, etc.). Withdrawal reactions are negative, whether displayed by mood expression (crying, fussing, grimacing, verbalizations, etc.) or motor activity (moving away, spitting out new food, pushing a new toy away, etc.).

4. *Adaptability* includes responses to new or altered situations. One is not concerned with the nature of the initial responses, but with the ease with which they are modified in desired directions.

5. *Threshold of responsiveness* covers the intensity level of stimulation that is necessary to evoke a discernible response, irrespective of the specific form that the response may take or the sensory modality affected. The behaviors utilized are those concerning reactions to sensory stimuli, environmental objects, and social contacts.

6. *Intensity of reaction* is the energy level of response, irrespective of its quality or direction.

7. *Quality of mood* includes the amount of pleasant, joyful, and friendly behavior, as contrasted with unpleasant, crying, and unfriendly behavior.

8. *Distractibility* is defined as the effectiveness of extraneous envi-

ronmental stimuli in interfering with or in altering the direction of the ongoing behavior.

9. *Persistence* refers to the continuation of an activity in the face of obstacles.

Thomas and Chess (1977) found among other things that a specific temperamental constellation (low approach, low adaptability, negative mood, and high intensity of reaction) implies an increase risk of behavior problems in the family or in school. The outcome was, of course, dependent on the way that parents and teachers were able to deal with this constellation, which has been referred to as a "difficult temperament."

The theoretical status of the concept of temperament or behavioral style has been and is a topic of vehement discussion. Because parents fill out the questionnaire concerning their perceptions of child behavior, many are concerned with the following issue: To what extent is temperament a perception of the parent, and to what extent is it a characteristic of the individual child (Plomin, 1983)? At the moment we assume that the results on the TTS are influenced both by characteristics of the child and how the child is seen by the parents. It is not necessary for the purposes of this study to see a specific temperamental constellation as a congenital, permanent trait of the child. It is sufficient to state that, from an interactionist point of view, certain aspects of the behavioral style of the child, as reported by the parents, may be a risk factor for the further development of the interaction. In other words, we became interested in temperament as a descriptive variable.

To be able to compare the TTS scores of the VLBW group with those of a normal group, we administered the TTS to a group of 130 parents of similar socioeconomic background, but with timely born children. This group was selected randomly from a number of well-baby clinics in the area surrounding Utrecht. The TTS was distributed by the well-baby clinic physicians to mothers, who were asked to return it by mail. Ninety percent of the mothers responded.

The first step in data analysis was to compare the temperament scores of children in the VLBW group with those of the control group (see Table 1). Except for mood and approach, all dimensions showed significant differences in favor of the control group.

As has been discussed, the VLBW children seem to present a behavioral style that makes them less easy for their parents to deal with. To portray this difference in style, we constructed a graphic comparison. The 16 children that the TTS manual stated could be considered as "difficult" were taken from the full-term comparison group and these were used as a third group. Then the specific patterns of the VLBW group, the modified full-term group, and the typical difficult group were com-

**Table 1.** TTS Scores from the VLBW Group Compared with Those from the Control Group ($N = 60$ and 130)

| | Mean | | *SD* | | Significance of *t* |
|---|---|---|---|---|---|
| | VLBW | Control | VLBW | Control | |
| Activity | 3.6 | 3.0 | .7 | .6 | $p < .001$ |
| Rhythmicity | 2.6 | 2.2 | .6 | .6 | $p < .001$ |
| Approach | 2.6 | 2.8 | 1.0 | .7 | — |
| Adaptability | 3.2 | 2.8 | .8 | .6 | $p < .001$ |
| Intensity | 3.7 | 3.4 | .6 | .7 | $p < .005$ |
| Mood | 2.9 | 2.8 | .6 | .5 | — |
| Persistence | 3.3 | 2.9 | .9 | .6 | $p < .004$ |
| Distractability | 4.5 | 4.0 | .9 | .6 | $p < .001$ |
| Threshold | 4.0 | 3.5 | .8 | .8 | $p < .001$ |

pared by converting the scores on the nine dimensions in standard scores. Figure 1 shows the three patterns that resulted.

If this figure can be considered a model, it appears that VLBW children have a temperamental profile that is different from that of the difficult child. VLBW children may be described as high in motor activity and distractability, with a low threshold of responding (i.e., irritable). Thinking of the effect these characteristics have on the parents, one could, in analogy to the difficult temperament, perhaps speak of a "fatiguing" temperament: The parent has to expend considerable emotional and physical energy to keep the restless, distractible child within the boundaries of an acceptable interaction.

The results of the TTS were confirmed by the pediatric examina-

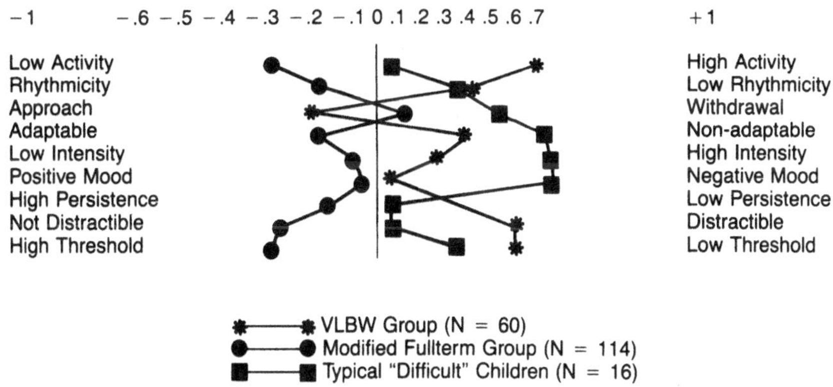


**Figure 1.** Temperament profile of VLBW children, the control group, and the typical "difficult" child.

tion. About 30% of the parents reported that bringing up their child was more difficult than they expected. In most cases, the children were described as overactive, distractible, and hot-tempered.

Some aspects of the behavior style described here are also reported in studies with infants. Field (1979) found that children who were 4 months premature were more distractible during feeding sessions with their mothers. In addition, prematures were found less attentive to their mothers in a face-to-face interaction situation (Field, 1977a). The higher activity level of the 2- to 4-year-old VLBW child seems to be in contradiction with the generally reported "fussiness" and low activity of the premature infant (Goldberg, 1979). The TTS activity subscale, however, has to do with nonfunctional motor activity like not sitting still while the parent reads from a book, and may best be described as restlessness. Thus, there may be the same style of nonfunctional activity in premature infants who are described as fussy and nonresponsive in interactive situations and the style of activity in our older 2- to 4-year-old VLBW children.

In conclusion, the VLBW status ($\leq$1,500 g) constitutes a serious risk factor for children. In addition to the risk of a severe handicap, the children who develop normally are described by their parents as having a behavioral style that may present problems in caregiving. These children and their parents certainly deserve our efforts in prevention and guidance in and after the neonatal period.

## REFERENCES

Cools, A., & Hermanns, J. (1979). *Vroegtijdige onderkenning van problemen in de ontwikkeling van jonge kinderen: Constructie en toepassing van een Denver ontwikkeling screening test.* Amsterdam: Swets & Zeitlinger.

DiVitto, B., & Goldberg, S. (1980). The development of early parent-infant interaction as a function of newborn medical status. In T. Field, S. Goldberg, S. Stern, & A. Sostek (Eds.), *High risk infants and children.* New York: Academic Press.

Field, T. (1977a). Effects of early separation interactive deficits and experimental manipulations on mother–infant interaction. *Child Development,* 48, 763–571.

Field, T. (1977b). Maternal stimulation during infant feeding. *Developmental Psychology, 13,* 539–540.

Field, T. (1979). Interaction patterns of preterm and term infants. In T. Field, A. Sostek, S. Goldberg, & H. Shuman (Eds.), *Infants born at risk.* New York, Spectrum.

Fullard, W., & McDevitt, S. (1978). *Toddler Temperament Scale.* Philadelphia: W. Carey.

Goldberg, S. (1979). Premature birth: Consequences for the parent-infant relationship. *American Scientist,* 67(2), 214–220.

Hunter, R. S., Kilstrom, A. C., Kraybill, E. N., & Loda, F. (1978). Antecedents of child abuse and neglect in premature infants: A prospective study in a newborn intensive care unit. *Pediatrics, 61,* 629–635.

Jeffcoate, J., Humphrey, M., & Loyd, J. (1979). Disturbance in parent-child relationship following preterm delivery. *Developmental Medicine and Child Neurology, 21*, 344–352.
Klein, M., & Stern, L. (1971). Low birth weight and the battered child syndrome. *American Journal of Disabled Children, 122*, 15–18.
Plomin, R. (1983). Childhood temperament. In B. Lakey & A. Kazdin (Eds.), *Advances in clinical child psychology* (Vol. 6, pp. 45–92). New York: Plenum.
Thomas, A., & Chess, S. (1977). *Temperament and development*. New York: Brunner/Mazel.
van Doornik, M., Cats, B., Versluys, C., de Saint Aulaire, E., & van de Woerd, H. (1980). Pasgeborenen met een zeer laag geboortegewicht. *Tijolschrift voor kindergeneeskunde, 48*, 470–485.

PART IV

# Regional and National Programs of Early Identification

CHAPTER 21

# Report of a Screening, Diagnosis, and Treatment Program for High-Risk Two-Year-Olds in Bermuda

*Elizabeth Hrncir, Amy Goldfarb, Sandra Scarr, and Kathleen McCartney*

Screening has attracted widespread attention in recent years as a means of detecting and subsequently treating developmental problems (Frankenburg & Dodds, 1967). Screening programs are based on evidence that early identification and treatment of children with developmental handicaps can reverse or ameliorate problems before they become entrenched, and before children come to view themselves (and others come to view them) as defective (Bronfenbrenner, 1975; Fandal, Kemper, & Frankenburg, 1978; Gerber & Heber, 1977; Ramey & Campbell, 1979). Early identification of developmental delay has been shown to improve children's responsiveness to treatment (Bronfenbrenner, 1975; Ramey & Brownlee, 1981).

In fact, the child's second year may be a particularly opportune time to identify and treat developmental problems, for disturbances in the acquisition of language and mild or borderline intellectual deficits may become pronounced around the second birthday (Knoblock & Pasamanick, 1953; Ramey & Haskins, 1981). The 2-year-old period is also a critical time for both children and parents with regard to behavior management, for the 2-year-old's increasing competence and mobility brings about increasing independence and assertion of autonomy (Atkeson &

***Elizabeth Hrncir*** • Child Development Project, Hamilton, Bermuda. ***Amy Goldfarb*** • Yale University, New Haven, Connecticut 06520. ***Sandra Scarr*** • University of Virginia, Charlottesville, Virginia 22903. ***Kathleen McCartney*** • Harvard University, Cambridge, Massachusetts 02138.

Forehand, 1981; Mrazek, Dowdney, Rutter, & Quinton, 1982). Finally, early identification of poor home environments can help prevent the downward spiral of learning difficulties typically experienced by children reared in disadvantaged conditions (Bradley & Caldwell, 1980; Zigler, Abelson, Trickett, & Seitz, 1982; Zigler & Butterfield, 1968).

In 1982, the government of Bermuda, in collaboration with psychologists from the United States, launched an island-wide Screening, Diagnosis, and Treatment (SDT) program for 2-year-olds. The program identified children at risk for the three most common early developmental problems in Bermuda: cognitive, language, and behavior management problems. In addition, children whose home environments placed them at risk for future delays in these areas were identified.

The multi-faceted focus of the SDT program evolved from an earlier intervention study conducted in a representative parish in Bermuda by Scarr and colleagues (Scarr, McCartney, & Schwarz, 1983). Twelve percent of the children in their sample were found to have significant developmental delays in the cognitive, language, and behavioral areas, and during this initial study were not receiving proper identification and treatment.

## SCREENING, DIAGNOSIS, AND TREATMENT PROGRAM

The SDT program focused first on an initial screening of the majority of 2-year-olds in Bermuda. A four-part screening battery was developed which combines well-established measures of child development with new screening measures developed especially for this project. Because screening tests require follow-up diagnostic evaluation of suspect children, a more comprehensive assessment battery was developed as a diagnostic tool. The battery covered cognitive, developmental language, behavioral, and environmental areas; the need to focus on children with problems has been verified by substantial evidence in the literature, as follows.

### Cognitive Delays

Estimates of the prevalence rate for mild intellectual retardation range from 2.5% to 6% and from 4% to 8% for borderline intellectual abilities. Socioeconomic conditions and age affect the prevalence rates among very poor school-aged children (Ginsberg, 1972; Stein & Susser, 1970; Tarjan, Eyman, & Meyers, 1973). Children with mild mental retardation show developmental delays in virtually every area of growth. These children benefit significantly from education and training for semi-independent living (Koch & Koch, 1975). Youngsters with borderline intelligence show minimal retardation in language, conceptual, and communicative development by age 5. School achievement is apt to become increasingly depressed (Sarason & Doris, 1979) despite relatively mild early impairments.

### Developmental Language Problems

The results of recent epidemiological studies indicate a prevalence rate of disturbance in language acquisition and speech for 2- and 3-year-olds to be between 3% and 8% (Allen & Bliss, 1978; Stevenson & Richman, 1976). The prevalence of mild language disruptions is greater in lower than in middle socioeconomic groups (Allen & Bliss, 1978), but moderate to severe language disabilities are found in 1 out of every 250 children (American Psychiatric Association, 1980) and occur at every socioeconomic level. Seventy percent of all children who have language disturbances remain handicapped through prepuberty, and a full 50% continue to have speech and language difficulties as young adults (Hall & Tomblin, 1978). Failure to receive appropriate early intervention has been associated with increasingly poor academic performance (Cantwell, Baker, & Mattison, 1979).

### Behavioral Problems

Although most investigators accept a prevalence rate for hyperactivity of between 3% and 5% for school-age children (Barkley, 1981), differing definitions of hyperactivity have led to varying reports of prevalence rates. England, for example, has fewer reported cases of hyperactivity than the United States. In their Isle of Wight survey, Rutter and colleagues (1977) diagnosed only 1.6% of children as hyperactive, but defined 54.4% as restless, 60.8% as fidgety, and 81.8% as having poor concentration. In the United States such children are usually labeled "hyperactive," whereas in England they are said to have "conduct disorders." For the purpose of the Bermuda study, hyperactivity was broadly defined to include the British description of conduct disorders.

Problem behaviors for children with severe conduct disorders will most likely continue through their life if left untreated (Robins, 1966). Poor school performance and disturbances in relationships with peers, parents, and family members become prominent during the school years. In adolescence, children with conduct disorders are at high risk for psychiatric disorder and juvenile delinquency (Mendelson, Johnson, & Stewart, 1971; Minde, Weiss, & Mendelson, 1972; Weiss, Minde, Werry, Douglas, & Nameth, 1971).

### Home Environment

The quality of stimulation in the home environment has been strongly linked with cognitive development in infants, young children, and school-age populations (Bradley & Caldwell, 1976a,b, 1977, 1978; Bradley, Caldwell, & Elardo, 1977; Elardo, Bradley, & Caldwell, 1975, 1977; Freund & Elardo, 1978). Indeed, specific environmental processes (Bradley & Caldwell, 1980) rather than gross index of socioeconomic status such as parental income, education, and IQ (Honzik, 1967; Kagan & Freeman, 1963) are strongly related to test performance and school achievement.

The goal of this research was to evaluate the screening and initial diagnostic components of the SDT Program. The evaluation focused on three criteria commonly used to evaluate programs of this kind: (a) comprehensiveness in reaching the target population; (b) detection accuracy; and (c) cost-effectiveness (Buck & Gart, 1966; Frankenburg, Camp, & Van Natta, 1971; Frankenburg & Dodds, 1967; Frankenburg, Goldstein, & Camp, 1971; Lichenstein, 1981; McCall, 1982; Ramey & Brownlee, 1981).

## METHOD

### Subjects

A total of 624 children turned 2 years of age in Bermuda between April of 1982 and February of 1983. Four hundred eighteen of these children were screened within a month of their second birthday. Their names were taken from hospital records obtained from health visitors.

### Measures

#### *Screening*

At the beginning of the screening interview, demographic data were collected, and mothers were asked to discuss any concerns they might have about their children. Mothers were rated as being either not concerned, concerned about an area that their children failed on the screening, or concerned about an area that their children did not fail on the screening.

As has been discussed, the screening measure covered four areas: cognitive, language, behavior, and environment. The cognitive section includes 21 consecutive items from the Bayley Mental Scales of Infant Development (Bayley, 1969). The items were chosen so that if a child did not pass at least 11 items, his or her IQ was estimated to be below 80.

Children who failed the cognitive screening were referred for a complete diagnostic evaluation.

The language section of the screening instrument included items from the language portion of the Portage Guide to Early Education Checklist (Bluma, Shearer, Frohman, & Hilliard, 1976). The checklist gives a comprehensive range of expected behaviors in expressive and receptive early language development. Children who did not pass at least 10 of 15 consecutive age-appropriate items were suspected of language delays and were referred for a complete diagnostic evaluation.

The behavior management section of the screening instrument included two parts: (a) observation of mother–child interaction; and (b) maternal rating of the child's overall manageability. In the observation portion, mothers were asked to teach their children a difficult visual-motor integration task (Beery & Buktenika, 1967). It was expected that this task would place the mother–child dyad under some stress, allowing for ratings on child attentiveness, cooperativeness, ability to remain seated at appropriate times, endurance for the testing situation, and ability to work happily with mother.

Mothers rated their children's overall manageability, using four items from Richman and Graham's Behavioral Screening Questionnaire (Richman & Graham, 1971). Children who did not receive positive ratings on at least 3 of the 5 dimensions rated by the observers, or who did not receive at least 5 of the possible 8 points on the maternal ratings, were considered to be potential behavior management problems and were referred for a complete diagnostic evaluation.

Environment was assessed as follows: Children who did not currently show developmental delays, but who were at risk for later delays because their home environments are lacking in stimulation, were identified with the Home Screening Questionnaire (HSQ) (Coons, Gay, Fandal, Ker, & Frankenburg, 1981). The pass–fail cutoff was based on the average score received by children falling in the lower 15th percentile (of possible scores) during the first 6 months of screening. Children who did not earn at least 28 of the possible 42 points on the HSQ were considered to be at risk because of deficient home environments, and were referred for a complete evaluation.

### *Diagnostic Evaluation*

Children who failed any part of the screening were offered a three-part, in-depth diagnostic evaluation. Children's cognitive functioning was assessed with the Bayley Mental Scales of Infant Development and/or Stanford–Binet Test of Intelligence (Terman & Merrill, 1973). A Bayley Mental Development Index or Stanford–Binet IQ score was obtained for each child.

Children's language development was assessed with the Sequenced Inventory of Communicative Development (Expressive Scale) (Hendrick, Prather, & Tobin, 1975). The diagnostic evaluation included items passed by 90% of children in the standardization sample at five age levels, beginning with 24 months and continuing up to 40 months. Testing began at the child's age level and continued until the child failed all of the items within an age level.

Behavior management difficulties were diagnosed with the Maternal Teaching Task, adapted from Hess and Shipman (1968). Mothers were asked to teach their children a difficult toy-sorting task while observers rated the children's manageability along three dimensions: cooperativeness, enthusiasm, and resistance. An overall "positiveness of child behaviors" score was computed by combining these three ratings. Observers also categorized mothers' discipline techniques as positive (i.e., encouragement or reasoning), neutral (i.e., bribe, pleading, or firm command), or negative (i.e., threat, physical restraint, or physical punishment).

Mothers also rated their children's behavior problems, using 104 items drawn from Conners' Parent Rating Scale (Conners, 1970) and the Werry–Weiss–Peters Activity Scale (Werry, 1968). Mothers were interviewed about their discipline techniques using the Maternal Discipline Interview, a measure developed by Scarr *et al.* (1983) for earlier research in Bermuda. Mothers were presented with five vignettes of typical child misbehaviors and asked what they would do if their child hit another child to get a toy; made a mess in the parents' closet; was rude to one of the grandparents; broke an important possession of the parents; or took an item from a store without paying. After the mothers gave one response, they were asked what they would do if the child did the same thing again—and a third time. On the basis of their responses, a second rating of the positiveness of their discipline techniques was made. An example of positive discipline is mild verbal punishment as contrasted with severe punishment (negative discipline).

In addition to the diagnostic measures described thus far, mothers also responded to 20 of the original 44 items on the Cain–Levine Social Competency Scale (Cain, Levine, & Elzey, 1977). They also rated their children on 20 of the original 48 items on the Childhood Personality Scale (CPS) (Cohen, Dibble, & Grawe, 1977). At the end of the evaluation, the staff member who assessed the children also rated them on the CPS.

**Assignment to Treatment Groups**

On completion of the diagnostic evaluation, a clinical case conference was held to determine their treatment needs. Assignment to treatment groups was made on the basis of the formal screening and diagnostic results, as well as the level and nature of the mother's concern and the child development project staff's more informal impressions of the family. Assignment was as follows:

1. Children with Bayley DQs or Stanford-Binet IQs ranging from 70 to 80 were assigned to the cognitive treatment group.

2. Children functioning below age-appropriate levels in expressive and/or receptive language on the Sequenced Inventory of Communicative Development were assigned to the language treatment group.

3. Children who had low ratings on cooperation and enthusiasm, who were often highly distractible and resistant (as reflected by the Maternal Teaching Task), and whose mothers often tended to use more physical, punitive types of control strategies (as reflected by the Maternal Discipline Interview) were assigned to the behavior management treatment group.

4. Children who scored below 28 on the Home Screening Questionnaire and who showed the potential for developmental delay in at least one other area were assigned to the Mother–Child Home Programme (MCHP).

5. Children who showed delays in more than one area, as 70% of the children did, were assigned to the treatment groups from which they were expected to receive the most benefit.

One-half of the children assigned to each of the tailored treatment groups were randomly assigned to a general educational enrichment program (i.e., the MCHP). The other half were randomly assigned to programs tailored to their specific needs.

Whenever possible, children were included in the SDT research model of comparison of tailored programs with a general educational enrichment program. However, it was not always ethically feasible to assign a child to the research model if it were known that the child's needs were so severe that she or he would benefit best from either a tailored program or the general educational enrichment program. Therefore, children with DQs or IQs below 70 and who often have severe and multiple handicaps (i.e., Down's syndrome, Aperts syndrome, toxoplasmosis) were assigned to a nonresearch cognitive group; children with no productive language were assigned to a nonresearch language group; and children exhibiting self-mutilating behaviors or severe emotional disorders were assigned to a nonresearch behavior management group. Children passing the diagnostic evaluation on measures of cognitive, language, and behavioral development, and with passing HSQ scores (i.e., above 28), but whose homes were still reported by health visitors and child development workers to be disadvantaged were assigned to a nonresearch MCHP.

## RESULTS AND DISCUSSION

### Comprehensiveness in Reaching the Target Population

The comprehensiveness of the screening and diagnostic program was assessed by computing the percentage of children eligible for services who actually received them. In the first 10 months that screening was conducted, 515 children (83%) of the 624 children who were eligible for screening were located. Of the children located, 418 (81%) were screened. The remaining 97 children (19% of the children found) were not screened. Only half of these children ($n$ = 49, or 10% of the children found) were not screened because of outright refusals. The other half were not screened because they had left Bermuda ($n$ = 40); because they spoke only Portuguese, creating a language barrier with the project staff, who spoke only English ($n$ = 4); or because they died before they had reached the age of 2 ($n$ = 4).

In light of these figures, the program's staff was concerned about the comprehensiveness of the SDT. The cooperation of the media was sought to increase the percentage of children on the island being reached by the screening. In addition, the staff worked to build a more effective liaison with the island's health visitors, because they see all the children born on the island and could be helpful in locating families. From April of 1982 through February of 1983, of the 104 children who were identified during that period as needing a diagnostic evaluation, all but 9 were either evaluated or scheduled for evaluation.

### Detection Accuracy

Ideal detection accuracy would result in all children who have serious developmental or home problems failing the screening and diagnostic evaluation, and being assigned to an appropriate treatment program. Children who do not have serious problems should pass the screening and diagnostic evaluation, and should not be assigned to a treatment program (McCall, 1982).

One of the first steps toward insuring that children are screened, diagnosed, and treated accurately is to chose measures with high validity. Tests that measure the same construct should correlate highly with each other. Tests that measure different constructs should not be highly correlated.

The cognitive screening in this program showed good discriminant validity. It correlated .61 with the cognitive assessment, but not nearly as well with the other diagnostic measures (Table 1). In contrast, the language, behavior management, and home screening measures fell short with regard to discriminant validity. The language screening cor-

**Table 1.** Correlations among Screening and Diagnostic Measures*

| | Cognitive | Language | Behavior management | | | |
|---|---|---|---|---|---|---|
| | IQ/MDI | SICD | Parent questionnaire | Positive maternal discipline (MTT) | Positive child behavior (MTT) | Positive maternal discipline (self-report) |
| Cognitive | .61 | .46 | −.03 | .16 | .18 | .19 |
| Language | .53 | .47 | −.20 | .03 | .02 | .10 |
| Behavior management observations | .15 | .06 | .15 | .17 | .27 | .10 |
| Behavior management mother | −.03 | −.12 | .50 | .08 | .24 | −.04 |
| Home questionnaire subtotal | .04 | −.03 | .13 | .14 | .13 | .27 |
| Home toy checklist subtotal | .07 | .06 | .23 | .24 | .11 | .15 |
| Home total | .08 | .03 | .20 | .24 | .14 | .30 |

*Because the number of subjects ranged from 98 to 104, all correlation values ⩾ .20 are significant at the .05 alpha level.

related more highly with the cognitive evaluation than it did with the language evaluation. In fact, scores on the language evaluation were predicted just as well by the cognitive screening as they were by the language screening. These results can be attributed, in part, to the high reliability of the Bayley and Stanford-Binet, which comprised the cognitive screening and diagnostic evaluation. The language measures are being examined in order to improve their discriminant validity.

The discriminant validity of the behavior management measures was also relatively weak. It was hypothesized that the four tests that measured child manageability would correlate highly with each other, and that the two tests that measure maternal discipline techniques would also correlate highly with each other. In addition, high correlations between child and maternal measures were expected.

The relationship among the behavior management measures was quite inconsistent. However, the correlation of .50 between two of the child manageability measures—mother's rating of the child at screening and her rating of the child on the parent questionnaire at assessment—is of particular importance. The behavior management measures are also being examined with the aim of improving their discriminant validity.

The discriminant validity of the HSQ was lower than expected. The HSQ showed low to moderate correlations with the two maternal discipline measures in the assessment (see Table 1). This result makes sense because maternal discipline is a key part of children's home environments. However, the HSQ also correlated reliably with the parent questionnaire, which measured children's current functioning. This occurred despite the fact that the HSQ is not designed to measure children's current status. The cultural relevancy of the HSQ is currently being examined; certain items that are not highly relevant to Bermudian culture are being modified or eliminated. This strategy, along with others, is expected to improve the discriminant validity of the HSQ.

In addition to discriminant validity, the relationship between screening results and assignment to treatment groups was examined. Here also the cognitive portion of the program worked well, whereas the language, behavior management, and home portions needed improvement.

Two kinds of screening errors hindered detection accuracy: Children falsely suspected as having a problem who did not, and children falsely suspected as not having a problem when in fact they did. The SDT program produced only one child who passed the screening but was diagnosed as having a problem in that area (the behavior management program) and ultimately was assigned to that treatment group. Unlike many early intervention programs in which children are only assessed in the screening areas they fail, the SDT program provides a three-part assesssment to all children, even if they fail only one part of the screening. Although this approach is not highly cost-effective, it does increase the accurate identification of children with developmental disabilities.

In contrast, the SDT program produced a relatively large number of children who failed the screening in a certain area, but ultimately were not assigned to that treatment group. The low predictive value of a positive in the language (50 children), behavior management (41 children), and home (50 children) areas was troublesome. These data suggest that the screening may be too liberal. Higher screening cutoffs will be tested to assess whether or not this strategy will lessen the number of children falsely identified on screening without significantly increasing the number of children with problems who are missed.

### Cost-Effectiveness

In order for a program to be cost-effective, the benefits for children must be maximized while the expenditure of government funds and staff time must be held to a minimum. The number of children in the SDT program who failed a part of the screening but were not assigned to any treatment group were as follows: There were 6 in the cognitive area, 24 in the language area, 18 in the behavior management area, and 23 in the home area. In the future, special attention will be paid to the predictive value of a positive (children who are falsely suspect on screening), for such an error represents a large drain on government resources.

## SIGNIFICANCE OF THE STUDY

Since 1977, the government of Bermuda has established a history of commitment to the welfare and development of its children. The ongoing evaluation of the SDT program was designed to help the government evaluate, and thereby streamline, the screening and diagnostic batteries. Thus, the Bermuda government is better able to wisely allocate its resources to serve the maximum number of children at minimum cost. In addition, the SDT program contributes new measures for 2-year-olds to the screening and diagnostic literature, and offers a methodology that might be useful for other professionals attempting to identify children at risk for cognitive, language, or behavioral problems and/or poor home environments. Finally, evaluation of the SDT model in Bermuda will eventually help answer central questions regarding the plasticity of human development and the role of experience in shaping development.

The authors of this project conceive of it as a pilot or preliminary study, as the final evaluation of its accuracy will require follow-up of a large number of screening nonsuspects to determine the sensitivity or accuracy of these procedures in identifying all of the problem cases. Furthermore, some of the diagnostic procedures or criteria were created for this project promoted the development of Bermuda's children. The current findings are very promising.

## REFERENCES

Allen, D., & Bliss, L. (1978). *Report of Project No. No1-NS-6-2355.* Bethesda: NINCDS. NIH, DEW.

American Psychiatric Association. (1980). *Diagnostic and statistical manual of mental disorders* (3rd ed.). Washington: Publisher.

Atkeson, B. M., & Forehand, R. (1981). Conduct disorders. In E. J. Mash & L. G. Terdal (Eds.), *Behavioural assessment of childhood disorders.* New York: Guilford Press.

Bayley, N. (1969). *Bayley scales of infant development: Manual.* New York: Psychological Corp.

Barkley, R. A. (1981). *Hyperactive children: A handbook for diagnosis and treatment.* New York: The Guilford Press.

Beery, K. E., & Buktenika, N. A. (1967). *Developmental Test of Visual-Motor Integration.* Chicago: Follett.

Bluma, S., Shearer, M., Frohman, A., & Hilliard, J. (1976). *Portage Guide to Early Education Checklist* (CESA 12). Portage, Wisconsin: Cooperative Educational Service Agency 12.

Bradley, R. H., & Caldwell, B. M. (1967a). Early home environment and changes in mental test performance in children from 6 to 36 months. *Developmental Psychology, 12,* 93–97.

Bradley, R. H., & Caldwell, B. M. (1976b). The relation of infants' home environment to mental test performance at 54 months: A follow-up study. *Child Development, 47,* 1172–1174.

Bradley, R. H., & Caldwell, B. M. (1977). Home observation for measurement of the environment: A validation study of screening efficiency. *American Journal of Mental Deficiency, 81,* 417–420.

Bradley, R. H., & Caldwell, B. M. (1978). Screening the environment. *American Journal of Orthopsychiatry, 48,* 114–130.

Bradley, R. H., & Caldwell, B. M. (1980). The relation of home environment, cognitive competence, and IQ among males and females. *Child Development, 51,* 1140–1148.

Bradley, R. H., Caldwell, B. M., & Elardo, R. (1977). Home environment, social status, and mental test performance. *Journal of Educational Psychology, 69,* 697–701.

Bronfenbrenner, U. (1975). Is early intervention effective? In M. Guttentag & E. L. Struening (Eds.), *Handbook of evaluation research* (Vol. 2). Beverly Hills, CA: Sage Publications.

Buck, A. A., & Gart, J. J. (1966). Comparison of a screening test and a reference test in epidemiologic studies: Indices of agreement and their relation to prevalence. *American Journal of Epidemiology, 83,* 586–592.

Cain, L. F., Levine, S., & Elzey, F. F. (1977). *Manual for the Cain–Levine social competency scale.* Palo Alto, CA: Consulting Psychologists Press.

Cantwell, D., Baker, L., & Mattison, R. (1979). Psychiatric disorders in children with speech and language disorders: Factors associated with development. *Journal of the American Academy of Child Psychiatry, 450,* 423–426.

Cohen, D. J., Dibble, E., & Grawe, J. M. (1977). Fathers' and mothers' perceptions of children's personality. *Archives of General Psychiatry, 34,* 480–487.

Conners, C. K. (1970). Symptom patterns in hyperkinetic, neurotic, and normal children. *Child Development, 41,* 667–682.

Coons, C. E., Gay, E. C., Fandal, A. W., Ker, C., & Frankenburg, W. K. (1981). *The Home Screening Questionnaire: Reference Manual.* Denver, Colorado: John F. Kennedy Child Development Center, School of Medicine, University of Colorado Health Sciences Center.

Elardo, R., Bradley, R., & Caldwell, B. M. (1975). The relation of infants' home environment to mental test performance from 6 to 36 months: A longitudinal analysis. *Child Development, 46,* 71–76.

Elardo, R., Bradley, R., & Caldwell, B. M. (1977). A longitudinal study of the relation of infants' home environments to language development at age three. *Child Development, 48,* 595–603.

Fandal, A. W., Kemper, M. B., & Frankenburg, W. K. (1978). Needed: Routine developmental screening for all children. *Pediatric Basics.* Fremont, MI: Gerber Products.

Frankenburg, W. K., Camp, B. W., & Van Natta, P. A. (1971). Validity of the Denver Developmental Screening Test. *Child Development, 42,* 475–485.

Frankenburg, W. K., & Dodds, J. B. (1967). The Denver Developmental Screening Test. *The Journal of Pediatrics, 71,* 181–191.

Frankenburg, W. K., Goldstein, A. D., & Camp, B. W. (1971). The revised Denver Developmental Screening Test: Its accuracy as a screening instrument. *The Journal of Pediatrics, 79,* 988–995.

Freund, J. H., & Elardo, R. (1978). Maternal behavior and family constellation as predictors of social competence among learning disabled children. *Learning Disability Quarterly, 1,* 80–86.

Gerber, H., & Heber, F. (1977). The Milwaukee Project: Indications of the effectiveness of early intervention in preventing mental retardation. In P. Mittler (Ed.), *Research to practice in mental retardation: Care and intervention* (Vol. 1). Baltimore: University Park Press.

Ginsberg, H. (1972). *The myth of the deprived child: Poor children, intellect, and education.* Englewood Cliffs, NJ: Prentice Hall.

Hall, P., & Tomblin, J. (1978). A follow-up study of children with articulation and language disorders. *Journal of Speech and Hearing Disorders, 43,* pp. 227–241.

Hendrick, D. L., Prather, E. M., & Tobin, A. R. (1975). *Sequenced Inventory of Communicative Development.* Seattle: Univ. of Washington Press.

Hess, R. D., & Shipman, V. (1968). Maternal influences upon early learning: The cognitive environments of urban preschool children. In R. D. Hess & R. M. Bear (Eds.), *Early education.* Chicago: Aldin Press.

Honzik, M. (1967). Environmental correlates of mental growth: Prediction from the family setting at 21 months. *Child Development, 38,* 337–364.

Kagan, J., & Freeman, M. (1963). Relation of childhood intelligence, maternal behaviours, and social class to behaviour during adolescence. *Child Development, 34,* 899–911.

Knoblock, H., & Pasamanick, B. (1953). Further observation on the behavioural development of Negro children. *Journal of Genetic Psychology, 83,* 137–157.

Koch, R., & Koch, K. (1975). *Understanding the mentally retarded child.* New York: Random House.

Lichenstein, R. (1981). Comparative validity of two preschool screening tests: Correlational and classificational approaches. *Journal of Learning Disabilities, 14,* 68–72.

McCall, R. B. (1982). Issues in the early development of intelligence and its assessment. In M. L. Lewis & L. T. Taft (Eds.), *Developmental disabilities: Theory, assessment, and intervention*. New York: Spectrum.

Mendelson, W., Johnson, N., & Stewart, M. A. (1971). Hyperactive children as teenagers: A follow-up study. *Journal of Nervous and Mental Disease, 153,* 273–279.

Minde, K., Weiss, G., & Mendelson, N. (1972). A five-year follow-up study of 91 hyperactive school children. *Journal of the American Academy of Child Psychiatry, 11,* 595–610.

Mrazek, D. A., Dowdney, M. A., Rutter, K. L., & Quinton, D. L. (1982). Mother and preschool child interaction: A sequential approach. *Journal of the American Academy of Child Psychiatry, 21,* 453–464.

Ramey, C. T., & Brownlee, J. R. (1981). Improving the identification of high-risk infants. *American Journal of Mental Deficiency, 85*(5), 504–511.

Ramey, C. T., & Campbell, F. A. (1979). Compensatory education for disadvantaged children. *School Review, 87,* 171–189.

Ramey, C. T., & Haskins, R. (1981). The causes and treatment of school failure: Insights from the Carolina Abecedarian Project. In M. Begab (Ed.), *Psychosocial influences and retarded performance: Strategies for improving social competence* (Vol. 2). Baltimore: University Park Press.

Richman, N., & Graham, P. J. (1971). A behavioural screening questionnaire for use with three-year-old children: Preliminary findings. *Journal of Child Psychology and Psychiatry, 12,* 5–33.

Robins, L. N. (1966). *Deviant children grown up: A sociological and psychiatric study of sociopathic personality.* Baltimore: Williams & Wilkins.

Rutter, M. (1977). Brain damage syndromes in childhood: Concepts and findings. *Journal of Child Psychology and Psychiatry, 18,* 1–21.

Sarason, S., & Doris, J. (1979). *Educational handicap, public policy, and social history.* New York: Free Press.

Scarr, S., McCartney, K., & Schwarz, J. C. (1983). *Report to the Bermuda Government on the Mother-Child Home Programme.* Sponsored by the Child Development Project of the Ministries of Health and Social Services and Education of the Bermuda Government, Unpublished manuscript, Yale University.

Stein, Z., & Susser, M. (1970). Mutability of intelligence and epidemiology of mild mental retardation. *Review of Educational Research, 40,* 29–67.

Stevenson, J., & Richman, N. (1976). *Developmental Medicine and Child Neurology, 431.*

Tarjan, G., Eyman, C., & Meyers, C. (1973). *Socio-behavioural studies in mental retardation: Monograph I.* Washington, DC: American Association on Mental Deficiency.

Terman, L., & Merrill, M. (1973). *Stanford–Binet Intelligence Scale: Manual for the third revision, Form L-M.* Boston: Houghton-Mifflin.

Weiss, G., Minde, K., Werry, J., Douglas, V., & Nameth, E. (1971). Studies on the hyperactive child: VIII. Five-year follow-up. *Archives of General Psychiatry, 24,* 409–414.

Werry, J. S. (1968). Developmental hyperactivity. *Pediatric Clinics of North America, 15,* 581–600.

Zigler, E., Abelson, W. D., Trickett, P. K., & Seitz, V. (1982). Is an early intervention programme necessary in order to improve economically disadvantaged children's IQ scores? *Child Development, 53,* 340–348.

Zigler, E., & Butterfield, E. C. (1968). Motivational aspects of changes in IQ test performance of culturally deprived nursery school children. *Child Development, 39,* 1–14.

*CHAPTER 22*

# The Denver Developmental Screening Test in Population Studies

## DESIGN AND METHODS

*Antonio Berdasco and José R. Jordan*

---

Since 1960, when the National Health System was established, major progress has been made in the health of Cuba's children. The system's first priority was to reduce infant and maternal mortality and morbidity, improve nutrition, and combat infectious diseases. These efforts have resulted in a decline in the infant mortality rate from 46.7 per 1,000 live births in 1969 to 17.3 in 1982. Life expectancy in Cuba is now 73.5 years, and malaria, poliomyelitis, diphtheria, and tetanus of the newborn have been eradicated.

As part of its effort to improve child health, Cuba conducted a National Child Growth Study in 1972. This study sampled 55,000 children ranging in age from birth to 20 years. Results (Jordan, 1973, 1979, 1980; Jordan, Bebelagua, Ruben, & Hernandez, 1980; Jordan, Ruben, Bebelagua, & Hernandez, 1977; Jordan, Ruben, Hernandez, Bebelagua, Tanner, & Goldstein, 1975) show that Cuban children grow and develop very similarly to children in developed countries (Eveleth & Tanners, 1976). Similar studies have been planned to take place every 10 years (the year after each national census) to monitor physical growth and nutrition. Thus, the second National Child Growth Study was conducted in 1982. The standardization project on which this chapter reports was a part of that larger 1982 Growth Study.

---

***Antonio Berdasco and José R. Jordan*** • Instituto de Desarrollo de la Salud, Havana, Cuba.

## PROJECT DESIGN

### Sampling Procedure

In May of 1982, a random (probability) sampling of the entire population of Cuba under the age of 20 was undertaken to study the growth of Cuban children. This sampling was based on the national census conducted in 1981, which put the population of Cuba at 9.7 million, of which approximately 4 million were under age 20 (Censo, 1983). The census divided the country into 14,150 districts, which were then grouped into macrodistricts each having a population of about 3,500 inhabitants. For the purposes of the study, 98 macrodistricts were randomly selected, yielding a set of 128,800 eligible children.

The size of the sample that was needed to allow adequate information about the growth of Cuba's children was estimated to be 30,000, but the sample was increased to 35,000 to allow for nonrespondents. Maps of the randomly selected 98 macrodistricts and lists of their residents were supplied by the census office, and members of the Women's Federation (with the help of the Small Farmer's Association for rural areas) visited every house. They updated the lists to include all children under 20 and every woman more than 6 months pregnant. These lists were then sent to a central office in Havana where a computer calculated decimal age, classified individuals into age groups, and randomly selected children to be examined from those who were eligible. The selection ratio was one in 3.6, for a total of 35,000 out of 128,800. The entire procedure (listing residents, processing data, and selecting children to be examined) took about 50 days. All children born during this interval were included in the sample.

### Subjects

Two special subsamples were randomly selected from the main sample. These included a group of 9,000 children under the age of $6\frac{1}{2}$ years who would be involved in the standardization of the Denver Developmental Screening Test (DDST) (Frankenburg & Dodds, 1967; Frankenburg, Goldstein, & Camp, 1971), and another group of children from 3.5 to 20 years who would receive physical fitness and functional capacity tests recommended by the International Biological Program (Weiner & Lourie, 1969). Of the 9,000 children selected for the DDST subsample, 8,246 were examined. Because this was a random sample of children from Cuba's entire population, no attempt was made to exclude apparently deviant children from the survey. Thus, children who were small for gestational age at birth, who were preterm, twins, breech deliveries, and so on, were also included; they will be separated in a later stage for comparison with children regarded as strictly normal, but will not be included in the final standardizing procedure unless they show no apparent departure from the rest. Children with gross sensorial defects, sickle cell anemia, cardiac anomalies, and so on were not included in the study.

Information gathered about the children included locality (urban/rural), province, sex, ethnic group, parents' educational levels, experience with other children, living with older siblings, attending day care nurseries, etc.

## METHODS

The first step in the standardization study involved translating the DDST, which resulted in the inevitable change in some words. For example, the word for *hedge* in Spanish is *seto*, which is never used in Cuba. Therefore, the word *cerca*, which means *fence*, was used.

### Training of Technicians

Two 6-week courses with 25 female participants each were begun in February of 1982. These were taught by two instructors (a psychometrist and a technician) along with a specially trained pediatrician with broad experience in using the DDST. The participants learned the theories and principles behind screening, watched training videocassettes, and had practice testing sessions with children from day care nurseries. All participants had completed, at a minimum, ninth grade. Both courses ended with administration of a proficiency test (test–retest, comparison with the instructor) from which the best 10 candidates were selected (from a total of 50). Each participant had practiced the DDST on more than 200 children by the conclusion of the course, and reliability was 95% in all cases.

### Preliminary Data-Gathering

A questionnaire developed for use in this study was completed by the child's parent or a care provider (such as a grandmother) prior to testing with the DDST. Data requested from the parents included duration of gestation, twinning, type of delivery, and other perinatal events. A history of infection of the nervous system and such identified problems as mental retardation and vision, hearing, and speech problems were recorded. Possible answers (as well as the 105 items of the DDST) were precoded for easy transcription to keypunching.

## Testing of Subjects

Examination of the children, which began in May and ended in December of 1982, was conducted by eight teams operating simultaneously in different areas. All children selected to receive the DDST were first submitted to this screening test and then were examined for anthropometry. Two of the DDST technicians were kept as substitutes in the event that another tester became ill; these two reserve test administrators alternated in performing the DDST with the local teams in order to maintain proficiency. All of the technicians worked in plain clothing and avoided white gowns, so as to put the children as much at ease as possible.

The DDST technicians used test kits of their own construction that were exact replicas of the original. Because raisins are not available in Cuba, black paper balls of about the same size and texture as raisins were substituted.

During this standardization testing, all items to the left of the age line on the DDST were explored, a procedure that resulted in many passes. Next, all age-appropriate items were tested, and then items far to the right of the age line were administered—until all items had been failed. All of this information was recorded in detail, and will be used to establish standards for scoring Cuban children; these standards will later be compared to those obtained in United States standardization studies with the DDST.

## Quality Control Sessions

Two quality control sessions were conducted during the period of the study. The first was held 2 months into the study, and the second was conducted at 4 months. During these quality control sessions, all the teams met in a day care nursery and examined the same group of children. While one technician tested a child, another would observe and rate the test. A pediatrician in charge supervised this process and evaluated both technicians.

On 3 consecutive mornings, each technician examined 4 children, 2 as an active tester and 2 as an observer–rater. In the afternoons, the technicians participated in an exercise in which they formulated questions for the mother or caregiver. The way the technicians calculated the child's age and the way they asked questions (including phrasing and vocabulary used) were analyzed. At each quality control session, each technician went through between 171 and 201 child tests and questions.

In the first quality control session, the percentage of questions formulated correctly ranged from 91% to 100%, and correct interpretation of the answers on the questionnaire ranged from 93% to 100%. Performing the test correctly with children ranged from 94% to 100%. In the second quality control session, results were even better. Ninety-six percent to 100% of the technicians formulated the questions correctly and interpreted the answers well; tests administered to the child were carried out correctly 97% to 100% of the time. All results from both sessions were compared with results obtained by the pediatrician who trained the teams.

## SAMPLE RESPONSE

The overall sample response for the DDST study (Table 1) was well over 90%, ensuring a representative probability sample of the entire country. The exact reason for the nonrespondent rate is not known, but we do not believe it is related to parents' fears of learning their child might be mentally retarded. This belief is based on the parents' perceiving the study as one of child nutrition and anthropometry; children tested with the DDST were only a small subsample of the larger study. However, some of the nonrespondents are being traced to see whether any departure from normality could exist that could introduce bias into the standardization study.

As can be seen from Table 1, there were sufficient children in each age group to draw conclusions even if different combinations of variables were to be analyzed. In addition, the inclusion of every child randomly selected (including children who were small for gestational age, twins, preterm, breech delivery, etc.) is justified because the sample is so large that those children can be deleted later and, in a second stage, can also be compared with children regarded as normal in order to avoid "contaminating" the sample.

**Table 1.** Distribution of Subjects by Age

| Age in months | Number of groups | Number of children per group | Total number of children |
|---|---|---|---|
| .5 to 14 | 42 | 110 | 4,260 |
| 15 to 17 | 3 | 151 | 453 |
| 18 to 22 | 6 | 213 | 1,278 |
| 23 to 30 | 3 | 155 | 465 |
| 31 to 54 | 15 | 76 | 1,140 |
| 55 to 72 | 6 | 53 | 318 |
| Totals | 75 | | 8,274 |

## CONCLUSIONS

The National Health System strategy of Cuba has been evolving for the past two decades. From 1960 to 1970, planning and organization were the country's main child-health thrust. In the decade from 1970 to 1980, mother–child morbidity and mortality programs were undertaken, efforts were made to combat infectious disease rates, and the physical growth and development of Cuba's children were studied. From 1980 to 1990, Cuba will focus on the prevention and treatment of chronic diseases, developmental handicaps, and accidents in children.

As part of this latter effort, the DDST is being standardized with Cuban children under the age of 6 years. It is hoped that this standardization effort will furnish invaluable information about the early detection of developmental problems in children. No ethical problems related to lack of follow-up are envisaged when the standardized DDST is placed into widespread use in the health system; we are already preparing proper stimulation programs for children with delayed development; we are planning for adequate facilities for these stimulation programs, and are training specialized personnel.

## REFERENCES

Censo de Poblacion y Viviendas, 1981. (1983). *Comité estatal de estadísticas oficina national del censo*. La Habana: Publicacion oficial.

Eveleth, P. B., & Tanner J. M. (1976). *Worldwide variations in human growth*. London: Cambridge Univ. Press.

Frankenburg, W. K., & Dodds, J. B. (1967). The Denver Developmental Screening Test. *Journal of Pediatrics, 71*, 181.

Frankenburg, W. K., Goldstein, A. D., & Camp, B. W. (1971). The Revised Denver Developmental Screening Test: Its accuracy as a screening instrument. *Journal of Pediatrics, 79*, 988.

Jordan, J. R. (1973). Los estudios sobre el Crecimiento del Niño en los paises en Desarrollo. *UNICEF Assignment Children, 23*, 46.

Jordan, J. R. (1979). Desarrollo humano en Cuba. La Habana: Instituto de la Infancia, Ministerio de Cultura.

Jordan, J. R. (1980). *The Cuban national child growth study*. Proceedings of the International Pediatric Congress, Barcelona, Spain.

Jordan, J. R., Bebelagua, A., Ruben, M., & Hernandez, J. (1980). Credimiento y Desarrollo del Niño en Cuba. *Boletín Médico del Hospital Infantil de Mexico, 37*, 599.

Jordan, J. R., Ruben, M., Bebelagua, A., & Hernandez, J. (1977). Investigacíon nacional, Credimiento y Desarrollo, Cuba 1972–1974: II. Técnica de las mediciones y controles de Calidad. *Revista Cubana de Pediatria, 49*, 513.

Jordan, J. R., Ruben, M., Hernandez, J., Bebelagua, A., Tanner, J. M., & Goldstein, H. (1975). The 1972 Cuban National Child Growth Study as an example of population health monitoring: Design and methods. *Annals of Human Biology, 2*, 153.

Weiner, J. S., & Lourie, J. A. (1969). *Human biology: A guide to field methods*. Oxford: Blackwell.

CHAPTER 23

# Early Identification of the Child at Risk

## A PHILIPPINE PERSPECTIVE

*Corazon V. Madrazo and Phoebe Dauz Williams*

In 1968 Wilson and Junger wrote:

> As communicable disease comes under control in the developing countries ... the chronic diseases that occupy the limelight in the developed countries may be expected to increase in importance in them; in some of the developing countries this trend has already become apparent. It may ... be expected that screening for disease will grow in importance. (p. 8)

Screening is the presumptive identification of an unrecognized disease or defect by the application of tests, examinations, or other procedure that can be applied rapidly. Screening tests sort out apparently well persons who probably have the problem from those who probably do not, permitting those with positive or suspicious findings to be referred for diagnosis and necessary treatment as early as possible. This early detection model is also called secondary prevention and applies to developmental disabilities as well as to detection of disease.

The early detection and intervention model for developmental disabilities has been shown to be operational in countries with well-developed health care delivery systems, such as Sweden (Sundelin, Mellbin, & Vuille, 1982), the Netherlands (Cools & Hermanns, 1977), and the United States (Frankenburg, Dodds, Fandal, Kazuk, & Cohrs, 1975;

***Corazon V. Madrazo*** • Philippine Nurses' Association, Malate, Manila, Philippines. ***Phoebe Dauz Williams*** • College of Nursing, University of Florida, Gainesville, Florida 32610. The study received in part joint funding from the Association of Christian Schools and Colleges, the National Research Council of the Philippines, and the University of the Philippines Graduate School.

Pierson, Levine, & Wolman, 1982; Scheiner & Abroms, 1980). The present study was designed to explore the existing mechanism for detection and diagnosis of children with certain developmental disabilities in Metropolitan Manila, the Philippines. Specifically, the study focused on (a) the circumstances leading to the detection and diagnosis of two kinds of disabilities (i.e., deafness and mental retardation); and (b) the general development of these disabled children as compared to that of a normal control group.

## METHODOLOGY

### Sample

This preliminary study sample consisted of 47 mothers of 28 deaf and 19 mentally retarded children and 50 mothers of apparently normal children. The subjects were from middle-class families whose longest place of residence was in Metro-Manila, although many parents originally came from other cities or from rural areas of the Philippines.

The mean age of the children was 7 years, 7 months. Age ranges were as follows: 3 to 12 years, deaf; 3 to 20 years, mentally retarded; and 3 to 8.7 years, apparently normal. (Although age limits of 3–8 years were set initially, only 11 deaf and 4 mentally retarded children could be located; hence, the inclusion of older subjects and the wider age ranges.)

When 9 directors of schools for the mentally retarded were asked to participate in the study, 6 agreed. Letters were then sent to parents of the children attending the 6 schools. The 37 letters sent resulted in 19 (51.4%) of the families agreeing to take part in the study.

The directors of two schools for the deaf and one diagnostic center for hearing impaired children all agreed to participate. Of 39 letters sent to parents of the schools' children, 26 (66.7%) agreed to participate. Of 10 letters sent to parents of children attending the diagnostic center, only 2 agreed to take part in the study.

The apparently normal group consisted of mothers who brought their children to a pediatric clinic at a 300-bed general hospital, and of mothers who were also staff nurses, midwives, nursing instructors, and married nursing students at the same hospital. Informed consent was obtained from all subjects.

### Data Collection

#### *Instruments*

Two instruments—an interview schedule and a screening tool—were used. The interview schedule covered sociodemographic information; child-rearing practices in relation to activities of daily living, sleep patterns, discipline, and affectional relationships; and related experiences (particularly initial concerns and actions, neighbor and kin relations, and mothers' thoughts and feelings at the time of the interview). The instrument was modified from Barsch's (1968) study on the rearing of children who were deaf, were blind, had cerebral palsy, had organic brain damage, or were born with Down's syndrome. A similar instrument was used by Quimbo (1979) in her Philippine study of children with cerebral palsy.

The screening tool used was the Metro-Manila Prescreening Developmental Questionnaire (MMPDQ). This tool evaluates development in gross motor, fine motor-adaptive, language, and personal-social behavior of children by maternal report. No other locally standardized test was available that evaluated the same aspects of behavior. The MMPDQ was developed from the 90th percentile norms of the Metro-Manila Development Screening Test (MMDST), which was standardized on 6,006 Metro-Manila children between the ages of 2 weeks and $6\frac{1}{2}$ years with supporting studies on reliability, validity, and cross-cultural identity (Williams, 1980a,b; 1984).

The MMPDQ consists of 97 items arranged to correspond with chronological ages starting from 2 months to 6.5 years. Each age range has 10 items. A mother may give 1 of 4 possible answers to a question: "yes," "no," "refuses," and "no opportunity." If a child passes all 10 items in his or her chronologic age range, items in the next age range are given, and so on, until the child passes less than 8 of the 10 items in a particular age range. On the other hand, if the child passes less than 8 items in his or her own chronologic age range, items on the preceding age range are asked, until the child passes at least 8 of 10 items in a particular age range. A child with normal performance passes at least 8 items in his or her own age range. A child who fails more than 2 items in his or her age range is considered to be nonnormal or abnormal.

The MMPDQ was administered to children between the ages of 3 and 6.9 years, who were tested on levels appropriate for their chronological age. Older children were given the 10 items of the upper age limit of the test, which is 6.6 to 6.9 years.

One of the authors (Madrazo) was assisted in data collection by two well-trained nurses. Administration of the MMPDQ and the interview schedule was conducted either in homes or in schools so as to be convenient for the mothers.

### Data Analysis

Frequency and percentage distributions were obtained for response to items in the interview schedule. Chi-square tests were done to determine differences among the groups on certain parameters of child behavior.

The child's performance on the MMPDQ was rated as normal or not normal, as described earlier. Age subgroups were created for the 3 comparison groups to tabulate the data: 3.0 to 6.9 years, 6.10 to 8.11 years (for all 3 groups), 9.0 to 13.11 years (for the deaf and mentally retarded groups), and 14.0 to 20 years (for the mentally retarded group only). Because several cells had zero frequencies, however, the age subgroups were collapsed for a chi-square test to be done.

## RESULTS

### Detection of Developmental Disabilities

*Age and Manner of Detection.* The age ranges at which deafness or mental retardation were detected were 7 months to $5\frac{1}{2}$ years, and birth (Down's syndrome) to 7 years, respectively (Table 1). The earliest signs recalled by mothers of deaf children were lack of response to sounds, "always silent," lack of startle, weak cry, and nonimitation of sounds produced by the mothers. The earliest signs recalled by mothers of mentally retarded children were lack of head control, inability to crawl or walk at expected ages, and poor motor coordination.

*Initial Reactions.* Three-fourths of the parents in both groups reacted with worry and concern, fear, disbelief, sadness, and pity. However, only 6 parents from both groups sought immediate medical consultation; the rest waited. Nevertheless, the first persons consulted were a physician or a kin-parent or sibling. The mothers consulted various physicians to obtain a diagnosis (Table 2). The majority (89.2% of parents in the deaf group and 78.95% of parents with mentally retarded children) sought a second opinion. Some of the parents consulted another physician, whereas others consulted an acupuncturist or a faith healer.

**Table 1.** Age of Child When Handicap Was First Noticed

| | Deaf ($N$ = 28) | | Mentally retarded ($N$ = 19) | |
|---|---|---|---|---|
| Age | No. | Percentage | No. | Percentage |
| Infant (0–12 months) | 10 | 35.71 | 5 | 26.31 |
| Toddler (1.1–3 years) | 15 | 53.57 | 10 | 52.63 |
| Preschool (3.1–6 years) | 2 | 7.14 | 2 | 10.53 |
| School (6.1–15 years) | — | — | 2 | 10.53 |
| Not applicable[a] | 1 | 3.57 | — | — |

[a]Mother was abroad at the time.

**Table 2.** Persons to Whom Mothers Took Child for Diagnosis

| | Deaf ($N$ = 28) | | Mentally retarded ($N$ = 19) | |
|---|---|---|---|---|
| Person consulted | No. | Percentage | No. | Percentage |
| Pediatrician | 3 | 10.71 | 9 | 47.37 |
| ENT specialist | 19 | 67.86 | — | — |
| Neurologist | 1 | 3.57 | 1 | 5.26 |
| Other MD[a] | 3 | 10.71 | 8 | 42.11 |
| Others, not MDs[b] | 2 | 7.14 | 1 | 5.26 |
| Total | 28 | 99.99 | 19 | 100.00 |

[a]Geneticist, obstetrician, general practitioner.
[b]Special school, hearing aid agency.

## Diagnosis

Initial diagnoses ranged from specific (i.e., profound hearing loss) to broad (i.e., "Your child is special"). Among the deaf children, diagnosis was ascertained mostly between the ages of 7 months and 3 years. Except for the child with Down's syndrome, the mentally retarded group was generally diagnosed later (after age 3).

## General Development

***The MMPDQ.*** In the control group, only 1 of 50 children's performance on the MMPDQ was not normal, compared to 6 of 28 in the deaf group and 15 of the 19 children in the mentally retarded group. Table 3 shows the results ($p < .001$) of the chi-square test.

**Table 3.** Results Comparing MMPDQ Performance of 3 Groups of Children

| | MMPDQ scores | | |
|---|---|---|---|
| Group | Not normal (passes < 8) | Normal (passes ⩾ 8) | Total |
| Normal | 1<br>(11.3) | 49<br>(36.7) | 50 |
| Deaf | 6<br>(6.4) | 22<br>(21.6) | 28 |
| Mentally retarded | 15<br>(4.3) | 4<br>(14.7) | 19 |
| Total | 22 | 75 | 97 |

*Note.* $\chi^2 = 47.97$ ($df = 2$). $p < .001$.

*Activities of Daily Living.* Comparisons were made of skills in bladder and bowel control, washing, feeding, and dressing by children in the three groups. The ages of attainment of bladder control were significantly different ($p < .05$) among comparison groups; more children in the normal and deaf groups achieved control before age 3. The ages of attainment of bowel control were also significantly different ($p < .01$) among comparison groups. Again, more children in the normal and deaf groups achieved control before age 3.

At the time of interview, more deaf than normal children in the 3- to 6-year age range performed tasks of washing, feeding, and dressing. Ninety percent of the deaf children could dress themselves in this age range, as compared with 76% of normal children; 100% of deaf children could wash themselves (vs. 84% of normal children); 100% of both groups fed themselves. One of 2 mentally retarded children in this age range could feed and wash (but not dress) herself—the rest achieved these tasks beyond the age of 6.

## DISCUSSION, IMPLICATIONS, AND RECOMMENDATIONS

The early identification model discussed earlier (Cools & Hermans, 1977; Frankenburg *et al.*, 1975; Pierson *et al.*, 1982; Scheiner & Abroms, 1980; Sundelin *et al.*, 1982; Whitby, 1974; Wilson & Jungner, 1968) does not seem to be operational in Metro-Manila, the Philippines, at this stage of development of its health care programs. The management of disabilities that children may receive depends mostly on individual parents' initiative and resources. Even among the study sample of middle-class families, only one mentally retarded child's and one deaf child's diagnoses were ascertained at 5 and 7 months, respectively. These children received optimum care from parents and kin who were themselves health care professionals. The rest of the sample's children were diagnosed later, generally before 3 years of age among deaf children and after 3 years of age among mentally retarded children. The latest final diagnosis for a mentally retarded child was 15 years, and 7 years for a deaf child.

Rubin (1980) has stated that a baby handicapped by a hearing deficit will exist in a state of sensory deprivation. This deprivation interferes with the reciprocal process of communication between baby and mother and prevents the infant from acquiring the auditory skills needed for language and speech development. Thus, it is little comfort to note McFarland and Simmons' (1982) observations from a review of studies that

1. Excepting children of the deaf, the impaired hearing of most

children with severely handicapping hearing deficits is not detected until they are between 2.2 and 2.9 years old;
2. A full year elapses on the average between the first suspicion of a hearing loss (usually by the parents) and a final confirmation of the loss;
3. If a child has only a mild to moderate loss (but a loss still great enough to require a hearing aid), the age of suspicion averages over 3 years, and the age of the child at diagnosis is 4.5 years.

The identification record for mentally retarded children is not much better. Kaminer and Jedrysek (1982) report, from their experience in a developmental evaluation clinic where the Denver Developmental Screening Test (DDST) is routinely used, that (a) mildly retarded children are identified in the preschool years; and (b) that screening has its greatest impact on the early identification of healthy, motorically intact, unstigmatized, mildly retarded children who, as a group, have shown the best response to intervention.

The Metro-Manila version of the DDST, the MMDST, would be appropriate both as a selective screening tool and a surveillance tool, particularly for high-risk groups of infant (or other children under $6\frac{1}{2}$ years). A prescreening questionnaire, the MMPDQ, has been constructed from the MMDST; it reduces screening time considerably, for the MMDST must be conducted only in cases of "positives" on the MMPDQ. Thus, both tools are potentially useful for a two-stage screening process similar to the Prescreening Development Questionnaire and DDST combination (Frankenburg *et al.*, 1975; Frankenburg, van Doorninck, Liddell, & Dick, 1976).

Kaminer and Jedrysek (1982) have noted that developmental screening by health care workers serves an additional purpose besides early identification. The act of screening states to the parent that the health care worker's role includes knowledge of and interest in the child's development and behavior. Even normal findings become an introduction to individualized anticipatory guidance. Similar observations about this added value of screening have been made by Williams (1984) and Morley (1979). In fact, with severe constraints in resources in a country like the Philippines, this screening benefit may be paramount at the present time.

In conclusion, the study indicates the need for (a) earlier identification and intervention for developmental disabilities; (b) training of more health professionals in the early identification and management of the same; (c) family involvement and support; and (d) greater public awareness about developmental disabilities. Although it is recognized that the study sample for the validation of the MMPDQ was a nonrandom sample, the results of this study reveal that the MMPDQ is a potentially useful tool in screening a random sample of children. With these promising preliminary results, it is hoped that a second study of the general population of 3 months to 6 years of age will be selected to determine if the preliminary scoring of the MMPDQ is valid when screening the general population. The MMPDQ and MMDST are screening tools that potentially may be used at the primary health care level. In the case of abnormal findings, diagnostic evaluations should be conducted in a tertiary health care center. On the other hand, nonsuspect findings may serve as a basis for anticipatory guidance, as well as a reinforcement to caregivers for a job well done. The results of this study have major implications for other developing countries.

## REFERENCES

Barsch, R. (1968). *The parent of the handicapped child.* Chicago, IL: Charles C Thomas.

Cools, A. T. M., & Hermanns, J. M. A. (1977). *Early detection of developmental problems in children.* The Netherlands: Univ. of Utrecht.

Frankenburg, W. K., Dodds, J. B., Fandal, A. W., Kazuk, E., & Cohrs, M. (1975). *The Denver Developmental Screening Test.* Denver, Colorado: Univ. of Colorado Press.

Frankenburg, W. K., van Doorninck, W. J., Liddell, T. N., & Dick, N. (1976). The Denver Prescreening Developmental Questionnaire (PDQ). *Pediatrics, 57,* 744–753.

Kaminer, R., & Jedrysek, E. (1982). Early identification of developmental disabilities. *Pediatric Annals, 11,* 5, 427–437.

McFarland, W. H., & Simmons, F. B. (1982). The importance of early intervention with severe childhood deafness. *Pediatric Annals, 9,* 1, 13–19.

Morley, D. (1979). *Pediatric priorities in the developing world.* London: Butterworths.

Pierson, D. E., Levine, M. D., & Wolman, R. (1982). Auditing multidisciplinary assessment procedures. In N. H. Anastasiow, W. K. Frankenburg, & A. W. Fandal (Eds.), *Identifying the developmentally delayed child.* Baltimore: University Park Press.

Quimbo, C. (1979). *The child with cerebral palsy: Effects on parental attitudes and on intrafamily and other relationships.* Unpublished thesis, University of the Philippines.

Rubin, M. (1980). Meeting the needs of hearing impaired infants. *Pediatric Annals, 9,* 1, 46–50.

Scheiner, A. P., & Abroms, I. F. (1980). *The practical management of the developmentally delayed child.* St. Louis: Mosby.

Sundelin, C., Mellbin, T., & Vuille, J. (1982). From 4 to 10: An overall evaluation of the general health screening of 4-year-olds. In N. J. Anastasiow, W. K. Frankenburg, & A. W. Fandal (Eds.), *Identifying the developmentally delayed child.* Baltimore: University Park Press.

Whitby, L. (1974). Screening for disease-definitions and criteria. *The Lancet,* October 5.

Williams, P. D. (1980a). A comparative study of DDST norms developed in five locales. In P. D. Williams (Ed.), *Nursing research in the Philippines: A sourcebook.* Quezon City: JMC Press.

Williams, P. D. (1980b, August 26). *Predictive validity of the Metro-Manila Developmental Screening Test.* Paper presented at the Philippine Psychological Association Convention, Manila.

Williams, P. D. (1984). The Metro-Manila Developmental Screening Test (MMDST): A normative study. *Nursing Research, 33,* 4, 208–212.

Wilson, J. M. G., & Jungner, G. (1968). *Principles and practice of screening for disease.* Public Health Papers #34. Geneva: World Health Organization.

CHAPTER 24

# Adapting and Translating the Denver Prescreening Developmental Questionnaire for the Sudan

*Babiker Badri and Edith H. Grotberg*

The Sudan, as a developing country, is increasingly concerned about the development of its young children. For example, a Kindergarten Institute promotes the development and education of young children, and a Directorate of Special Education in the Ministry of Education provides staff and resources to young children with disabilities. The Sudan's efforts are broad, but do not include screening to determine developmental status, highlighting areas of underdevelopment, or undertaking intervention strategies to stimulate the total development and education of young children. However, the Sudan has a private university in Omdurman, Ahfad University for Women, which is addressing the screening and early intervention issues.

Ahfad University is a focal point for introducing new programs, techniques, and materials to the country. As a private university, Ahfad is quite free to experiment and test new ideas, with the frequent result that the central government of the Sudan adopts the ideas for national use.

One of the current areas of innovation at Ahfad is training students in the area of special education. Students take courses in child development and special education in which they learn how to screen children to determine overall developmental status and how to organize

***Babiker Badri and Edith K. Grotberg*** • Department of Psychology and Special Education, Ahfad University College for Women, Omdurman, Sudan.

activities to stimulate further development, especially in areas of developmental lag.

In order to train Ahfad students, it was necessary to (a) select a screening instrument; (b) instruct students in its content and use; (c) provide an Arabic version of the instrument; (d) test the Arabic version; and (e) prepare students to organize activities to stimulate further child development. This chapter reports on how those activities were conducted.

## SELECTION OF A SCREENING INSTRUMENT

It was not difficult to decide that one of the screening instruments developed by the Denver group was appropriate for use in the Sudan. The tests had been carefully field tested among different populations within the United States and in other countries, such as Jamaica (UNESCO, 1981) and sections of China. Furthermore, the test items generally have universal application as they involve developmental areas and levels common to all children. The cultural hurdles were not insurmountable.

The question, then, became one of selecting either the Denver Developmental Screening Test (DDST) or the Denver Prescreening Developmental Questionnaire (DPDQ). The considerations necessary to make that choice were the relative difficulty of administering the two tests, the desire to involve parents in the testing, the ease of translating the tests into Arabic, and the interest in promoting the development of all children rather than focusing just on screening for children at risk. After consideration of these issues, the DPDQ was selected (Frankenburg, van Doorninck, Liddel, & Dick, 1976; Rosenbaum, Chua-Lim, Whilhite, & Mankead, 1983). At some later date, the DDST may be used to train professionals in the Sudan, and an Arabic version is expected to be developed.

## INSTRUCTION OF STUDENTS

In a third year undergraduate course on exceptional children at Ahfad University, students who had earlier courses in child development were trained in the content and use of the English version of the DPDQ. Twenty-five students were trained in the methods and procedures for administering the DPDQ, and an item analysis was conducted with the class to clarify what was being measured. Each item was recognized as part of a progression in one of the four developmental areas (gross motor, fine motor-adaptive, language, and personal-social). The students became skilled at recognizing the sequence of development from 3 months to 6 years and 3 months in each of the areas.

## PROVIDING AN ARABIC VERSION

Next the DPDQ was translated into Arabic. Two issues were critical to this translation. One was the appropriate standard of Arabic to be used, and the other was the adaptation of items to the different culture.

The first issue was addressed at the start of the translation. A group of assessors from the faculty of Ahfad University were consulted specifically on the suitability of the standard of the Arabic language to be used for the DPDQ. They all suggested that a middle course between classical and colloquial standards be followed if a universal application of the DPDQ were desired. The Sudan is a large country where many different dialects and levels of Arabic are in use. Moreover, the classical level is not fully understood by the large mass of the population, many of whom may be illiterate or semiliterate. Hence, even if the questions were read to many parents, the words might be too difficult for them to comprehend. Consideration was also given to the potential use of the Arabic version in other Arab-speaking countries.

The second issue addressed culturally appropriate items. An example of the kinds of changes required are as follows:

1. Item 57 on the DPDQ asks whether the child can go up and down stairs. A major change was required in this item, as stairs are not commonly found in Sudanese homes. An alternative response was adopted which asks if the child can walk on his or her tiptoes.

2. Item 73 on the DPDQ, which inquires about language ability, refers to putting an *s* at the end of words to pluralize them. In Arabic, the construction of plurals involves the addition of more than a single letter. Sometimes it requires a complete change of the word, whereas at other times it involves the addition of more than one letter. Therefore, the question was reformulated in Arabic with these considerations in mind. Nevertheless, the examples quoted in Arabic used the same words as in English (i.e., blocks, shoes, and toys). The first word (*blocks*) required the addition of two letters when put in plural. The other two words involved more changes.

## TESTING THE ARABIC VERSION

After the students demonstrated an understanding of the DPDQ in English, they formed small groups of five and compared the Arabic translation with the English original. They used a variety of techniques to do this. Some groups had 1 person read the Arabic while the others followed with the English. Other groups, especially where a member was not fluent in Arabic, had 1 person read in English while the others compared it with the Arabic version.

When there was general understanding of the Arabic translation, 5 students were assigned to field test the Arabic version to determine if parents understood the questions and could answer them easily. The students covered the age range of the DPDQ and conducted sessions with 25 parents. Parents' comments generally fell into three categories. One was the clarity of the questions; parents indicated that they had no difficulty understanding and answering the questions. Another was the length of some of the questions; parents often forgot the beginning of a question and it had to be repeated. The third involved questions directed to the children, where the Arabic word was not recognized and a more colloquial word was provided.

The class discussed these field experiences as they prepared for individual assignments to administer the DPDQ to parents. Where the parents spoke Arabic, the students administered the test in Arabic; where the parents spoke English, the English version was used. As there were insufficient copies of the test in Arabic, many of the students copied the appropriate 10 questions from the Arabic version and traced pictures or made the designs and colored blocks on their copy prior to testing an individual child.

The results of the field test and the class assignment became the basis for scoring and analyzing the responses. As more tests are administered, results will be analyzed to begin determining cultural patterns and to consider the value of standardization on the Sudanese population.

## PREPARATION OF STUDENTS TO STIMULATE CHILD DEVELOPMENT

The DPDQ was developed as a screening test, and was not designed to be used as a criterion for the need for early intervention. However, due to the lack of diagnostic services in the Sudan, we have designed an intervention program based on the results of the DPDQ. The intervention program consists of a series of activities designed to correspond to the items in the DPDQ. The intent is not to teach the test, but to promote development in the areas sampled by the DPDQ. These activities may be engaged in by parents or other family members, or by a trained outsider. They may be organized with the total development of the child in mind, and with special concern for those areas of development that are not at the expected level. It consists of teaching parents what to do to foster the development of children. This may not be the adequate or appropriate treatment, so the progress of children who are given such treatment will be monitored. The children who do not seem to make developmental gains from the program will receive what limited diagnostic services are available in the country.

## REFERENCES

Frankenburg, W. K., van Doorninck, W. J., Liddell, T. N., & Dick, N. P. (1976). The Denver Prescreening Developmental Questionnaire (PDQ). *Pediatrics, 57*, 744–753.

Rosenbaum, M. S., Chua-Lim, C., Whilhite, J., & Mankead, U. N. (1983). Applicability of the Denver Prescreening Developmental Questionnaire in a low-income population. *Pediatrics, 71*(3), 359–363.

UNESCO. (1981). *Early stimulation in Jamaica*. Special Education Unit.

CHAPTER 25

# Periodic Developmental Screening of Japanese Children from Three Months to Ten Years of Age

*Reiko Ueda*

Since 1977, child health check-ups have been carried out throughout Japan at 3 months, $1\frac{1}{2}$ years, and 3 years of age. The purpose of the current study was to discover how medical or developmental problems at 3 months of age may influence later development of the children, and to evaluate various screening methods.

## SUBJECTS AND METHODS

The 397 subjects were selected from 1,452 children who had been born in an urban area of Tokyo, and had been examined at a health center at 3 months of age in 1972. They were divided into three groups. Group 1 consisted of children with medical problems diagnosed by a pediatrician ($N$ = 147); Group 2 included children whose mothers had reported developmental and physical problems on a comprehensive developmental questionnaire ($N$ = 123); and Group 3 was a control group of children without known medical or developmental problems ($N$ = 127). The children were followed up with a developmental questionnaire at *4*, 6, *9 to 12*, 24, *36*, 48, 60, and 72 months, and at 10 years of age. At the key ages italicized, both medical and psychological screening were also conducted. At 10 years of age, information on each child concerning learning, behavioral, and physical problems and the results of an intelligence test were collected from the school.

***Reiko Ueda*** • Department of Maternal and Child Health, School of Health Sciences, University of Tokyo, Tokyo, Japan.

### Loss of Subjects

Unfortunately, loss of subjects was considerable. From the original 397 subjects, 279 (70.3%) were examined at 4 months. The number of the subjects who could be followed steadily decreased, until at 10 years of age, only 147 remained for examination. By that time, 2 subjects had died and 195 had moved from the area.

## RESULTS

At 4 months of age, the DQs of the children were measured with the Mother–Child Counseling Test, which was restandarized from the Cattell Developmental Test for Japanese children (Cattell, 1940). Developmental quotients (DQs) under 89 were found in 66 (55.0%) of Group 1, 44 (49.4%) of Group 2, and 25 (32.5%) of Group 3. There were statistically significant differences between Groups 3 and 2 ($p < .05$), and Groups 3 and 1 ($p < .01$). There was no statistical difference among the three groups at 1, 3, and 10 years of age.

Medical and developmental risk cases were identified by the questionnaires at 3 months, 1 year, and 3 years. Prevalence of risk cases was higher in Groups 1 and 2 than in Group 3 at each key age. However, there was no difference between the three groups at 10 years of age.

Cases more than 20% overweight were less prevalent in Group 1 than in Groups 2 and 3 at 3 months (cases more than 20% underweight were seen in higher percentages in Group 1 until 1 year of age) and at 3 and 10 years.

Table 1 shows changes in intelligence scores from 4 months to 10 years of age. Agreement between categories of DQs (problematic vs. normal) at 4 months and Intelligence Standard Scores (ISS) at 10 years

**Table 1.** Changes in Intelligence Scores: Relationships between 10 Years and 4 Months, 1 Year, and 3 Years

| ISS at 10 years | Above 45 | Under 44 | Total |
|---|---|---|---|
| DQ at 4 months | ($N$=60) | ($N$=19) | ($N$=79) |
| Above 90 | 46.7% | 31.6% | 43% |
| Under 89 | 53.3% | 68.4% | 57% |
| DQ at 1 year | ($N$=54) | $N$=17) | ($N$=71) |
| Above 90 | 75.9% | 76.5% | 76.1% |
| Under 89 | 24.1% | 23.5% | 23.9% |
| IQ at 3 years | ($N$=54) | ($N$=21) | ($N$=75) |
| Above 92 | 83.3% | 45% | 77.3% |
| Under 91 | 16.7% | 38.1% | 22.7% |

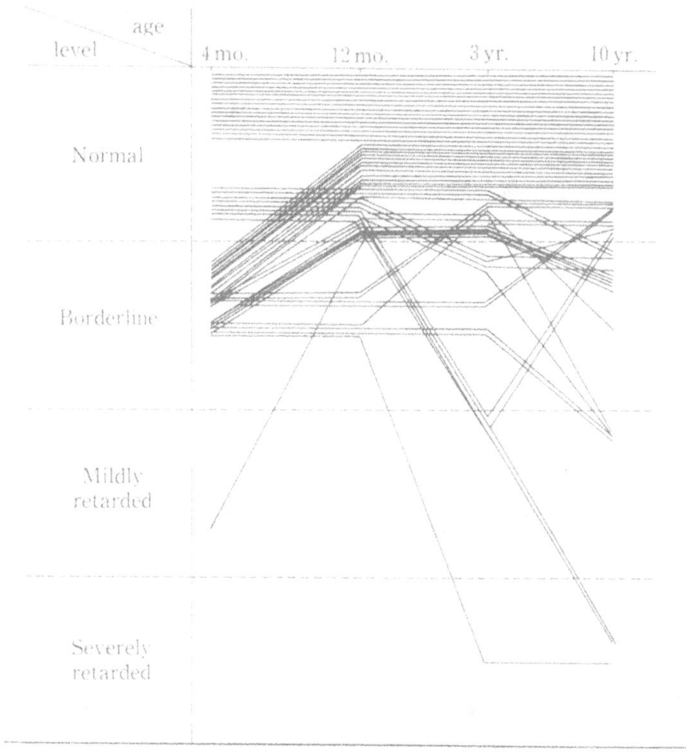


**Figure 1.** Long-term follow-up of intelligence from 4 months to 10 years.

was only 51.9%. However, the rate of agreement with 10-year outcome scores increased steadily with advancing age. Agreement between DQ at 1 year and ISS at 10 years was 63.4%, and between IQ at 3 years and ISS at 10 years was 70.7%.

Different courses of intelligence scores were revealed in the 58 cohort children who have complete records of medical and psychological tests at 4, 12, and 36 months, and at 10 years (Figure 1). Thirty-three percent of subjects were normal through these years, but 31% changed from borderline or mildly retarded to normal, whereas 10% changed from normal to borderline or severely retarded.

The strongest correlation with 10-year ISS and predictor variables of 58 special cohort children was with IQ at 3 years (.54). Interestingly, the only concurrent variable ( high-risk scores on questionnaires at 10 years) was correlated at a lesser strength, with neonatal problems almost set at the same level (−.38 and −.36, respectively). The correlation with problems during pregnancy and delivery was considerably lower.

Table 2 presents a stepwise linear multiple-regression analysis on

**Table 2.** Multiple Regression Analysis between Factors and Intelligence Standard Score at 10 Years of Age ($N = 49$)*

| Physical health variables–social factors | Multiple $R^2$ | Simple $R$ |
|---|---|---|
| IQ at 3 years | .22 | .4743 |
| Neonatal problem | .30 | −.4121 |
| Fathers' occupation | .38 | .1976 |
| Mother's work at 3 years | .45 | −.2540 |
| Illness and physical problem at 4 months | .52 | −.2955 |
| DQ at 1 year | .55 | .0346 |

*Nine cases were excluded because they were untestable at 4 months or 1 year of age although they came for a health checkup.

ISS at 10 years. As shown, the combination of physical health variables in early childhood and the socioeconomic status of the subjects yielded correlations of .55 with subsequent intellectual development.

## DISCUSSION

Continuity, and the predictability of child development have been discussed theoretically by many professionals (Emde & Harmon, 1984; McCall, 1981; Rutter, 1978; Thomas, 1981). However, there are very few long-term prospective studies from infancy to middle childhood on a community level. A few long-term follow-up studies are based on samples from specific socioeconomic status or institutions because of the ease of getting the subjects' cooperation to the study (Hanako, Nakajima, Umemoto, Okaya, Minakawa, & Miyake, 1981; Lubchenco, Delivoria-Papadopoulos, & Searls, 1972). The samples of the present study were drawn from a public health center where health check-ups of all the children in the district are carried out as a part of routine health services. The long-term prospective study was conducted from 3 months of age to 10 years.

Almost the same percentages of borderline and retarded 3-month-old infants were found in two separate groups: a group with medical problems diagnosed by a pediatrician and a group whose mothers had reported developmental and physical problems on a developmental questionnaire. At 4 months, there was a statistically significant difference between each of these groups and a control of infants without known medical or developmental problems. These results would suggest that both physicians' examinations and psychological examinations, together with questionnaires for the parents, are important as the primary step of developmental screening.

Only 33% of the 58 special cohort subjects were normal throughout (from 4 months to 10 years), and many cases changed either upward or downward (Figure 1). Seventy-seven percent of subjects changed from borderline or mildly retarded to normal within the first year. The DQ or IQ of 66.7% of subjects who changed from normal to borderline or retarded at 10 years decreased within the first 3 years. These results suggest that development during the first 3 years of life is both plastic and dynamic, as Kagan (1979) has stated.

The analysis of the agreement between DQ at infancy, IQ in preschool years, and ISS at 10 years showed that the closer to 10 years, the higher the agreement ratio. The result may mean that new functions unrelated to past events emerge as qualitative changes during infancy and influence the development of the infant. It also means that the present is as important as the past for child development. The predictive value of the DQ at 0 to 2 years for later childhood is not high, but the DQ score is useful as far at it represents the present development status. Therefore, periodic development screenings appear necessary.

Because there is little evidence for the view that DQs at 0 and 2 years provide a clear prediction of middle childhood, factors that may correlate with the outcome of intelligence development and variables in early childhood that would have predictive value in middle childhood were sought. From the analysis of 58 special cohort children, association was found between the ISS at 10 years and the physical health variable (neonatal problems and physical problems at 4 months) as well as the social variables (length of fathers' education and types of mothers' work).

A multiple regression analysis of the predictive factors seemed to address immediate as well as long-term effects on child development. In addition to socioeconomic variables, physical health variables such as neonatal problems, illness and phsyical problems at 4 months, were predictive of developmental outcome at 10 years.

## REFERENCES

Cattell, P. (1940). The measurement of intelligence of infants and young children. New York: The Psychological Corporation.

Emde, R. N., & Harmon, R. J. (Eds.). (1984). Continuities and discontinuities in development. New York: Plenum.

Hanako, F., Nakajima, M., Umemoto, Y., Okaya, E., Minakawa, T., & Miyake, K. (1981). Longitudinal study of child development. *Japanese Journal of Child Health, 40*(4), 361–373.

Kagan, K. (1979). The form of early development. *Archives of General Psychiatry, 36,* 1047–1054.

Lubchenco, L. O., Delivoria-Papadopoulos, M., & Searls, D. (1972). Long-term follow-up studies of prematurely born infants: II. Influence of birth weight and gestational age on sequelae. *Journal of Pediatrics, 80*(3), 509–512.

McCall, R. B. (1981). Nature–nurture and the two realms of development: A proposed integration with respect to mental development. *Child Development, 52*(1), 1–12.

Rutter, M. (1978). Early sources of seculity and competence. In J. S. Bruner & A. Garton (Eds.), *Human growth and development*. Oxford: Claredon Press, pp. 53–61.

Thomas, A. (1981). Current trends in developmental theory. *American Journal of Orthopsychiatry, 51*(4), 580–609.

CHAPTER 26

# Application of the Short DDST-R in Urban Districts of Shanghai

## A PRELIMINARY REPORT

*Sung Chieh, Yueh-mei Chu, Shih-ying Lu, Tsui-hung Tang, and Tze-tsai Wang*

The current study was undertaken to find an expedient and efficient method of determining the behavioral development of children in clinical practice and health programs in the Shanghai region. The authors sought a screening method that took less time than the original Denver Developmental Screening Test (DDST), and therefore focused research on the short (prescreening) version of the test. In this short version, only the 3 items immediately to the left of, but not touching, the age line are administered, which results in administration of only 12 items (3 from each of the four sectors) instead of the more usual 25 items. If the child fails even 1 of the items on the short version, the remaining items are administered while the child is still in the setting.

This study deals with the practicability of applying the short version of the DDST in screening the behavioral development of Chinese children, and the extent of agreement between full and short DDST results (Frankenburg, Dodds, Fandal, Kazuk, & Cohrs, 1975; Frankenburg, Fandal, Sciarillo, & Burgess, 1981; Song Jie, 1982). For this study, two different test forms were utilized: The Chinese revised DDST (DDST-R) form was used for administration of the short version of the test, and the original DDST form was used for administration of the full version of the test. On the DDST-R form, items are arranged in stepwise

*Sung Chieh, Yueh-mei Chu, Shih-ying Lu, Tsui-hung Tang, and Tze-tsai Wang* • Section on Intelligence Tests, Research Laboratory of Medical Genetics, Shanghai No. 6 People's Hospital, Shanghai, People's Republic of China.

fashion, like a growth chart. The items themselves and administration of the items are the same on the DDST and DDST-R forms; therefore, the current study could have been carried out on either form without affecting the validity of the results.

## SUBJECTS AND METHODS

A total of 1,911 children under 6 years of age were recruited from the municipal and private nurseries and kindergartens in the urban districts of Shanghai. They were divided into six age groups of 1 to 6 months, 7 to 12 months, 13 to 18 months, 19 to 24 months, 25 to 48 months, and 49 to 72 months. This division was based on Frankenburg *et al.* (1981). All the children received screening with the Chinese restandardized full DDST and the short version of the DDST-R; the items tested as well as the method of scoring were all taken from the reference manual of the DDST (Frankenburg, Dodds, Fandal, Kazuk, & Cohrs, 1975; Song Jie, 1982).

## RESULTS

The reliability of the test was determined by having two examiners, one performing the tests and the other observing, both scoring the tests independently. When the Denver scoring criteria was applied to the Chinese form of the DDST, the results revealed 100% agreement between the two forms in identifying children falling in the abnormal category. However, there was some disagreement for children placed in the questionable category. With the DDST-R, 397 cases (21%) were questionable, whereas 205 cases (11%) were questionable on the basis of the full DDST. Hence, 10% of the positive short DDST-R cases were false positives (Table 1). The paired independent scorings by the examiner and observer were compared in 164 cases (normal = 93% agreement, questionable = 94% agreement, abnormal = 91% agreement).

## DISCUSSION

Although a complete DDST had to be carried out in the 21% positive cases, the remaining 79% could be recognized conclusively as negative after brief (5–6 minutes) testing with a few selected items on the short DDST-R. In clinical use, then, much time could be saved by use of the short version of the test, and the short DDST-R is therefore con-

**Table 1.** Results of Full DDST and Short DDST-R in 6 Groups of Children

| | 1–6 Months | | 7–12 Months | | 13–18 Months | | 19–24 Months | | 25–48 Months | | 49–72 Months | | Total | |
|---|---|---|---|---|---|---|---|---|---|---|---|---|---|---|
| DDST score | Short DDST-R | Full DDST | Short DDST-R | Full DDST | Short DDST-R | Full DDST | Short DDST-R | Full DDST | Short DDST-R | Full DDST | Short DDST-R | Full DDST | Short DDST-R | Full DDST |
| Normal | 249 | 270 | 203 | 228 | 137 | 148 | 72 | 83 | 289 | 355 | 168 | 226 | 1,118 | 1,310 |
| Questionable | 48 | 27 | 66 | 41 | 36 | 25 | 17 | 6 | 124 | 58 | 106 | 48 | 397 | 205 |
| Abnormal | 14 | 14 | 31 | 31 | 43 | 43 | 28 | 28 | 106 | 106 | 174 | 174 | 396 | 396 |
| Total | 311 | 311 | 300 | 300 | 216 | 216 | 117 | 117 | 519 | 519 | 448 | 448 | 1,911 | 1,911 |

sidered valuable for clinical practice and large-scale screening. This manner of testing and scoring is therefore applicable to Chinese DDST norms. In China, it will permit assessment of the developmental status of children within a few minutes and will depict diagramatically the rate of their development over time. Hence, it can be generally used to evaluate relevant medicosocial data in clinical and health work.

## REFERENCES

Frankenburg, W. K., Dodds, J. B., Fandal, A. W., Kazuk, E., & Cohrs, M. (1975). *Denver Developmental Screening Test (DDST): Reference Manual, Revised.* Denver, Colorado: University of Colorado Medical Center.

Frankenburg, W. K., Fandal, A. W., Sciarillo, W., & Burgess, D. (1981). The newly abbreviated and revised Denver Developmental Screening Test (DDST-R). *Journal of Pediatrics, 99*(6), 995–999.

Song Jie. (1982). Restandardization of Denver Developmental Screening Test (DDST) for Shanghai children. *Chinese Medical Journal (English Edition), 95*(5), 375–380.

CHAPTER 27

# Development of 129 Chinese Children with Low Apgar Scores

*Xiang-yun Liu, Xi-ying Zhu, Mu-shi Zheng, Zhi-ping Kuo, and Ling-ying Feng*

Neonatal asphyxia is a common and serious complication at birth, often leading to neonatal death or later developmental defects. The development of 129 survivors of birth asphyxia (Apgar scores of 7 or less at 1 minute after birth) was assessed in this study by the American-normed Denver Developmental Screening Test (DDST).

## SUBJECTS AND METHODS

There were a total of 2,763 live births from two neighborhood regions delivered at Zhong-Shan Hospital between January of 1976 and July of 1980. Of these babies, 170 (6.15%) had birth asphyxia. Of the 170 infants, 6 died in the neonatal period, 35 could not be traced by 1980, and data were available only for 129 children. The distribution of their Apgar scores is listed in Table 1.

The 129 children included 83 boys and 46 girls. Eleven were born prematurely (9 with a birth weight less than 2,500 g), and 9 were born postmaturely. Seventy-five suffered from fetal distress, 26 from winding of the umbilical cord around the neck, and 4 from prolapsed cord at delivery. The major complications encountered during pregnancy of the mothers were as follows: 24 had toxemia of pregnancy, 4 had hypertension, 1 had severe heart disease, 11 had placental abnormalities, and 17 had prolonged labor. Fifty-nine of the babies were delivered sponta-

***Xiang-yun Liu, Xi-ying Zhu, Mu-shi Zheng, Zhi-ping Kuo, and Ling-ying Feng*** • Children's Hospital of Shanghai, First Medical College, Shanghai, People's Republic of China.

**Table 1.** Apgar Scores of 129 Children with Birth Asphyxia

| Time after birth (min.) | Total cases | Apgar scores 0–3 | 4–7 | 8–10 | No record |
|---|---|---|---|---|---|
| 1 | 129 | 52 | 77 | 0 | 0 |
| 5 | 129 | 1 | 6 | 111 | 11* |

*11 infants had no record at 5 minutes; however, 6 of the 11 attained scores of 8 to 10 at 7 minutes.

neously, 17 by cesarean section, 24 by applying forceps, 16 by aspiration, and 13 with breech presentation.

At a follow-up clinic, measurement of height, weight, and head circumferences and a complete physical examination were performed for each child. A developmental history including genetic background was obtained from the mother at the same clinic visit, and a DDST was administered. The children's age at the time of examination varied from 1 year to 5 years and 11 months.

Another 137 nonasphyxiated children with normal birth weight were selected at random from nurseries, kindergartens, and well-baby clinics as a control group. The distributions of age of the two groups were similar.

## RESULTS

Administration of the DDST revealed results as shown in Table 2. The difference of outcome between two groups was highly significant ($p < .01$).

There were 7 abnormal children within the birth asphyxia group, and they received further neurological and ophthalmologic examinations. Among these 7 children, there were 2 with cerebral palsy, 2 with epilepsy, and 3 with visual defects. Electroencephalograms showed epileptic waves in 3 children and slow electrical action in 4 children.

In the asphyxiated group, the development of children whose head

**Table 2.** Comparison of DDST Results between 2 Groups

| Group | Total cases | Results of DDST (no. of cases) Normal | Questionable | Abnormal | Questionable/Abnormal |
|---|---|---|---|---|---|
| Asphyxiated | 129 | 112 | 10 (7.8%) | 7 (5.4%) | 17 (13.2%) |
| Control | 137 | 132 | 4 (2.9%) | 1 (.7%) | 5 (3.6%) |

**Table 3.** The Relationship between Head Circumference and Development

| Head circumference | Total cases | Results of DDST (no. of cases) | | | |
|---|---|---|---|---|---|
| | | Normal | Questionable | Abnormal | Questionable/Abnormal |
| ⩾ $p3$* | 116 | 105 | 9 | 2 | 11 (9.5%) |
| < $p3$ | 13 | 7 | 1 | 5 | 6 (46.2%) |
| | 129 | | | | |

*$p3$ equals the 3rd percentile of Shanghai children at the same age

circumferences were below the 3rd percentile of normal were poorer than those above the same percentile (Table 3). The percentage of questionable and abnormal children was 46.2% versus 9.5%.

When influence of duration and severity of asphyxia on development was analyzed (Table 4), no significant difference in DDST scores were noticed between the mild group (1-minute Apgar scores of 4–7) and severe group (1-minute Apgar scores of 0–3). The number of questionable and abnormal children in the group with birth asphyxia persisting for 5 minutes or more was higher than in the group with asphyxia for less than 5 minutes, although the difference did not reach statistical significance.

## DISCUSSION

In our study of 129 children with birth asphyxia, 2 had cerebral palsy, and 1 of these also had epilepsy. The rates of cerebral palsy (1.3%

**Table 4.** The Relation between the Duration and Severity of Asphyxia and Development

| | Total cases | Results of DDST (no. of cases) | | | |
|---|---|---|---|---|---|
| | | Normal | Questionable | Abnormal | Questionable/ Abnormal |
| Severity of asphyxia* | | | | | |
| Mild | 77 | 68 | 6 | 3 | 9 (11.6%) |
| Severe | 52 | 44 | 4 | 4 | 8 (15.4%) |
| | 129 | | | | |
| Duration of asphyxia** | | | | | |
| < 5 minutes | 111 | 98 | 8 (7%) | 5 (5%) | 13 (11.7%) |
| ⩾ 5 minutes | 7 | 4 | 1 (14%) | 2 (29%) | 3 (42.9%) |
| | 118 | | | | |

*Mild case with Apgar scores of 4 to 7, and severe case of 0 to 3.
**11 babies had no record at 5 minutes.

with Apgar scores of 4–6 at 1 minute and 1.9% with Apgar scores of 0–3) were similar to those reported by Nelson (1979).

Most studies (Adamsons & Meyers, 1973; Ucko, 1965; Nelson, 1981) have shown that the risk of mental retardation on children with neonatal asphyxia is much higher than that of normal children. However, the incidence has varied a great deal, probably due to the difference of the samples selected. In our series of 129 asphyxiated children, 7 (5.4%) were mentally retarded, and 10 had developmental delay at least in one field on follow-up examinations.

The result of this investigation suggests that birth asphyxia might affect mental development, and has a close relationship to some later neurological sequelaes. Therefore, optimal obstetrical care, immediate newborn resuscitation, and skillful neonatal management are crucial to prevent birth asphyxia and improve the outcome of survivors.

## REFERENCES

Adamsons, K., & Myers, R. E. (1973). Perinatal asphyxia: Cause, detection, and neurologic sequelae. *Pediatric Clinics North America, 20,* 465.

Nelson, K. B. (1979). Neonatal signs as predictors of cerebral palsy. *Pediatrics, 64,* 225.

Nelson, K. B. (1981). Apgar score as predictors of chronic neurologic disability. *Pediatrics, 68,* 36.

Ucko, L. E. (1965). A comparative study of asphyxiated and nonasphyxiated boys from birth to five years. *Developmental Medicine and Child Neurology, 7,* 643.

CHAPTER 28

# A Survey and Follow-Up of the Development of Chinese Children Born of Mothers with Eclampsia and Preeclampsia

*Yueh-mei Chu, Tsui-hung Tang, Shih-ying Lu, Wei-ying Chen, and Ying-ying Shih*

---

Toxemia of pregnancy is a disease that seriously endangers the health of expectant mothers (Stembera, 1976). When toxemia has proceeded to preeclampsia and eclampsia, the health and lives of both the mothers and their infants are threatened. In order to ascertain the status of children born of these mothers, the development of 158 children was investigated. In addition, another 120 cases of normally delivered children were randomly selected as controls. All of the children were between 18 months and $6\frac{1}{2}$ years of age.

## SUBJECTS AND METHODS

During the 6 years from January of 1973 to December of 1978, 23,837 pregnant women gave birth to a total of 24,014 babies at the International Peace Maternity and Child Health Hospital of Shanghai. Among the 332 infants born of mothers with eclampsia and preeclampsia, 11

---

***Yueh-mei Chu, Tsui-hung Tang, and Shih-ying Lu*** • Section on Intelligence Tests, Research Laboratory of Medical Genetics, Shanghai No. 6 People's Hospital, Shanghai, People's Republic of China. ***Wei-ying Chen and Ying-ying Shih*** • The International Peace Maternity and Child Health Hospital of the China Welfare Institute, Shanghai, People's Republic of China.

were the product of multiple pregnancies, 18 were born to mothers with eclampsia, and 303 were born to mothers with preeclampsia. Among the 18 children born to eclamptic mothers, there were 2 fetal deaths, 1 neonatal death, and 15 infants who survived. Of the 314 infants born to 303 mothers with preeclampsia, there were 2 fetal deaths, 3 stillbirths (2 of them twins), 7 neonatal deaths, and 302 live births.

In April of 1980, a retrospective survey of development was made of 158 children. Seven of these had been born to mothers with eclampsia, and 151 had been born to mothers with preeclampsia (71 with severe preeclampsia and 80 with mild preeclampsia). The recently Chinese-normed Denver Developmental Screening Test (DDST) was administered to all the 158 children, and the results were interpreted as described in the DDST Manual (Frankenburg, Dodds, Fandal, Kazuk, & Cohrs, 1975). In addition, the Chinese adaptation of the Gesell Developmental Dianostic Survey (Gesell & Amatrude, 1947) was also given to those children under 3 years of age. Moreover, 120 uncomplicated, normally delivered children were randomly selected from nurseries and kindergartens as controls; the same methods were used to assess their development.

In April of 1983, another retrospective developmental survey was made with 72 children who were randomly sampled from the 158 children surveyed in 1980. The same test methods (DDST for all, and the Gesell for those under 3 years) were used for these 72 children. In addition, for children older than $6\frac{1}{2}$ years in this follow-up study, school test scores and scores from the Draw-A-Man test were also utilized.

## RESULTS OF THE 1980 SURVEY

Of the 158 children examined with the DDST, 73.42% were classified as normal in development, 22.15% were questionable, and only 4.43% were rated as abnormal. In the control group of 120 children, 89.26% were normal in development, only 10.74% were questionable, and none were abnormal. There was marked significant statistical difference ($p < .01$) between the two groups (Table 1).

When 7 children born of eclamptic mothers, 71 children born of severe preeclampsia mothers, and 80 children born of mild preeclampsia mothers were compared, no significant statistical differences could be found ($p > .05$).

However, a significant difference in development ($p < .01$) was found when the control group was compared with 110 children aged 3 to 7 years, born of mothers with complications. Among the latter, there were 66.36% normal children, 27.28% who were questionable, and 6.36%

**Table 1.** Capacity of Children Born 1973 to 1978 (Using the DDST)

| Classification | Status of children | | | |
|---|---|---|---|---|
| | Normal | Questionables | Abnormals | Total |
| Children born of eclamptic, pre-eclamptic pregnancies | 116 (73.42%) | 35 (22.15%) | 7 (4.43%) | 158 |
| Children born of normal pregnancies | 107 (89.26%) | 13 (10.74%) | 0 (0%) | 120 |

abnormal. In comparison, of the 75 children in the control group, 84% were classified as having normal development, 16% as questionable, and none abnormal (Table 2.)

When an additional DDST survey was conducted with 48 children under 3 years of age born of mothers with complications, no marked difference ($p > .05$) in development could be found between these children and children in the control group.

Similarly, no marked statistical differences ($p > .05$) was found as a result of investigating two groups of children under 3 years of age with the Gesell's Developmental Schedules. Table 3 summarizes the findings of this portion of the study.

## RESULTS OF THE 1983 RESURVEY

As was previously described, a resurvey was undertaken in 1983. It involved 72 children randomly sampled from the children born of preeclamptic and eclamptic mothers who were surveyed in 1980. Results are shown in Table 4; there was no statistical difference ($p > .05$) between the 1980 and 1983 results.

**Table 2.** Status of Children 3 to 7 Years of Age (Using the DDST)

| Classification | Status of children | | | |
|---|---|---|---|---|
| | Normal | Questionables | Abnormals | Total |
| Children born of eclamptic, pre-eclamptic pregnancies | 73 (66.36%) | 30 (27.28%) | 7 (6.36%) | 110 |
| Children born of normal pregnancies | 63 (84.0%) | 12 (16.0%) | 0 (0%) | 75 |

**Table 3.** Capacity of Children under 3 Years of Age (Using Gesell's Test)

| | Status of children | | | |
|---|---|---|---|---|
| Classification | DQ 86 | DQ 76–85 | DQ 75 | Total |
| Children born of eclamptic, pre-eclamptic pregnancies | 32 (67%) | 13 (27%) | 3 (6%) | 48 |
| Children born of normal pregnancies | 35 (78%) | 10 (22%) | 0 (0%) | 45 |

## DISCUSSION

Because it has been documented that eclampsia and pre-eclampsia may cause severe damage to both mothers and children, 158 children born with such complications were clinically evaluated with the DDST and Gesell's Developmental Schedules. They were compared with 120 randomly selected, full-term children of the same age who had had normal deliveries. Very significant differences were found between these two groups; however, comparison of the development of children whose mothers had had eclampsia, severe preeclampsia, and mild preeclampsia did not show any significant difference.

Second, the development of two groups of children, aged 3 to 7 years, was assessed. One group was comprised of 110 children born of mothers with complications, and another group consisted of 75 children born of mothers without complications. Here there also were found to exist significant differences.

Third, the development of two groups of children younger than 3 years was assessed with two methods, the DDST and the Gesell. This portion of the study showed that among children under 3 years of age, whether or not they were born of mothers with complications and

**Table 4.** Follow-up Survey of Development in 72 Children from Eclamptic and Preeclamptic Mothers

| | Results of 1980 survey | Results of 1983 survey |
|---|---|---|
| Normal | 49 (68%) | 54 (75%) |
| Questionable | 19 (26%) | 9 (12.5%) |
| Abnormal | 4 (6) | 9 (12.5%) |
| Total | 72 | 72 |

whether the DDST or Gesell's Developmental Schedules were used as the developmental assessment, the results were comparable and without any significant difference.

In the 110 high-risk children over 3 years of age, 37 children were found to be questionable or abnormal on the DDST. In the 48 high-risk children under 3 years of age, only 5 were questionable. Presumably this improvement came about because in recent years our hospital has enhanced the perinatal care of high-risk pregnancies, including those with eclampsia and preeclampsia. In addition to use of blood and urine for pretesting placental function, since 1977 the hospital has been utilizing electronic monitoring during high-risk deliveries. For high-risk infants born of high-risk mothers, intensive nursing care and proper medical treatment are also given. Littman (1978) has found little relationship between obstetric and neonatal events and developmental outcome. However, significant correlations were seen between medical events occurring in later infancy and mental development at 2 years of age. Although no severe medical complications were found in the high-risk children of the current study, some authors (Livingston, 1977) have suggested that such children should be followed up to school age, which in China is generally 6 years.

The resurvey of 1983 found several things. First, there were very apparent differences in mental development between children born of preeclamptic and eclamptic mothers and of normal partum. Second, a comparison of the development of the children born of mothers with these complications made 3 years apart did not demonstrate any statistical difference. We therefore have concluded that the DDST can be used in our setting as a valid developmental evaluation for children between 3 and $6\frac{1}{2}$ years of age.

## CONCLUSIONS

Surveys of mental development (using the DDST) of 158 children born of mothers with eclampsia and preeclampsia and of 120 children born of mothers without eclampsia showed a difference of great statistical significance. In addition, a follow-up survey of 72 randomly selected children from the eclampsia series 3 years later (using the DDST or the Draw-A-Man test) corresponded well with the primary survey. These data together suggests that the DDST can be utilized not only for the correct evaluation of development of children at a particular age, but to predict later development as well.

## REFERENCES

Frankenburg, W. K., Dodds, J. B., Fandal, A. W., Kazuk, E., & Cohrs, M (1975). *Denver Developmental Screening Test Reference Manual.* Denver, CO: University of Colorado Medical Center.

Gesell, A., & Amatrude, C. (1947). Developmental diagnosis. Boston: Hoeber.

Littman, B. (1978). Medical correlates of infant development. *Pediatrics, 61*(3), 470–474.

Livingston, C. (1977). *The development of the infant and young child* (7th ed.). Edinburgh: Churchill Livingstone, pp. 28–61.

Stembera, E. (1976). High-risk pregnancy and the child. The Hague: Martinus Nijhoff/ Medical Division, pp. 180–183

CHAPTER 29

# Examination of the Development of 63 Full-Term, Small-for-Date Chinese Children

*Xiang-yun Liu, Xi-ying Zhu, Mu-shi Zheng, Zhi-ping Kuo, and Ling-ying Feng*

This study was undertaken to offer some information on the development of small-for-date (SFD) children with intrauterine growth retardation.

## SUBJECTS AND METHODS

The 63 full-term SFD children selected for the study (14 male and 49 female) were born between November of 1974 and December of 1979. All were delivered between 37 and 43 weeks of gestation, with 54.2% being delivered at 39 to 40 weeks. (Gestational age was calculated from the first date of the last menstrual period reported by the mothers of the SFD infants to the maternity hospital.) The birth weights of the SFD children varied from 1,520 to 2,700 g; all were in the 10th percentile or less according to the Shanghai Intrauterine Growth Chart (Qian, 1980). At 1 minute after birth, the majority of the children (76.2%) had Apgar scores of 8 to 10, 15.9% had scores of 4 to 7, and 7.9% had scores of 0 to 3. Following resuscitation, all of the children's Apgar scores improved within several minutes. The range of ages of follow-up examination was from 10 months to 5 years and 10 months.

The average maternal age at the time of delivery was 28.6 years,

***Xiang-yun Liu, Xi-ying Zhu, Mu-shi Zheng, Zhi-ping Kuo, and Ling-ying Feng*** • Children's Hospital of Shanghai, First Medical College, Shanghai, People's Republic of China.

**Table 1.** Age Distribution of the 2 Groups

| | | Age (Years) | | | | | |
|---|---|---|---|---|---|---|---|
| Groups | Total | 0 | 1 | 2 | 3 | 4 | 5–6 |
| SFD | 63 | 5 | 35 | 18 | 1 | 3 | 1 |
| Control | 58 | 2 | 32 | 18 | 1 | 3 | 1 |

with a range of 24 to 38 years. This was the first pregnancy for 44 of the mothers,and the second or more pregnancy for 19 of the mothers. The modes of delivery were spontaneous vaginal 71.4%, vaginal with forceps 1.6%, and caesarean section 27%. Of 26 mothers who had complications of pregnancy, 18 had toxemia and 3 of these came to have preeclampsia. Other maternal complications included secondary anemia and 1st and 3rd trimester bleeding. Of the maternal chronic diseases, hypertension was comparatively common (7 cases), and there were 3 cases of congenital malformation (2 cases of malformation of the womb, and 1 case of congenital heart diseases with atrial septal defect). In addition, there were 3 cases of hyperthyroidism and 2 cases of nephritis. The majority of the mothers had received middle school education (2 had 6 years of schooling, 52 had 9 years, 7 had 12 years, 1 had 15 years, and 1 had 16 years).

Growth was evaluated by measuring the children's height, weight, and head circumference. Each child's development was evaluated by the newly established Chinese norms for the Denver Developmental Screening Test (DDST). The Denver criteria for normal, questionable, and abnormal were then applied to the children evaluated against the Chinese-normed DDST.

A control group of 58 children, 28 male and 30 female with normal birth weight (ranging from 2,800–3,900 g), was selected at random from nurseries, kindergartens, and well-baby clinics. For age distribution of the SFD children and those in the control group, see Table 1.

The chi-square test was used in the statistical analyses.

## RESULTS

Development as measured with the Chinese DDST was found to be as follows. When the development of 63 full-term SFD children was compared (through use of a chi-square) with those in the control group, 85.7% were scored as normal, 12.7% questionable, and 1.6% as abnormal. In contrast, of the 58 children in the control group, 96.6% were scored as normal, 3.4% as questionable, and none as abnormal (see Ta-

**Table 2.** Comparison of DDST Scores between the 2 Groups

| | | Result of developmental screening | | | |
|---|---|---|---|---|---|
| Weight | Total *N* | Normal | Questionable | Abnormal | Questionable/ Abnormal |
| SFD | 63 | 54 | 8 | 1 | 9 (14.3%) |
| Control | 58 | 56 | 2 | 0 | 2 (3.4%) |

ble 2). The percentage of the questionable and abnormal children in the SFD group (14.3%) was higher than that in the control group (3.4%), with the difference being marginally significant ($p = .074$).

To study the influence of birth weight on development, the SFD children were divided into two groups according to the degree of their deficient birth weight (i.e., low birth weight and very low birth weight). The development of the SFD children whose birth weight was severely low (below the 10th percentile for the month of gestation minus 500 g), showed definite retardation in comparison with those in the control group. The difference, $p < .01$, was of high significance.

The relation of developmental status to gravida in the SFD group was also examined. In the SFD group, the development of children of multiple gravida was poorer than those of prima gravida. The difference was significant with $p < .05$. The same applies to the influence of maternal ages. In the SFD group, the development of children whose mothers were 31 years of age or older was more delayed than those whose mothers were 30 years of age or younger.

The relation of physical growth to development was studied by dividing the SFD children into two groups according to current weight (above or below the 3rd percentile of the Shanghai Growth Standards for their peers). For the results of their developmental screening, see Table 3. The development of children with weights below the 3rd per-

**Table 3.** The Relation of Present Weight to Development

| | | Result of developmental screening | | | |
|---|---|---|---|---|---|
| Weight | Total *N* | Normal | Questionable | Abnormal | Questionable/ Abnormal |
| $\geq P_3$* | 50 | 47 | 3 | 0 | 0 (6.0%) |
| $< P_3$ | 13 | 7 | 5 | 1 | 6 (46.2%) |

*Note. p* .01.
*$P_3$ = The 3rd percentile of the Shanghai Growth Standards for their peers.

centile was much more retarded than the development of children who weighed above the 3rd percentile.

## DISCUSSION

Researchers have not agreed on the prognosis for development of SFD versus normal birth weight children. Most studies have shown that SFD children have slower developmental rates in the areas of early development, intelligence, and the ability to study at school (Fitzhardinge & Steven, 1972; Low, 1978). However, other studies have compared IQs of SFD to normal birth weight children and have not found any great difference; in fact, these studies have found that the development of the SFD children as well as their level of maturity was close to normal (Babson & Kangas, 1969; Neligan, 1967).

In this study, the numbers of questionable and abnormal children in the SFD group were found to be comparatively high but the probability ($p = < .074$) was in the marginal range. Perhaps because the majority of the SFD children were under 3 years of age in this study, the differences in development had not been completely distinct and the slight injuries to the nervous system suffered during early childhood not yet easily noticed.

This current study reminds us of the importance of perinatal care. In order to ensure not only normal fetal growth but also healthy development after birth, child health care providers must cooperate with obstetricians, and perinatal care must be reinforced to secure the robust growth of children.

## REFERENCES

Babson, S. G., & Kangas, J. (1969). Preschool intelligence of under-sized term infants. *American Journal of Diseases of Children, 117,* 553.

Fitzhardinge, P. M., & Steven, E. M. (1972). The small-for-date infant: Neurological and intellectual sequelae. *Pediatrics, 50,* 50.

Low, J. A. (1978). Intrauterine growth retardation: A preliminary report of long-term morbidity. *American Journal of Obstetrics and Gynecology, 130,* 534.

Neligan, G. A. (1967). The clinical effects of being "light for dates." *Proceedings of the Royal Society of Medicine, 60,* 881.

Qian, Shuei-gun. (1980). The distribution of newborns' weights in Shanghai (28–44 gestation weeks). *Chinese Journal of Obstetrics and Gynecology, 15,* 198.

CHAPTER 30

# Predictive Value of a Combined Health Score at Four Years with Respect to Behavioral and Learning Problems at Age Ten

*Jean-Claude Vuille, Claes Sundelin, and Tore Mellbin*

---

A program of comprehensive health screening of 4-year-olds was introduced in Sweden in 1968, and rapidly expanded until 95% of all 4-year-olds in the country are screened today (Socialstyrelsen, 1968, 1979). The steps in the screening program are presented in Table 1 (Sundelin & Vuille, 1975b).

The effectiveness of such a screening program has been evaluated by several teams (Köhler, 1973; Lagerkvist, Lauritzen, & Olin, 1975; Sundelin & Vuille, 1975a). In Uppsala, the authors reexamined three cohorts containing a total of 3,607 children when they reached 10 years of age, including a control group which had not been screened at 4 years. The main finding from that 1982 study was that, with the exception of overweight, the program had not helped to reduce the prevalence of developmental problems (Mellbin, Sundelin, & Vuille, 1982; Sundelin, Mellbin, & Vuille, 1982).

However, during that study we observed a number of significant, unspecific correlations between physiologically unrelated health problems. This suggested the hypothesis that an aggregate measure of ill health (taking into account physical and mental deviations as well as

---

*Jean-Claude Vuille* • School Health Service, Bern, Switzerland. *Claes Sundelin* • Department of Pediatrics, University Hospital, Uppsala, Sweden. *Tore Mellbin* • School Health Service, Uppsala, Sweden.

**Table 1.** Steps in Sweden's Screening Program for 4-Year-Olds

| Source of information/ examination | Performed by | Comment |
|---|---|---|
| Questionnaire | Parents | Replacing conventional pediatric history. Contains a few very simple questions about child's mental and emotional development. |
| Interview concerning child's behavior and development | Nurse | |
| Assessment of mental development | Nurse/ Physician | Draw a man, count 3 objects, participation at examination, observed behavior. |
| Test of speech development | Nurse/ Physician Auxiliary | 1969–1970. Simple observation (conversation). Since 1971, specific test: pronunciation of 10 key words (pictures). |
| Hearing test | Auxiliary | Audiogram at 250, 500, 1000, 2000, 4000, and 8000 c/s. Pass level = 25 dB. |
| Vision test | Nurse/ Auxiliary | Single symbol. Snellen's E or Bostrom's hook. Each eye tested separately. |
| Test for bacteriuria | Auxiliary | Uriglox |
| Height and weight | Auxiliary | |
| Physical examination | Physician | Special emphasis on motor coordination: 11 items in 1969–1970. Three items since 1971. |
| Dental examination | Dentist | Orthodontic abnormalities. Caries. Oral hygiene and gingival disease. |

social problems) might provide a more effective way of defining children at risk for later learning and behavior problems. To test this hypothesis, the authors studied results of all the children who had been screened at 4 years of age and who still resided in Uppsala when they were 10.

To obtain information about the 10-year-olds' health status and their learning and behavioral characteristics, the authors reviewed school health charts and held standardized interviews with school nurses and teachers.

For this analysis, two measures of outcome were used:

**Table 2.** Discriminant Analysis of Subgroup Membership*

| Step | Variable entered | Wilks' Lambda** | Significance |
|---|---|---|---|
| 1 | Developmental screening | 0.9336 | 0.0000 |
| 2 | Unmarried mother | 0.9164 | 0.0000 |
| 3 | Speech screening | 0.9046 | 0.0000 |
| 4 | Social class (lowest) | 0.8937 | 0.0000 |
| 5 | Diagnosis of mental retardation | 0.8852 | 0.0000 |
| 6 | Diagnosis of motor retardation | 0.8775 | 0.0000 |
| 7 | Fine motor screening | 0.8707 | 0.0000 |
| 8 | Diagnosis of speech retardation | 0.8659 | 0.0000 |
| 9 | Diagnosis of physical disease | 0.8613 | 0.0000 |
| 10 | Diagnosis of visual problem | 0.8575 | 0.0000 |
| 11 | Diagnosis of neurological problem | 0.8539 | 0.0000 |
| 12 | Hyperactivity during examination | 0.8510 | 0.0000 |
| 13 | Physician's general impression | 0.8487 | 0.0000 |

*A further 13 variables entered the equations as significant predictors of subgroup membership, but their contribution to the discriminant power of the equations was negligible; see Footnote 1.
**All values are significant at less than $10^{-4}$.

1. A behavior score derived from the teacher interview (the sum of six items, with a possible score of 0, 1, or 2);
2. Subgroups categorized as to whether they had one or more severe behavioral, social, or learning problems.

## RESULTS

As a result of subgroup categorization, 82.3% of boys ($N$ = 1,828) and 91% of girls ($N$ = 1,799) were found to have no serious developmental or social problems. Significant behavior disorders without severe social problems were found in 13.4% of the boys and 6% of the girls. Severe learning difficulties without severe behavior disorders or social problems were found in 2.6% of the boys ansd 2.2% of the girls. Other combined-problem categories ranged from an incidence of .4% to 1%.

### Predictor Variables

Multiple stepwise regression, with the behavior score as the dependent variable, and discriminant analysis with respect to subgroup membership, yielded similar heirarchies (Tables 2 and 3). (For an explanation

**Table 3.** Multiple Stepwise Regression with the Behavior Source as the Dependent Variable*

| Step | Variable entered | $R^2$ |
|---|---|---|
| 1 | Development screening | 0.0652 |
| 2 | Unmarried mother | 0.0787 |
| 3 | Speech screening | 0.0893 |
| 4 | Diagnosis of mental retardation | 0.0992 |
| 5 | Diagnosis of motor retardation | 0.1074 |
| 6 | Fine motor screening | 0.1136 |
| 7 | Social class 3 (lowest) | 0.1190 |
| 8 | Hyperactivity during examination | 0.1234 |
| 9 | Diagnosis of physical disease | 0.1271 |
| 10 | Behavior interview | 0.1301 |

*Results of first 10 steps.

of definitions and subgroup classification used, see Footnote 1.) Results of a simple test of mental development had the strongest statistical relationship with the dependent variables, followed by descriptors of the social situation, results of speech development screening, motor/neurological problems, and physical problems—in that order.

It is interesting to note that the parents' own observations, communicated to the examining team in the form of a questionnaire and an interview in the home, contributed very little to the prediction of future problems. This is in sharp contrast to our original hypothesis, which strongly emphasized the parents' perception of their child's strengths and difficulties.

## Predictive Value of a Combined Score

The question answered next was what is the practical predictive value of a score derived from previously identified variables? Could such a score be used as a basis for the definition of an at-risk group of children at 4 years of age who should be followed more closely over the years? For a scoring procedure to be applicable in practice, it must be

[1]Definitions used in the study were as follows: A behavioral problem was defined to include children who had a score of 4 or more on a teacher rating scale developed in Sweden by the authors. A social problem included such severe family social problems as drug abuse, child abuse, or parental criminal behavior. A severe learning problem included children who required special teaching in school. The subgroups were categorized as follows: (a) no serious behavioral or social problem; (b) significant behavioral disorders without social problems in the family; (c) significant behavioral disorders with social problems in the family; (d) severe learning difficulties without social problems in the family; and (e) severe learning difficulties with social problems in the family.

**Table 4.** Scoring Sheet

| | | Weight |
|---|---|---|
| Development screening | (0–6) | × 3 = |
| Speech screening | (0–2) | × 3 = |
| Unmarried mother | (yes = 1) | × 3 = |
| Social Class 3 | (yes = 1) | × 3 = |
| Diagnosis* of mental retardation | (yes = 1) | × 2 = |
| Diagnosis* of motor retardation | (yes = 1) | × 2 = |
| Diagnosis* of speech retardation | (yes = 1) | × 2 = |
| Fine motor screening | (0–2) | × 2 = |
| Diagnosis* of physical disease | (yes = 1) | × 1 = |
| Diagnosis* of neurological problem | (yes = 1) | × 1 = |
| Diagnosis* of visual problem | (yes = 1) | × 1 = |
| Hyperactivity during examination | (0–2) | × 1 = |
| Physician's general impression | (0–2) | × 1 = |
| Total score | | |

*Diagnosis was used to mean that the problem had been verified by special examination from birth to age 4, or after the 4-year-old screening.

simple and straightforward. Therefore, the results of a computer analysis were simplified as shown in Table 4.

The effectiveness of the resulting score in identifying children with future problems was evaluated by determining its sensitivity and percentage of children falsely identified with respect to severe behavioral, social or learning problems at 10 years of age. The sensitivity of the combined score, as shown on Table 5, is about twice as high as that of any single specific variable. At the same time, however, the predictive value of a positive is important, for more than half the children falsely identified as positives are already in the 10% at-risk group.

**Table 5.** Predictive Value of a Total Health Score at 4 Years of Age

| Size of high-risk group (defined on the basis of the total score) | Sensitivity* | | Predictive value of a positive (%) | |
|---|---|---|---|---|
| | Boys | Girls | Boys | Girls |
| 10% | .26 | .38 | 45 | 34 |
| 20% | .41 | .52 | 37 | 24 |
| 33% | .57 | .69 | 31 | 19 |
| 50% | .72 | .81 | 28 | 15 |

*Fraction of all children with severe developmental problems at 10 years included in the high-risk group.

### Prediction of Different Types of Problems

The various problem subgroups of 10-year-olds can be identified with varying accuracy on the basis of the combined score. As expected, the most seriously disturbed children (those with severe behavior and social problems) could be identified most accurately; about 80% of them were included in a 20% at-risk group. The discrimination is less satisfactory for children with learning or behavior difficulties without serious social problems. Obviously, a more precise prediction of the probable type of problem—beyond the trivial statement "the higher the score, the more probable the future existence of a severe problem"—is not possible. Before trying to interpret these results, two words of caution are warranted.

1. Two of the subgroups (significant behavior disorder with severe social problem and severe social problems without significant behavior disorders) were very small in absolute numbers, so that presentation in the form of percentages is hazardous. It may well be that the bulk of preventive resources should be concentrated on the small but cumbersome multiproblem group.
2. This study's analysis of the possible effectiveness of the combined score is only a preliminary one, as it is based on the same population from which the scoring system was derived. For a true proof of effectiveness new information must be used; however, it will be many years before such new data will be available.

## DISCUSSION

Following our 1982 study (Mellbin *et al.*, 1982; Sundelin *et al.*, 1982), we were pessimistic about the possibility of predicting health problems in school children at 10 years from the general screening of 4-year-olds. Our findings were especially disappointing concerning prediction of behavior problems and signs of social maladjustment. Certainly, it was possible to show that the risk of presenting a health problem at 10 years of age was higher when the same problem existing at 4, but sensitivity and specificity were so limited that many of the screening procedures seemed questionable. It became so obvious to us that periodic health examinations of the whole population are necessary after 4 years, mainly to detect psychosocial problems (most somatic disorders are known by the age of 4).

However, following the current study, we are more optimistic. The results point to the existence of correlations between the state of health at 4 years (measured with a screening examination) and the state of psychosocial health at age 10. Above all, the analyses shown that there is a crossover between the problems of one subgroup at 4 years to a different subgroup at 10. These crossover phenomena should be studied further to yield a better understanding of the dynamics of health patterns during childhood. Although the current study still has far-from-satisfactory predictive ability, the authors believe that prediction can be improved if there is access to data of a higher quality from the preschool period, especially better data relating to the family's social background and to parent–child interactions.

Considering the limited long-term value of Sweden's screening program for 4-year-olds and the limited health resources of every country, perhaps it would be rational to limit routine prescreening to only those children who have serious problems at 4, or who have a multiplicity of problems. Ending routine rescreening of the majority of children would free additional resources for children truly at risk. In Sweden, for example, where 100,000 children are born each year, approximately 10,000 to 15,000 physicians' hours and the same number of hours for nurses could be saved each year by reducing the program by one visit for the low-score children.

A risk-group strategy of this kind would benefit children most at risk and would have other benefits as well. One advantage is that the responsibility for the health of children not at risk would be given back to the parents; during recent years, many persons taking part in the political debates in Sweden have been increasingly concerned about the responsibility-reducing effects of the increasing dominance of experts. Another advantage is that preventive work would be more problem-oriented, which would strengthen the role of health professionals, improve their self-satisfaction, and enhance their status in the community.

A serious disadvantage to this risk-group approach would be the implication of special treatment for certain children. This might be perceived by some parents as discriminating; others might feel that their children were in a less successful subgroup. These latter drawbacks are of great importance in Sweden, where there is strong tradition of emphasis for generality and overall applicability in all support systems (Berfenstam & William-Olsson, 1973).

In summary, the risk-group scoring should primarily be viewed as a source of warning for preventive health workers, and an indication that developmental and family issues should be examined in more depth. The scoring system should be combined with a flexible working method based on traditional clinical assessments.

## REFERENCES

Berfenstam, R., & William-Olsson, I. (1973). *Early child care in Sweden.* London: Gordon & Breach.

Köhler, L. (1973). Health control of 4-year-old children: An epidemiological study of child health. *Acta Paediatrica Scandinavia, 235.*

Lagerkvist, B., Lauritzen, S., & Olin, P. (1975). Four-year-olds in a new suburb: The need for medical and social care. *Acta Paediatrica Scandinavia, 64,* 413–420.

Mellbin, T., Sundelin, C., & Vuille, J.-C. (1982). *Från 4 år till 10. Hälsa och anpassning mellan lekålder och förpubertet (From four years to ten: Health and adjustment from play period to preadolescence).* Liber, Stockholm: Socialstyrelsen redovisar, p. 10.

Socialstyrelsen (Swedish National Board of Health and Welfare). (1968). *Allmän hälsokontroll av 4-åringar.* Stockholm: Socialstyrelsen redovisar, p. 2.

Socialstyrelsen (Swedish National Board of Health and Welfare). (1979). *Modra-och barnhälsovård. Forslag till principprogram (Organization of Mother and Child Health Care).* Stockholm: Socialstyrelsen redovisor, p. 4.

Sundelin, C., Mellbin, T., & Vuille, J.-C. (1982). From 4 to 10: An overall evaluation of the general health screening of 4-year-olds. In N. J. Anastasiow, W. K. Frankenburg, & A. W. Fandal (Eds.), *Identifying the developmentally delayed child.* Baltimore: University Park Press.

Sundelin, C., & Vuille, J.-C. (1975a). Health screening of 4-year-olds in a Swedish county: II. Effectiveness in detecting health problems. *Acat Paediatrica Scandinavia, 64,* 801–806.

Sundelin, C., & Vuille, J. C. (1975b). Health screening of 4-year-olds in a Swedish county: I. Organization, methods, and participation. *Acta Paediatrica Scandinavia, 64,* 795–800.

CHAPTER 31

# Methodologic Guides for the Evaluation of Community Developmental Screening Programs

*David Cadman, Larry Chambers, Steven Walter, David Sackett, and William Feldman*

---

A *screening program* is an organized effort to detect, among presumably developmentally normal children in the community, disabilities that were previously undetected. Such a program also includes all the events that must occur after screening if it is to benefit a community's children. These include diagnostic confirmation, therapeutic and preventive intervention, and follow-up.

The authors were approached by public health and education policymakers from a geographically well-defined community in Ontario, Canada, who asked assistance in determining if the preschool developmental screening program conducted in their community was both effective and worthwhile. The screening was targeted at all 4-year-olds and used the Denver Developmental Screening Test. The community wished to know if the program *did* work in their real-life situation rather than if a program *could* work in an ideal, highly controlled, experimental situation. The former research question is one of "effectiveness," the latter one of "efficacy" (Cochrane, 1972).

To answer the policymakers' questions, the authors have developed and used guidelines in the planning and execution of the Niagara Screening and Prevention Study (NSPS). In order to reach conclusions that are likely to be both valid (true) and generalizable (applicable else-

---

***David Cadman, Larry Chambers, Steven Walter, and David Sackett*** • Departments of Pediatrics and Clinical Epidemiology and Biostatistics, McMaster University, Hamilton, Ontario Canada L8N 325. ***William Feldman*** • Children's Hospital of Eastern Ontario, Ottawa, Ontario, Canada.

where), one should commence studies of the effectiveness of community developmental screening that meet six methodologic standards. These guidelines may prove useful not only to those who conduct research, but to consumers of clinical research who read journals and to those who teach students to critically appraise health care literature.

These six guidelines are as follows:

1. Is the basic study architecture appropriate?
2. Is the study sample representative of all individuals eligible for the screening program in the community?
3. Is the screening program feasible in other communities?
4. Are all clinically relevant outcomes reported?
5. Are the outcomes of all individuals who entered the study appropriately dealt with at the conclusion of the study?
6. Are both statistical and social significance considered?

## APPLICATION OF SIX GUIDELINES TO SCREENING PROGRAMS

### Appropriate Basic Study Architecture

This first criterion is paramount. Although other study designs such as before/after evaluations and cohort studies can generate useful hypotheses, only a well-executed, randomized controlled trial (where children are selected to be screened or not screened by a method analogous to the toss of a coin) can clearly answer research questions of screening program effectiveness.

Most clinicians know patients who have done well after early detection of disorders. However, clinical experience, even when based on prospective cohort or case-control studies, can be misleading. In fact, nonexperimental studies of screening can often spuriously appear to improve outcomes. There are two reasons for this phenomenon. First, those who come forward for screening and adhere to subsequent recommendations have better prognoses before they start. Thus, women in the New York randomized controlled trial of mammography plus clinical breast examination who accepted invitations for screening had only half the mortality from other causes (for which they were not screened) than experimental women who rejected screening invitations (Shapiro, 1977).

The second reason is that screening and early diagnosis of progressive disorders can appear to improve outcomes even when intervention is worthless. This arises from the failure to correct for the time shift that rises when early diagnosis is achieved (Sackett, 1980). If this lead time is not subtracted from the early diagnosed group, indexes such as the

5-year morbidity rate can be spuriously reduced, and the apparently improved outcomes are merely reflections of longer intervals during which the problem has been recognized.

Thus, in responding to the community's question, we undertook a randomized controlled trial of the NSPS screening program. After obtaining informed consent from 99% of more than 4,000 eligible parents, we randomly allocated children to one of the three study groups as follows.

1. Group 1 received the Denver Developmental Screening Test (DDST); in addition, children with positive results received public health, nurse-initiated follow-up with the child's family, physician, and school.
2. Group 2 received the DDST but no organized public health, physician, or school follow-up.
3. Group 3 had no DDST administered.

NSPS has had exceptional community support and will be completed during 1984. Although such studies may be costly, their expense is usually trivial compared to the costs incurred in a mass community-wide developmental screening program.

## Representative Study Sample

In a screening trial, the study sample should be representative of all individuals offered (or likely to be offered) the program in the entire community, not just a subgroup of those at highest risk or those with the greatest likelihood of responding to intervention. Unless there are clear exclusion and inclusion criteria (such as sociodemographic variables), it is impossible to judge whether the study sample and results are generalizable to the entire study community (or anywhere else). Conclusions based on volunteer samples are especially unlikely to be applicable elsewhere.

All children registering for kindergarten in three of the Niagara region's four school districts were eligible for inclusion in the NSPS with one exception: 19 recent Indo-Chinese immigrants who were non-English-speaking were ruled ineligible for inclusion in the study. In addition, children known by education officials to have a developmental disability so severe as to preclude admission to regular or special education school programs were not brought to school registration and were thus excluded from the study.

The sociodemographic characteristics of the community will be described based on 1981 Census of Canada data. Thus, when the NSPS is completed, readers will be able to judge whether the study's results are likely to be relevant to their own community.

## Feasibility of the Screening Program in Other Communities

The details of the screening program must be documented and described in sufficient detail so as to be replicable elsewhere. The costs of the program should be ascertained as well, because this is germane to judgments of feasibility.

In order to assist in explaining the results of the trial, one should address three issues:

1. In addition to the screening program, did the experimental group receive any cointerventions (which were extraneous to the research question) not available to control children and families?
2. Did control children receive any interventions similar to the experimental maneuver ("contamination")?
3. How well did parents and community professionals comply with the recommendations generated by the screening program?

Because an effectiveness study attempts to answer the research question in a real-life community, it is inevitable that noncompliance and perhaps even cointervention or contamination will occur. Their occurrence does not invalidate study conclusions, but documentation does help planners understand the results, and suggest methods for improvement.

## Reporting All Clinically Relevant Outcomes

An effectiveness study must go beyond highly specific outcome events (such as academic performance) to consider broader outcomes of child and family well-being, including social, behavioral, and emotional functioning. Because the purpose of a screening program evaluation is to assist in making management decisions (to implement or not implement the program in an actual community), both specific and more general outcomes are germane. Whenever possible, outcome measure should be made by an observer unaware of a child's study group to avoid potential bias.

The NSPS uses a broad range of outcome measures, including teacher reports through second grade, group academic achievement testing, and, for a sample of children, individual developmental and school achievement testing at the end of Grade 2. For this latter group, a parent-completed questionnaire of demonstrated reliability and validity (Eisen, Donald, Ware, & Brook, 1980) is used to measure the child's behavioral, social, and emotional function as well as the parent's perception of the child's school and developmental progress. Sociodemographic and family functioning covariables are also measured using this questionnaire.

## Analysis of Outcomes

Because implementing a community developmental screening program involves a decision to offer a service, the outcomes of individuals randomized to be screened who decline the offer, drop out, or who do not comply with recommendations must be included in the analysis for the screened group. Moreover, because the issue is whether or not an organized program adds anything to existing community services for case-finding and diagnosis, control individuals detected and treated by other means must be included in the analysis for their original randomly allocated control group.

## Considerations of Statistical and Social Significance

The level of statistical significance is an index of whether or not any differences in outcome found between experimental and control groups could have occurred by chance alone. Studies with large sample sizes may lead to substantively trivial but statistically significant differences. Studies with small samples may fail to show statistically significant effects even when the differences between groups is substantively large. A more detailed discussion of this issue may be found in Frieman, Chalmers, Smith, and Kuebber (1978).

Statistical significance is not directly concerned with the substantive importance or magnitude of differences in outcome between individuals who received the screening program and control individuals. A community screening effectiveness study should explicitly consider whether any differences in outcome are large enough to be judged important and worthwhile by citizens and public policymakers in the face of competing alternative uses for limited resources.

Measures of social value are becoming increasingly available and feasible for use (Kaplan, Bush & Berry, 1976; Sackett & Torrance, 1978). For example, Kaplan and his colleagues (1976) determined the social value of health states (defined in terms of physical function, mobility, social function, and medical symptoms) by asking a sample of the general public to rate their desirability (Kaplan *et al.*, 1976). These social values were applied to the health outcomes found in a study of serum thyroxine (T4) screening, and led to the conclusion that this screening was a worthwhile procedure (Epstein, Schneiderman, & Bush, 1981). Other approaches to measuring social significance described in the literature include measures of individuals' willingness to pay for various magnitudes of health benefits (Thompson, Read, & Liang, 1982).

In the NSPS, we plan to determine the decision threshold of public health and education policymakers prior to their knowing the study outcomes. We hope to aggregate the diverse types of outcome measures into a single quantified child well-being index using (a) the policymakers' own measured social preferences, and (b) the measured costs of the program. These will be used to determine the magnitude of outcome difference between experimental and control groups that would have to be found to justify a subsequent decision to continue, abandon, or modify a community preschool developmental screening program. The investigators will observe the actual decision made when the study results are presented with great interest.

## SUMMARY

Six commonsense methodologic guidelines have been proposed. Adherence to these in screening effectiveness studies will increase the likelihood that an evaluation will reach conclusions that are valid, generalizable, and useful to community public policymakers.

## REFERENCES

Cochrane, A. L. (1972). *Effectiveness and efficiency.* Oxford, England: The Nuffield Provincial Hospitals Trust.

Eisen, M., Donald, C., Ware, J. E, & Brook, R. H. (1980). *Conceptualization and measurement for children in the Health Insurance study.* Rand Publication R-2313-HEW. Santa Monica, CA.

Frieman, K., Chalmers, T., Smith, W., & Kuebber, F. Design and interpretation of randomized control trial: Survey of "negative" trials. *New England Journal of Medicine, 299,* 690–694.

Kaplan, R. M., Bush, J. W., & Berry, C. C. (1976). Health status: Types of validity and the index of well-being. *Health Services Research, 11,* 478–507.

Sackett, D. L. (1980). Evaluation of health services. In J. Last (Ed.), *Public health and preventive medicine* (11th ed., pp. 1800–1823). New York: Appleton-Century-Crofts.

Sackett, D. L., & Torrance,G. W. (1978). The utility of different health states as perceived by the general public. *Journal of Chronic Disease, 31,* 175–190.

Shapiro, S. (1977). Evidence on screening for breast cancer from a randomized trial. *Cancer, 39,* 2772–2779.

Thompson, M. S., Read, J. L., & Liang, M. (1982). Willingness-to-pay concepts for societal decisions in health. In R. L. Kane & R. A.Kane (Eds.), *Values and long-term care* (pp. 103–126). Toronto: Lexington Books.

CHAPTER 32

# Classification of Handicapped Dependents and Service Facilities in the U.S. Army

## A COMPREHENSIVE APPROACH

*Philip F. LoPiccolo*

Personnel in the United States Army currently have 662,000 dependent children (Sample Survey, 1982), of which 140,000 reside in Europe (Worldwide Manpower, 1980). In addition, there are more than 50,000 children born each year to active duty Army personnel (Medical Summary Report, 1983). A conservative estimate is that 10% of these children are in need of services for handicapping conditions (Pless, Satterwhite, & Van Vechten, 1976).

In the United States, legal mandates have given public schools the responsibility for providing education and related services to children with handicapping conditions (Public Law 94-142, 1975). However, for military dependents outside the continental U.S., the appropriate military medical departments have been mandated to provide needed services (Department of Defense Instruction 1342.12, 1981; Public Law 95-561, 1978).

When given what can be seen to be an enormous responsibility, the Army was concerned, for it was not geared or equipped—nor did it have the expertise in the pediatric field—to provide the required kinds and volume of services. It became clear that a systematized plan would have to be developed if the Army were to effectively meet the needs of handicapped dependents. The result was a new program, the Exceptional Family Member Program.

***Philip F. LoPiccolo*** • Seventh Medical Command, Heidelberg, West Germany.

## DESCRIPTION OF THE PROGRAM

The Exceptional Family Member Program includes the following elements: (a) an identification system, (b) a screening system, (c) guidelines for evaluation, and (d) a coding/classification system.

Procedures and guidelines have been established for the identification, screening, and evaluation of children. In addition, existing resources have beem mobilized and additional professional personnel have been added both within and outside the continental United States.

## THE PROGRAM'S CODING SYSTEM

The most unique element of the Exceptional Family Member Program is its coding and classification system. The system is designed to place exceptional family members into categories that reflect their medical and educational needs, and into levels that reflect the intensity of the care they need.

In addition, all of the Army's medical and educational facilities throughout the world have been coded using the same schema, so that the facilities' abilities to provide care in each of the categories and the level of care that can be provided is known. In other words, using this system, the Army not only knows the need of a given patient, but also which facility can provide the needed type and level of care.

There are four steps in the coding sytem: a Special Needs Medical questionnaire, an Educational Questionnaire, coding teams, and utilization of the coding/classification system.

### The Special Needs Medical Questionnaire

This questionnaire is unique in that it obtains a functional assessment of the individual being coded into the Exceptional Family Member Program. The questionnaire, which is 10 pages long, includes such areas as demographic data, diagnoses, prior and anticipated hospitalizations, historical medical data, services the dependent is presently receiving, current treatment programs and the professionals presently providing care, current evaluations, specific problem areas, medications, payment source, assignment/transfer information (for the Army member), and physician's review and signature.

This questionnaire is so comprehensive that it appears to elicit the necessary information in all problem areas; at least, in the vast majority of cases coded, the coding team has not needed to seek further information. Problems encountered with the form include physician not signing, evaluations that are not current, evaluations that are not included with the form, and occasionally, a striking difference between the parents' and the professionals' perception of the problem.

### The Educational Questionnaire

The Educational Questionnaire used in the program is similar to what many school districts use. If the child is of school age, the parents are required to bring the questionnaire to the school for completion and for the signature of a school official.

This questionnaire addresses four primary areas: (a) types of special education placement; (b) related services that are required; (c) required services for sensory and physical impairments (including visual, auditory, and orthopedic disabilities); and (d) grade level.

### The Coding Team

An integral aspect of the program is the coding team concept. The coding team (eight teams in the United States and one in Europe) consist of a pediatrician (sometimes a developmental pediatrician), a child psychologist or psychiatrist, and a physical medicine specialist. (The latter could be a physiatrist, or occupational or physical therapist.) All members of the teams were trained in a week-long conference in 1983. At this conference, the Army learned that when individuals from each of the disciplines mentioned were involved in coding a case, the accuracy of the coding increased substantially (Exceptional Family, 1983). Therefore, the concept of utilizing 3 professionals functioning as a team to code each case has been continued.

The coding/classification system was designed to reflect as accurately as possible the needs of the exceptional family member. The system has 22 categories, 21 of which are problem-oriented. (The final category indicates additional specialists who may be needed, but who have not been included in the other categories.) Each of the 21 problem-oriented categories is divided into levels that correspond to the level of care needed by each client.

The coding/classification system has gone through several revisions. The final 21 categories evolved are

1. High-risk newborn
2. Delayed development
3. Delayed cognitive development
4. Oral-motor deficit
5. Compromised respiratory function

6. Restricted mobility
7. Sensory integration deficit
8. Upper extremity deficit
8. Activity of daily living
10. Adaptive equipment needs
11. Architectural/environmental adaptations
12. Vision
13. Speech/language deficits
14. Hearing deficits
15. Learning problems
16. Behavioral/emotional disorders
17. Drug/alcohol abuse
18. Special care inside/outside home
19. Medical social work
20. Community health nurse
21. Functional disabilities

As has been discussed previously, levels of care needed have been developed for each of the 21 categories. An example of the levels for Category 1 ( high-risk newborn, 0–18 months) is as follows:

Level A: Follow-up care by a neonatologist, pediatrician, or family practitioner. Consultation with developmental pediatrician and/or pediatric PT/OT at 6-month intervals.

Level B: Follow-up care by a developmental pediatrician, and pediatric PT/OT every 2 to 4 months. Consultation to other specialists or child resource team as needed.

Level C: Follow-up care by developmental pediatrician and PT/OT every month. Consultation to other specialists and child resource team as needed.

Level D: An abnormality of movement or tone exists. Follow-up by developmental pediatrician, audiologist, speech/language pathologist, and/or child resource team will be frequent. Pediatric PT is indicated once or twice a week.

Another example of the content of levels can be seen in Category 16, behavioral and emotional disorders:

Level A: Primary care physician can manage alone or with occasional consultation to child guidance team.

Level B: Evaluation and management is needed by a child guidance team for short-term therapy with referral back to the primary physician for continued monitoring.

Level C: Long-term outpatient management by a child guidance team. No hospitalization is anticipated.
Level D: Short-term inpatient milieu management is anticipated or may be required.
Level E: Residential treatment program or long-term inpatient care is anticipated or required.

## IMPLEMENTATION OF THE PROGRAM

The phased implementation of the Exceptional Family Member Program began in January of 1983. Orientation programs were conducted at all of the Army's major medical centers, and service members who were registered in the Handicapped Dependent Program received a letter informing them of the new program and requesting that they fill out the appropriate forms. The result was that 1,043 service members responded; their forms were sent to a collection point. Coding teams were appointed and trained, and coding began.

## FINDINGS

The majority of the 1,043 responses involved dependents of enlisted service members. Of the dependents involved, 9.2% were under 3 years, 23% were between 3 and 6 years of age, and 54% were between 6 and 18 years. An additional 2% were in the 18- to 21-year range, 11% were over 21 years, and the ages of .8% were unknown. Of the total, 27% needed health services only 7% needed educational services only, and 66% needed both health and education services.

When the data from one region (the Walter Reed Army Medical Center region) were analyzed, 31% of the children were found to have a single diagnosis, whereas multiple diagnoses occurred in 68.6% of the cases. At times it was difficult for the team to determine which disability should be the primary diagnosis. When this occurred, it was decided that the condition requiring the most specialized treatment program would be designated the primary diagnosis. For example, a child with cerbral palsy and blindness would have a primary diagnosis of blindness because the treatment for this condition would be most specialized, and it would be the most limiting factor in the assignment process.

Table 1 indicates the levels of care required. It is interesting to note that the most frequently used of the 21 categories was the learning problem category. Only 46 children were diagnosed as having a learning disability, yet 146 (56%) were identified as having a need for evaluation,

**Table 1.** The Exceptional Family Member Program's Categorical and Level of Care Results for the Walter Reed Regional Area

| Category | Total no. children in each category* | Percentage of total in each level of care** | | | | |
|---|---|---|---|---|---|---|
| | | A | B | C | | |
| Speech/language deficits | 108 | 13.9 | 21.3 | 64.8 | | |
| Sensory integration deficit | 88 | 56.8 | 30.7 | 12.5 | | |
| Hearing deficit | 64 | 43.8 | 18.8 | 37.5 | | |
| Oral-motor deficits | 45 | 33.3 | 37.8 | 28.9 | | |
| | | A | B | C | D | |
| Learning problems | 146 | 48.6 | 27.4 | 21.2 | 2.7 | |
| Activity of daily living | 116 | 37.1 | 39.7 | 20.7 | 2.6 | |
| Medical social work | 98 | 81.6 | 16.3 | 2.0 | 0.0 | |
| Vision | 87 | 59.8 | 23.0 | 10.3 | 6.9 | |
| Restricted mobility | 82 | 37.8 | 4.9 | 18.3 | 39.0 | |
| Adaptive equipment needs | 72 | 20.8 | 45.8 | 22.2 | 11.1 | |
| Functional disabilities | 61 | 9.8 | 27.9 | 29.5 | 32.8 | |
| Delayed development | 61 | 1.6 | 6.6 | 6.6 | 85.2 | |
| Delayed cognitive development | 52 | 57.7 | 17.3 | 21.2 | 3.8 | |
| Architectural/environmental adaptations | 13 | 23.1 | 38.5 | 7.7 | 30.8 | |
| High-risk newborn | 2 | 0.0 | 50.0 | 50.0 | 0.0 | |
| | | A | B | C | D | E |
| Behavioral/emotional disorders | 90 | 48.9 | 26.7 | 18.9 | 5.6 | 0.0 |

*No children were classified into the following categories: special care inside/outside home, community health nurse, drug/acohol abuse, upper extremity deficit, and compromised respiratory function.
**Level A is the lowest level of care, level E the highest; individual categories go to the highest level of care shown.

monitoring, or active intervention. Nearly half of these children were coded into Level A, meaning that the coders felt from the information obtained that the children needed an initial psychoeducational evaluation, and that, depending on the results, they should be reevaluated at least every 3 years.

Data that could be extrapolated from examination of Table 1 include patient volume for each type of service; the number and kinds of professionals needed; the amount of time required to provide these services; the levels of expertise required; the need for new programs; the need for new or strengthened services; and space requirements.

## SUMMARY

Thus far, every identified individual who has a special need has been codable into the system, and the codes have been found to reflect accurately the condition and the level of care that each individual requires. This means that service members can feel secure in knowing that when they are reassigned, the needs of their exceptional family member will be taken into consideration. In the future, when the program is fully operational and all families are coded, service members could be given an accompanied tour only where appropriate facilities are available for their exceptional family member. For the United States Army, this policy reflects a genuine commitment to soldiers and their families. In the economic sphere, this program will save millions of dollars for the government by avoiding incompatible or inappropriate assignments.

The whole concept of the Exceptional Family Member Program is very simple: Know and document the needs of the exceptional family member and assign the service member to an area where those needs can be met. This policy preserves the family unit and makes for a more effective service member. Although the program has been developed to meet the needs of families of U.S. Army personnel, the concept has wide applicability and could be used successfully and meaningfully in the civilian sector.

## REFERENCES

Instruction 1342.12 Department of Defense (1981, December 17). "Education of Handicapped Children in the DoD Dependents Schools."

*Exceptional Family Member Coding Conference summary report.* (1983, March). Tacoma, Washington.

*Medical summary report #302.* (1983). DASG-PSA, Pentagon, Washington, D.C.

Pless, I. B., Satterwhite, B., & Van Vechten, D. (1976). Chronic illness in childhood. *Pediatrics, 58,* 37.

*Public Law 95–561: Defense Dependents' Education Act of 1978* (1978). (20 U.S.C. SS 921–232; Supp. II).

*Public Law 94–142: Education for All Handicapped Children Act of 1975* (1975). (20 U.S.C. 551401 et seq., 1976 and Supp. II 1978).

*Sample survey of military personnel.* (1982, August). DASG-PSA, Pentagon, Washington, D.C.

*Worldwide manpower distribution by geographic area.* (1980). Report, Washington Headquarters Services, Office of Secretary of Defense, Washington, D.C.

CHAPTER 33

# Longitudinal Data Collection

## A PREREQUISITE FOR EFFICIENT MASS SCREENING PROGRAMS

*Victor Weidtman*

Since the time when the goals of an effective screening program were defined (Frankenburg & Camp, 1975), most European countries have organized comprehensive screening programs. The organization and effectiveness of these programs are influenced by differing socioeconomic systems, national structures of medical care, and so on.

In West Germany, a national screening program was introduced in 1972 and has involved between 400,000 and 600,000 preschool children annually. Since 1977, screening has consisted of 8 examinations during the first 4 years of life, with 4 to 5 million screening examinations conducted per year. The timing of these examinations, from minutes after birth to 4 years, is shown in Figure 1. The figure also shows that participation in the program has improved between 1974 and 1978.

In such a large program, difficulties exist in monitoring the quality and efficiency of screening (Weidtman & Schwartz, 1980). Still, quality control is essential if weaknesses are to be identified and corrected. Only by providing data from an effective program can society influence health policy decisions. The purpose of this chapter is to show how longitudinal data collection can be an important tool for improving the efficiency of a nationwide screening program.

*Victor Weidtman* • Institute for Medical Documentation and Statistics, University of Cologne, Cologne, Federal Republic of Germany.

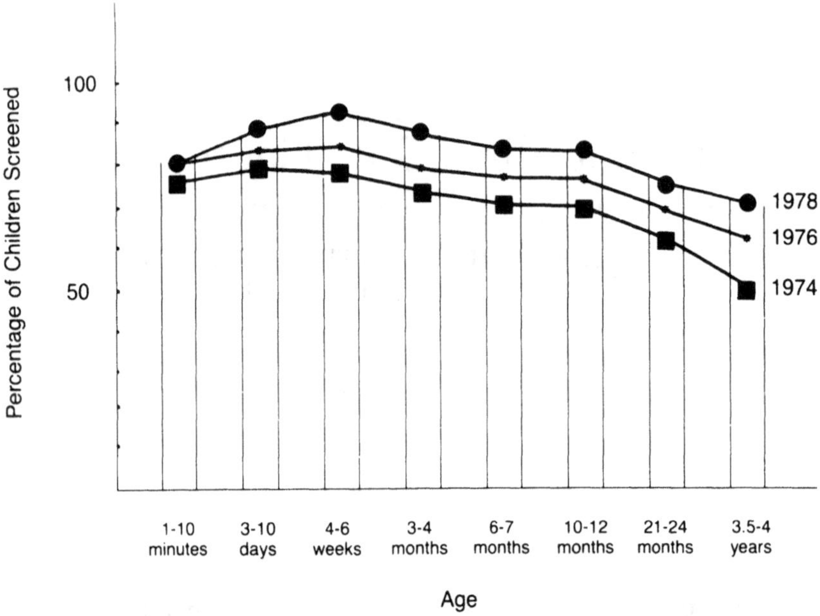


**Figure 1.** Participation in periodic health examinations under West Germany's National Health Insurance Plan.

## DIFFICULTIES ENCOUNTERED IN MASS SCREENING PROGRAMS

Following analysis of approximately 35 million screening protocols conducted over 10 years in West Germany, the following problems were found in the program's efficiency:

1. Lack of compliance, especially in the high-risk population;
2. Inadequate performance of some screening procedures; and
3. Inadequate additional diagnostic procedures and unnecessary treatment.

Cross-sectional statistics from the West German program have been published annually. These statistics have led to critical hypotheses, but have not provided detailed information about the program's shortcomings. As there is no supervision of the physicians performing the screening, statistical evaluation of screening records remains the only way to monitor efficiency. Recognizing the limited information available, West German health planners have considered ways to improve the screening program by introducing follow-up statistics through records linkage.

## RECORDS LINKAGE AND STIMULATION OF COMPLIANCE

Investigations by Collatz, Maltzahn, and Schmidt (1979), who analyzed a sample of 1,000 children living in the Duesseldorf region, have shown that the compliance rate of the families of children at risk of developing developmental delays is lower than the compliance rate of the population at large.

Some European countries have recognized the importance of some external stimulus or incentive even before implementation of a mass screening program. In Austria and the German Democratic Republic, for example, additional family allowances are paid conditional on regular participation of a family's child in screening examinations. In the Federal Republic of Germany, a strong feeling exists against this type of approach, and so a different set of strategies have been adopted, with differing degrees of success.

For example, one strategy was developed and implemented by a pediatrician in the city of Essen. He took the initiative and registered all newborns classified by obstetricians and pediatricians as being at risk. While still in the maternity wards, the mothers of these children were asked which physician they intended to visit for their children's screening, and were asked for their permission to inform the physician of this intent through the Medical Association. The physicians were then asked to report to the central registry when and whether the child was presented. If the child was not presented during the scheduled time, several attempts were made to urge the parents to have the child screened (Herpertz, 1976).

Because the data from the Essen study could not be analyzed systematically, a similar project was started in the area around Koblenz. Results from this study showed clearly that compliance can be increased with close follow-up (Allhoff & Selbmann, 1983). Very strict laws regarding personal data protection in the Federal Republic severely impede this type of work, because they require the written consent of the parents. Nevertheless, this model is the subject of much discussion centered around whether a similar approach should be generalized to other communities in the near future.

A similar approach was described in an editorial of the French journal, *Le Concours Médical* (Editorial, 1981). The French Department of Health proposed to use a "premier certificat de santé," which records the medical and socioeconomic status of mother and child shortly after delivery to select children at risk (via computer). These children were to be followed regarding regular screening and therapy. The system was rejected by the French Commission Nationale de L'Informatique et Libertés, and was never implemented.

## MONITORING THE OUTCOME OF SCREENING

When screening is less than optimal, too many children without problems are falsely identified as having a delay. This overidentification leads to costly additional diagnostic measures and, in some cases, unnecessary therapy.

To avoid the problem of overidentificaton, one must make regular comparisons of the outcome of the screening program with epidemiological data. Unfortunately, reliable epidemiological data on morbidity are seldom available, and often depend on social and geographic factors. Consequently, the only efficient control of an existing general screening program is the constant monitoring of validity and reliability. Regular information must be obtained about the development of the child after screening. As screening must be repeated during the developmental period to discover age-specific disorders, the needed information can be obtained if, and only if, there is a record linkage ready for evaluation by data processing techniques. Besides adding information about screening quality and a program's weak points, such data can provide more accurate information about morbidity rates than currently exists.

To assess the accuracy of screening, researchers made an attempt to link screening findings for each child with the results of follow-up diagnostic evaluations. Thirty-thousand linked records of 5,530 children who did not miss any of their first five or six screening appointments in Bremen were examined. Presumptive identification of childhood problems was heavily overrepresented in the cross-sectional statistics. Using linkage of records from screening through diagnosis, researchers avoided unwanted multiple counting, and derived more accurate morbidity data (Lajosi & Weidtman, 1983).

## DATA PROCESSING AND DATA PROTECTION

When record linkage is introduced and large numbers of children's files are recorded (half a million in the case of West Germany), data processing becomes a key concern. However, as incoming records are processed in regional computer centers, sorting and merging processes can be used that lessen the cost of the project.

The problem of data protection will be addressed in West Germany by giving each child an identification number and avoiding the use of a child's name. Only the parents or the child's physician will be able to recombine a number in such a way that the name of the patient can be known.

This will be done as follows: At the time of the first screening immediately after birth, the parents are currently given a booklet in which the results of this first and all subsequent screenings are recorded by the child's physician. A copy of this record has always been sent to a central agency for statistic evaluation; however, until now the records did not have any entry relating to the identity of the child, making record linkage impossible. In the future (based on a successful pilot study in the Bremen region), all booklets in which screening results are recorded will be numbered. The booklets will be distributed randomly so that the number of the child's record will be known only to the parents and physician. However, because all incoming records from each child will bear the same number over time, record linkage will be feasible.

It is hoped that use of this record-linkage method will permit us to avoid the rather time-consuming process of obtaining the written consent of the parents of each child, while still protecting the privacy of children. The identification numbers will have an additional function: A random sample of the population can be obtained merely by selecting numbers consisting of certain combinations of digits.

In conclusion, there is no doubt among health planners that mass screening programs must be monitored to preserve high standards of quality and efficiency. Cross-sectional statistics are of limited value to obtain reliable information about screening. Follow-up statistics using record linkage have proven more useful in providing information that can be used to strengthen a screening program.

## REFERENCES

Allhoff, P., & Selbmann, H. K. (1983). Früherkennungsuntersuchungen bei Kindern. *Muenchener Medizinische Wochenschrift, 46,* 1071–1076.

Collatz, J., Maltzahn, P., & Schmidt, E. (1979). Erreichen die gesetzlichen Früherkennungsuntersuchungen für Säuglinge und Kleinkinder ihre Zielgruppe? *Oeffentliche Gesundheitswesen, 41,* 173–190.

Editorial. (1981). Le traitement automatisé des certificats de santé dans les services de la PMI. *Le Concours Médical, 29,* 4645–4646.

Frankenburg, W. K. & Camp, B. W. (1975). *Pediatric screening tests.* Springfield, IL: Charles C Thomas.

Herpertz, H. (1976), Das Oberhausener Modell. *Der Kinderarzt, 5,* 606–610.

Lajosi, F., & Weidtman, V. (1983). Die Bedeutung der Längsschnittauswertung für die Evaluation der Früherkennungsuntersuchung im Kindesalter. *Monatsschrift Kinderheilkunde, 131,* 594–598.

Weidtman, V., & Schwartz, Fr. W. (1980). The organization and administration of follow-up studies to evaluate the results of screening in the "at risk infant." In S. Harel (Ed.), *The at-risk infant.* Amsterdam-Oxford-Princeton: Excerpta Medica.

CHAPTER 34

# Effectiveness of a Perinatal High-Risk Follow-Up Program in the Early Identification of Cerebral Palsy

*Margaret Cox, Ann Johnson, Edna McKim, and Gourdas Pal*

---

Newfoundland is the most easterly of Canada's Atlantic provinces, with a population of 500,000 scattered over an island 500 mi across, and even more sparsely over the large mainland section of Labrador. The area was settled 400 years ago predominantly by English and Irish emigrants who joined the native Inuit and Indian populations. The province's birth rate and family size formerly was the highest in Canada, and remains high (average family size is still 3.8 persons). Family ties are strong in Newfoundland, and the divorce rate is low. The perinatal mortality rate, previously considerably higher than the Canadian average, has declined to 11.5 per 1,000 births, as compared with 10.9 for Canada as a whole (Statistics Canada, 1983).

The current study examines the effectiveness of a High-Risk Follow-Up Program in the early identification of cerebral palsy. This program is part of Newfoundland's Provincial Perinatal Program, which began in 1979. It has four aims:

1. To follow high-risk infants in order to enhance early diagnosis and intervention for neurodevelopmental problems.
2. To collect morbidity and mortality statistics

***Margaret Cox, Ann Johnson, and Edna McKim*** • Newfoundland and Labrador Provincial Perinatal Program, St. John's, Newfoundland, Canada A1A 1R8. ***Gourdas Pal*** • Children's Rehabilitation Center, St. John's, Newfoundland, Canada A1A 1R8.

3. To upgrade standards of obstetric and neonatal care
4. To improve perinatal education programs

*High-risk*[1] is defined for the purposes of this study as an increased susceptibility to neurological and developmental handicaps. Follow-up is arranged through discussion with the parents, the child's physician, the Perinatal Program's director, nurse-coordinator, and nursing staff.

## METHODS

The nurse-coordinator of the Perinatal Program establishes contact with the parents of high-risk babies, who are recalled for follow-up at 3, 6, 9, 12, 18, and 36 months of age. Traveling clinics held at six sites once or twice a year facilitate the examination of babies living at distances of up to 700 mi from St. John's, where the program is based in the children's hospital. At the clinics, neurodevelopmental evaluations are emphasized, and the physicians, nurses, and physiotherapists involved obtain consultations as needed with neurology, audiology, ophthalmology and other disciplines. The Griffiths Development Scales (Griffiths, 1976) are employed. Babies with evidence of cerebral palsy or other physical handicaps are eventually referred to the Children's Rehabilitation Centre, which is the sole provincial agency for management of these problems. The Centre's team is multidisciplinary, travels across the province, and exchanges data with the Perinatal Program.

## RESULTS

In 1980, there were 9,981 births in Newfoundland (Health Statistics, 1980). Of these, 74 were referred by 1983 when they were 3 years of age

[1]At-risk criteria utilized by the High-Risk Follow-Up Program are as follows: birth weight 1500 g or less, and birth weight greater than 1500 g *if* (a) small for gestational age (less than 2000 g, 2 standard deviations or more *below* the mean weight or head circumference for gestation age), or large for gestational age (2 standard deviations or more *above* the mean); (b) twin of infant under 1500 g; (c) perinatal asphyxia—clinical evidence of fetal asphyxia in labor and delivery, apgar 6 or less at 5 minutes, neonatal (first month) asphyxia requiring resuscitation; (d) seizure activity or abnormal neurological activity in the neonatal period (first month); (e) respiratory distress, requiring mechanical ventilation, with "air leak" (e.g., pneumothorax or pneunomediastinum), oxygen more than 50% for 24 hours, chronic lung changes; (f) confirmed septicemia/meningitis; (g) negrotizing enerocolitis; (h) recurrent apnea (more than three episodes/24 hours); (i) recognizable social risk factors (e.g., maternal age of 16 or less); or (j) other (e.g., any baby who gives rise to concern in the prenatal, intranatal, or postnatal period up to 1 month of life).

to the Children's Rehabilitation Centre, and 25 were found to have cerebral palsy, an incidence of 0.25% for the province. The 1980 intake for the High-Risk Follow-Up Program was 204, and of these, 17 (8.33%) now have cerebral palsy. Comparing the Program's total of 17 with the Centre's total of 25, it is apparent that 8 cases of children with cerebral palsy escaped being tagged with the Program's high-risk criteria. The histories of these 8 children were reviewed from the records of the Rehabilitation Centre, and it was found that 7 were considered normal at birth. Of the 7, 1 developed seizures at 10 days, and 2 apparently developed cerebral palsy as a result of later illness (post-vaccinial encephalitis and hemophilus meningitis). The eighth child had hydrocephalus at birth.

(The Children's Rehabilitation Centre is the only such referral center in Newfoundland. Although it is possible that some children might have been referred to another province for treatment, thus making it possible that additional cases could have been missed, it is extremely unlikely. Special medical insurance coverage would be needed for such a referral, and usually a referral to another province would occur only after the child was seen at the Children's Rehabilitation Centre.)

The high-risk criteria recorded in the babies identified at birth are shown in Table 1. The most common associated finding was severe respiratory distress, defined as the need for ventilation and/or presence of chronic lung changes; this was present in 76% of the cerebral palsy group of 17 followed (as compared with 28% of the total high-risk population of 204, or 23.5% of the non-cerebral palsy, high-risk population of 187). Neonatal seizures occurred in 52% of the palsy groups (as compared with 7% of the total group, or 2.7% of the non-cerebral palsy group). Eight infants (47%) in the birth weight group between 1500 g

**Table 1.** Perinatal High-Risk Criteria Associated with Cerebral Palsy

| | Cerebral palsy group* ($N$ = 17) | Total high-risk group* ($N$ = 204) |
|---|---|---|
| Respiratory distress | 76% | 28% |
| Seizures | 52% | 7% |
| SGA > 1500 g | 47% | 40% |
| Asphyxia | 35% | 40% |
| 1500 g or less | 18% | 17% |
| NEC ENT | 18% | — |
| Hypotonia | 12% | — |
| Hyperbilirubinemia | 12% | — |
| Maternal age 16 or less | 12% | — |
| Septicemia | 6% | — |

*Total equals more than 100% because some children had more than one high-risk factor.

and 2000 g were small for gestational age (more than 2 standard deviations below the mean of the Atlantic Growth Chart) compared with 40% of the total high-risk group; asphyxia (Apgar score less than 6 at 5 minutes) (38% of the non-cerebral palsy group) was present in 35% of the cerebral palsy group, which was similar to the 40% found in the total high-risk group. Only 3 of the 17 babies (18%) with cerebral palsy weighed 1500 g or less at birth. This was a finding similar to the incidence (17%) of this weight group in the total high-risk population (or 16.5% in the non-cerebral palsy high risk group).

Of the total 25 children born in 1980 who have cerebral palsy, 22 are multiply handicapped. Spastic quadriplegia occurred in 17 (including 2 with diplegia); of these, 15 are developmentally retarded (the 2 diplegics are not), 8 have severe visual impairment, 2 have epilepsy, 1 has severe hearing loss, and 4 have strabismus. Spastic hemiplegia occurred in 3 children, annd of these, 1 is retarded, 1 has epilepsy, and 1 had a squint (now corrected). Extrapyramidal cerebral palsy occurred in 5 children; all of these have developmental retardation and severe visual impairment, and 3 have epilepsy and 1 has a severe hearing loss.

The severity of impairment is proportional to the number of disabilities. The 8 children with 4 or 5 handicaps each have developmental quotients (DQs) below 30 on the Griffiths Scale (Griffiths, 1976). Children with 2 or 3 handicaps have DQs between 40 and 66. Only the 3 children with single handicaps have "normal" DQs of 80 or above.

The age of diagnosis of cerebral palsy averaged 6 to 9 months in those babies in the High-Risk Program, although physiotherapy was begun in all suspect infants before diagnosis was confirmed. Babies with cerebral palsy not in the program averaged 18 months of age at time of referral to the Children's Rehabilitation Centre (except those severely affected with postnatal encephalitis or meningitis). The infants in the high-risk group therefore had the advantage of the earliest intervention.

A further 5 children born in 1980 and followed in the High-Risk Follow-Up program had neurological signs suggestive of cerebral palsy that resolved after 6 months of age. At age 2 to 3 years, 3 of these children show significant global delay or behavior disorder.

## DISCUSSION

In summary, the purpose of the study was to examine the effectiveness of the High-Risk Follow-up Program in identifying children with cerebral palsy. The Program followed all but 8 of the 25 children born in 1980 who have this condition. Two infants who were missed by the High-

Risk Program and were served by other agencies because of other dominant disorders are discounted; in addition, 2 infants not identified by the program presumably acquired cerebral palsy after the neonatal period.

We believe that the effectiveness of the program could be further improved if high-risk criteria received periodic reevaluation to focus attention on those babies most likely to benefit from early neurological diagnosis. One of the "missed" cases resulted from a pregnancy with several risks (maternal diabetes, toxemia, breech presentation, and cesarian section), each of which alone did not qualify for inclusion in the High-Risk Program. Perhaps inclusion of children with cumulative risk factors, as described by Parkyn in Chapter 13, would increase the program's usefulness.

Preliminary figures for 1981 births indicate that 15 children born that year have so far been referred to the Children's Rehabilitation Centre with cerebral palsy; of these 11 are in the High-Risk Follow-Up Program. Because children born in 1981 are still only $2\frac{1}{2}$ to $3\frac{1}{2}$ years of age, it might be expected that some children with cerebral palsy may not yet have been diagnosed, especially if they missed the 18-month visit. It is hoped that the addition of information from 1981 and subsequent births to the study will further elucidate the effectiveness of the High-Risk Follow-up Program in the early identification of cerebral palsy.

## REFERENCES

Griffiths, R. (1976). *Griffiths Mental Development Scales*. Amershan Bucks, U.K.: Eden House.

Health statistics. (1980). Newfoundland: Department of Health Statistics.

Statistics Canada. (1983, February). *Births and deaths*. Ottawa: Health Division, *1*.

CHAPTER 35

# Etiology and Clinical Features of Cerebral Palsy in Saudi Arabia

## IMPLICATIONS FOR PREVENTION AND TREATMENT

*Salah Ali Taha and Amad Hassan Mahdi*

Data from developing countries regarding cerebral palsy (CP) are still less than definitive, and such information is completely lacking in Saudi Arabia. This paper reports a study of 102 Saudi children severely affected with CP. The objective of the study, which was carried out from 1980 to 1983, was to identify etiological factors and clinical types of CP, and to determine how this information might affect prevention and treatment.

## SUBJECTS AND METHODS

The subjects were selected from among approximately 1,200 children attending the Pediatric Neurology Clinic of the University Hospitals at King Saud University in Riyadh during the 3 years of the study. The children came in large part from the Riyadh area and the central region of Saudi Arabia in which Riyadh is located, and represented all socioeconomic levels. Children were included in the study only if they exhibited the pivotal disorder of movement and posture according to the definition of the Little Club (MacKeith, MacKenzie, & Polani, 1959) and Bax (1964). Hereditary syndromes and acquired disorders that were phenocopies of CP were excluded, leaving 102 cases to be studied. Of

***Salah Ali Taha and Amad Hassan Mahdi*** • Department of Pediatrics, King Saud University, Riyadh, Saudi Arabia.

the children involved in the study, 75 were less than 1 year of age, and 6 were less than 2 years; male-to-female ratio was 3:2.

Family and pregnancy histories were obtained for each child, birth and other relevant medical records were reviewed, and the children were evaluated by pediatric neurologists and other professionals, including an audiologist, speech pathologist, and psychologist. Because no interdisciplinary team exists at the Pediatric Neurology Clinic or in Saudi Arabia, not all the children in the study were seen by all of these other professionals.

Following this evaluation, the children were grouped according to etiology. The presumed etiology of each case of CP was based on the likely time of onset. When there was no positive, documented history of insult at birth through the first 5 years of life, the cause was presumed to be prenatal; allocation to this group was further supported by the presence of the congenital abnormalities or of siblings with CP.

The final step in the study was classifying the subjects by the clinical type of CP they displayed (pyramidal, extrapyramidal, cerebellar, hypotonia, or mixed). Terminology used for CP in the medical literature to describe the specific signs of CP is confusing. The terminology applied in this chapter is a commonly used modification of those developed by Perlstein (1952) and by Vining, Accardo, Rubenstein, Farrell, & Roizen, 1976).

## RESULTS

The etiology of CP was found to be as follows: 23.5% was prenatal (before birth), 48% was perinatal (through or during birth), and 28.4% was postnatally (after birth) acquired. Details are provided in Table 1, and the results are compared to a United States series (Holm, 1982) in Table 2.

It is interesting to note that the prenatal group ($N$ = 24) included

**Table 1.** Etiology of CP by Timing of Onset in Saudi Arabia ($N$ = 102)

| Prenatal | | $N$(%) | Perinatal | $N$(%) | Postnatal | $N$(%) |
|---|---|---|---|---|---|---|
| Known | | 11 | Asphyxia | 18 | Infection | 26 |
| Siblings | 7 | | Injury | 14 | Trauma | 2 |
| Congenital abnormality | 1 | | Preterm | 10 | Near drowning | 1 |
| Brain malformation | 1 | | SGA | 7 | | |
| Intrauterine infection | 2 | | | | | |
| Unknown | | 13 | | | | |
| Totals | | 24(23.5) | | 49(48) | | 29(28.4) |

**Table 2.** Etiology of CP in Saudi Arabia Compared with a United States Series

| | Percentage | |
|---|---|---|
| | This series ($N$ = 102) | Holm (1982) ($N$ = 142) |
| Prenatal | 23.5 | 50.0 |
| Perinatal | 48.0 | 33.0 |
| Postnatal | 28.4 | 10.0 |
| Mixed | — | 7.0 |
| Totals | 99.9 | 100.0 |

7 (6.9%) children whose siblings had identical syndromes. In the perinatal group ($N$ = 49), 65.3% of cases were due to obstetric complications, whereas 34.7% were due to low birth weight (below 2500 g); of the latter, 58.8% were preterm infants and 41.2% were small for gestational age (SGA). Postnatally acquired CP ($N$ = 29) was mainly due to infection. Details of postnatal etiologies and comparison with a study from Western Australia (Blair & Stanley, 1982) appear in Table 3.

**Table 3.** Etiology of Postnatal CP in Saudi Arabia Compared with an Australian Study

| Apparent cause | This study ($N$ = 29) $N$(%) | Blair and Stanley (1982) ($N$ = 89) $N$(%) |
|---|---|---|
| Infection | 26(89.7) | 54(60.7) |
| Neonatal septicemia | 3 | 45 |
| Meningo-encephalitis | 7 | — |
| Respiratory tract | 3 | |
| Gastroenteritis & dehydration | 6 | 6 |
| Rubeola (measles) | 3 | 3 |
| Pertussis (whooping cough) | 4 | — |
| Post vaccination | 0 | 2(2.2) |
| Malnutrition | 0 | 2(2.2) |
| Anoxia | 1(3.4) | 7(7.9) |
| Near drowning | 1 | |
| Trauma | 2(6.9) | 20(22.5) |
| Home accident | 2 | 9 |
| Traffic accident | — | 11 |
| Cerebrovascular | — | 4(4.4) |
| Total postnatal CP | 29(100.0) | 89(99.9) |
| Total of all CP cases | 102(28.4) | 802(11.1) |

**Table 4.** Clinical Types of CP in Saudi Arabian Study ($N$ = 102)

| Clinical type | | N(%) |
|---|---|---|
| Pyramidal (spastic) | | 63(61.8) |
| Quadriplegia | 36(57.1) | |
| Diplegia | 12(19.0) | |
| Hemiplegia | 15(23.8) | |
| | 63(99.9) | |
| Extrapyramidal (Dyskinetic syndromes) | | 3(02.9) |
| Choreo-athetosis | 2 | |
| Dystonia | 1 | |
| Cerebellar | | 2(02.0) |
| Mixed cases | | 14(13.7) |
| Hypotonia | | 20(19.6) |
| Totals | | 102(100.0) |

The clinical types depicted by this study are shown in Table 4. Although all the known types of CP were represented in this study, hypotonics constituted nearly 20% of cases. There was no significant difference in the type of CP found in males as opposed to females.

Associated neurological defects were frequent. These are shown on Table 5.

## DISCUSSION

Improvements in medical practice in Western countries have resulted in a shift toward prenatal etiologies for CP (Hagberg, Hagberg,

**Table 5.** Associated Handicapping Conditions in Saudi Arabian Study ($N$ = 102)

| Defect | | N(%) |
|---|---|---|
| Mentally retarded (IQ below 70%) | | 82(80.4) |
| Seizures | | 25(24.5) |
| Ocular-visual | | 24(23.5) |
| Blindness | 10 | |
| Cataract | 1 | |
| Squint | 12 | |
| Complete ophthalmoplegia | 1 | |
| Language deficit (comprehension) | | 72(70.6) |
| Speech impairment (expression) | | 9(8.8) |
| Deafness (below 50 dB) | | 21(20.6) |

& Olow, 1975; Holm, 1982). The situation in Saudi Arabia today, as in many other developing countries, resembles pre-1950 Europe (Skatvedt, 1958). Consequently, the etiology of CP differs from Western countries in three important aspects. First, the majority of CP cases in Saudi Arabia originate in the perinatal and postnatal periods, both of which lend themselves to effective preventive measures. In fact if Saudi Arabia sets a goal equal to the present-day morbidity levels of Western countries as shown in Holm's study (1982), at least 30% of all CP cases would be prevented.

Second, low birth weight is a major cause of CP in Western countries, accounting for 30% to 40% of all cases (and 70% of the perinatal cases). In our study, low birth weight accounted for only 16.7% of the total cases, and 34% of those in the perinatal group. Further breakdown of the low birth weight patients shows that 41.2% of them were SGA—yet another potentially preventable cause. Third, in this series there were 7 (6.9%) affected children who had siblings with identical syndromes; they belonged to 3 families. This feature is considered very rare in Western countries (Gustavson, Hagberg, & Sanner, 1969) but it is likely to be an important etiological factor in traditional societies due to consanguineous marriages.

In developing countries, therefore, priority in prevention should be given to perinatal and postnatal etiological factors. Control of infectious diseases is an obvious goal and one which is relatively easy to achieve. One major approach to such primary prevention is through universal immunizations against infectious diseases. Improvement of obstetric and neonatal care, however, is hampered by the fact that in Saudi Arabia, 75% of pregnant women are delivered in the mother's home by untrained women (Department of Statistics, 1978). Under the circumstances, prevention is envisaged at three levels. The first, and most important, involves training the existing illiterate birth attendants (Williams & Jelliffe, 1972) so that they will be able to perform safer deliveries and refer problem pregnancies prior to delivery. The second involves the gradual development of district hospitals with obstetric and nonintensive neonatal care facilities, each catering to a population of a quarter of a million. This is the Swedish model which was found very effective in reduction of CP (Hagberg, Hagberg, & Olow, 1982). The third level consists of developing tertiary facilities to provide obstetric and intensive neonatal care.

All the known clinical types of CP were represented in this study. The high frequency of hypotonics, also reported by Holm (1982), is a function of age as the condition is known to be a transitory phase.

The brain insult that results in CP is not discrete and limited to the motor area. Other areas of the brain may be involved, resulting in additional neurological deficits that could be more handicapping to the child with CP than just the limitation of motility. The high frequency of associated defects leads to the conclusion that an accurate and complete diagnosis and proper rehabilitation of children with CP and other developmental disabilities require the combined effort of integrated, interdisciplinary teams. Such professional teams are sadly lacking in Saudi Arabia, a country that can afford and is working to provide the costly treatment of the handicapped as well as attending to other health problems.

## REFERENCES

Bax, M. C. O. (1964). Terminology and classification of cerebral palsy. *Developmental Medicine and Child Neurology, 6,* 295–297.

Blair, E., & Stanley, F. G. (1982). An epidemiological study of cerebral palsy in Western Austrialia, 1956–1975, Part III: Postnatal aetiology. *Developmental Medicine and Child Neurology, 24,* 575–585.

Department of Statistics. (1978). *Report on population survey, 1967/7.* Saudi Arabia, Ministry of Finance.

Gustavson, K. H., Hagberg, B. V., & Sanner, G. (1969). Identical syndromes of cerebral palsy in the same family. *Acta Paediatrica Scandinavica, 58,* 330–340.

Hagberg, B., Hagberg, T., & Olow, I. (1975). The changing panorama of cerebral palsy in Sweden, 1954–1970: Analysis of the general changes. *Acta Paediatrica Scandinavica, 64,* 187–192.

Hagberg, B., Hagberg, L. G., & Olow, I. (1982). Gains and hazards of intensive neonatal care: An analysis from cerebral palsy epidemiology. *Developmental Medicine and Child Neurology, 24,* 13–19.

Holm, V. A. (1982). The causes of cerebral palsy—A contemporary perspective. *Journal of American Medical Association, 247*(10), 1473–1477.

MacKeith, R. C., MacKenzie, I. C. K., & Polani, P. E. (1959). The Little Club memorandum on terminology and classification of cerebral palsy. *Cerebral Palsy Bulletin, 5,* 27–35.

Perlstein, M. A. (1952). Infantile cerebral palsy, classification, and clinical correlations. *Journal of American Medical Association, 149*(1), 30–34.

Skatvedt, M. (1958). Cerebral palsy: A clinical study of 370 cases. *Acta Paediatrica Scandinavica, 46*(Suppl. 3), 1–101.

Vining, E. P. G., Accardo, P. J., Rubenstein, J. E., Farrell, S. E., & Roizen, N. J. (1976). Cerebral palsy: A pediatric developmentalist's view. *American Journal of Diseases of Childhood, 130,* 643–649.

Williams, C. D., & Jelliffe, D. B. (1972). *Mother and child health: Developing the service.* London: Oxford Univ. Press, pp. 84–92, 129–145, 146–155.

# INDEX

www.ingramcontent.com/pod-product-compliance
Lightning Source LLC
LaVergne TN
LVHW052220200926
848481LV00001B/167
* 9 7 8 1 4 8 9 9 0 5 3 8 3 *